Augmentative and
Alternative Communication
Developmental Issues

Augmentative and Alternative Communication Developmental Issues

Edited by

STEPHEN VON TETZCHNER
University of Oslo

and

NICOLA GROVE
City University, London

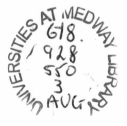

W
WHURR PUBLISHERS
LONDON AND PHILADELPHIA

© 2003 Whurr Publishers Ltd
First published 2003
by Whurr Publishers Ltd
19b Compton Terrace London N1 2UN England and
325 Chestnut Street, Philadelphia PA 19106 USA

British Library Cataloguing in Publication Data

A catalogue record for this book
is available from the British Library.

ISBN 1 86156 331 0

Contents

Contributors

Erna Alant, Centre for AAC, Department of Communication Pathology, University of Pretoria, 0002 Pretoria, South Africa. alant@libarts.up.ac.za

Kari Merete Brekke, Pedagogisk-psykologisk tjeneste, Alsteinsgata 7, N-4077 Stavanger, Norway. kari.merete.brekke. ppt@stavanger.kommune.no

John Clibbens, Centre for Thinking and Language, Department of Psychology, University of Plymouth, Drake Circus, Plymouth PL4 8AA, UK. j.clibbens@plymouth.ac.uk

Nicola Grove, Department of Language and Communication Science, City University, Northampton Square, London EC10 0HB, UK. n.c.grove@city.ac.uk

Kaisa Launonen, Department of Phonetics, University of Helsinki, PO Box 35, FIN-00014 University of Helsinki, Finland. kaisa.launonen@helsinki.fi

Shirley McNaughton, Department of Speech-Language Pathology, Faculty of Medicine, University of Toronto, Tanz Neuroscience Building, 6 Queen's Park Crescent West, Toronto, Ontario M5S 3H2, Canada. smcn@freespace.net

David A. O'Mara, Department of Applied Computing, University of Dundee, Dundee DD1 4HN, UK. domara@computing.dundee.ac.uk

Judith D. Oxley, Department of Communication Disorders, Louisiana State University Medical Center, 1900 Gravier Street, New Orleans, Louisiana 70112-2262, USA. oxley@lsumc.edu

Ana Peixoto, Centre for Habilitation of Cerebral Palsy, Tr. Maceda 160, P-4300 Porto, Portugal. ana.peixoto@clix.pt

Gaye Powell, College of St Mark and St John, Human Communication Studies, Derriford Road, Plymouth PL6 8BH, UK. gpowell@marjon.ac.uk

Gregor Renner, Sprengelstrasse 22, DE-13353 Berlin, Germany. gregor.renner@tu-berlin.de

Judy Seligman-Wine, PO Box 40012, Mevasseret Zion 90805, Israel. winej@netvision.net.il

Martine Smith, School of Clinical Speech and Language Studies, Trinity College, 184 Pearse Street, Dublin 2, Ireland. mmsmith@mail.tcd.ie

Gloria Soto, Department of Special Education and Communication Disorders, San Francisco State University, San Francisco, California 94132, USA. gsoto@sfsu.edu

Lourdes Tavares, Centre for Habilitation of Cerebral Palsy, Tr. Maceda 160, P-4300 Porto, Portugal. lourdes.tavares@operamail.com

Sukey Tucker, Haringey Primary Care Trust, Children's SLT Service, St Ann's Hospital, London N8 8PH, UK.

Stephen von Tetzchner, Institute of Psychology, University of Oslo, PO Box 1094 Blindern, N-0317 Oslo, Norway. s.v.tetzchner@psykologi.uio.no

Annalu Waller, Department of Applied Computing, University of Dundee, Dundee DD1 4HN, UK. awaller@computing.dundee.ac.uk

Notation

Naturally spoken utterances are italicized.

'Words and sentences in machine produced, digitized or synthesized speech' are in quotation marks.

MANUAL SIGNS are in capital letters.

GRAPHIC SIGNS and *PICTURES* are in capital letters and italicized.

Some manual or graphic signs need more than one word in translation. When the gloss of a single sign contains two or more words, these will be hyphenated, for example, YOU-AND-ME.

<u>Indications of whole words and written ready-made sentences</u> are underlined.

<u>S-p-e-l-l-i-n-g</u> is underlined and has hyphens between letters.

'Interpretations or translations of meaning' are used for interpretations of gestures and manual or graphic sign utterances. They are also used when giving the meaning of facial expressions, gestures, pointing, and so forth, for example, 'yes' (nodding) and 'no' (shaking the head).

{. . .} indicates simultaneous expressive forms, for example, speech and manual signs, or manual and graphic signs. {I GLAD *I am glad*} means that the manual signs for I and GLAD are produced simultaneously with the naturally spoken sentence *I am glad.*

CHAPTER 1

The development of alternative language forms

STEPHEN VON TETZCHNER AND NICOLA GROVE

Since the late 1960s, augmentative and alternative communication systems have gradually become more important as a supplement to, or a substitute for, spoken language, supporting the development of language and communication in motor-impaired, language-disordered, learning-disabled, autistic and other children. The experiences and skills of people who, through the years, have been using alternative language forms have provided insights into these means of communication, including the social and cultural situations of individuals who use alternative communication forms. Many of them grew up at a time when augmentative and alternative communication was an emerging field. For example, the personal history of Kari Harrington closely parallels the history of the field in Canada (see McNaughton, this volume). Most of the manual and the graphic systems that exist today have been in use for only 20 to 30 years. For individuals with limited or no speech for a period early in life, or throughout life, the systems have changed their lives dramatically: they develop means to share their interests, ideas and feelings with others, and some also develop means with which they can understand others. This has changed their pattern of social relations and has given them the opportunity to participate in society. At the same time, there has been a movement in many cultures towards a socially constructed view of disability that emphasizes the need to adjust to the abilities of individuals, and to remove barriers to participation (see Oliver, 1996; Renner, this volume). Alternative communication systems provide access to a functional means of constructing and sharing ideas with others but barriers may still need to be identified and removed. These barriers include limited understanding of how best to support users of alternative communication, and the attitudes that privilege spoken languages and deny the value of alternatives.

In addition to the users' own active participation in this process, it is the efforts of their families and of dedicated professionals that have made this

1

change possible – professionals who themselves learned about alternative communication as they were implementing it (see Brekke and von Tetzchner, this volume; McNaughton, this volume).

Alternative language development is the acquisition of non-speech language forms. The acquisition of such forms suggests not only deficits (in spoken language) but also achievements. The children's functioning abilities are reflected both in the failure to acquire spoken language and the ability to learn alternative communication modes. A large number of clinical studies have demonstrated the usefulness of such systems: children have learned to use and understand the communicative functions of manual and graphic signs, even if they failed to develop spoken language in a normal language environment and with intensive speech therapy. Some of them also started to speak or improved their limited speech skills following the introduction of alternative language forms (for reviews, see Bonvillian and Blackburn, 1991; Carr, Kologinsky and Leff-Simon, 1987; von Tetzchner and Martinsen, 2000).

The acquisition of alternative and augmentative communication may also provide insights into the nature of the underlying processes of language development in general. Alternative communication is not simply a non-vocal expression of spoken language, but has its own characteristics (Smith and Grove, 1999; von Tetzchner, 1985; Yoder and Kraat, 1983). For example, for aided communicators the highest level of communicative competence may be achieved through the acquisition of reading and writing skills for everyday communication. This developmental path, from the use of pictograms and photographs via Blissymbols to orthographic script, implies discontinuities in form not present in the acquisition of spoken language, and thus can help to elucidate the interaction between language meaning, language structure and language form.

A critical distinction between the acquisition of spoken or sign language and that of alternative communication is that they originate in different ways. The introduction of alternative communication systems came from speech therapists and teachers (see Arvidson and Lloyd, 1997; von Tetzchner and Jensen, 1996; Zangari, Lloyd and Vicker, 1994) and hence has been conceptualized mainly as a process of intervention. In the literature on augmentative and alternative communication, the acquisition of language in children who use non-speech systems to augment or substitute for speech is almost exclusively related to the intervention itself, on the efficiency of instructional strategies aimed at compensating for the deficits of disabled individuals. The users are rarely called 'children', but 'subjects', 'clients' or 'students', emphasizing the complementary role of the authors: researchers, speech therapists, psychologists or teachers.

Moreover, there are no detailed descriptions of the development of children who use alternative communication systems from a language perspective that are similar to the early diary studies of young children learning to speak (such as Bloom, 1973; Darwin, 1877; Lange and Larson, 1973; Leopold, 1939, 1947; Tiedeman, 1787). Similar studies exist of deaf children acquiring sign language (Ellenberger and Steyaert, 1978; Loew, 1980; McIntire, 1977; Morgan and Woll, in press; Stoloff and Dennis, 1978; Volterra and Erting, 1990; von Tetzchner, 1984a; Woll and Kyle, 1989). There are also very few studies describing aspects of semantics, syntax or pragmatics in children's comprehension and use of alternative language forms, which are so abundant in the traditional language development literature (for example, Fletcher and McWhinney, 1995; Krasnegor et al., 1991; Kuczaj, 1982; Lock, 1978; Slobin, 1985a; Snow and Ferguson, 1977; Tomasello and Merriman, 1995; Wanner and Gleitman, 1982). There are many detailed studies of the spoken language of children with language disorders (for example, Bishop, 1997; Grunwell, 1990; Morehead, 1976; Morton and Marshall, 1977; Ruder and Smith, 1984; Watkins and Rice, 1994; Wyke, 1978), yet there is to our knowledge no published longitudinal description of language development in hearing children using manual signing as their main form of communication. For example, despite the many studies on manual sign intervention with children who have Down syndrome (for example, Launonen, 1996, 1998; le Prevost, 1983; Remington and Clarke, 1996), there is no detailed description of how manual and spoken language evolves in this group of children over an extended period of time, although Abrahamsen and associates (1990) and Kouri (1989) provide accounts of the transition from sign to speech in pre-school children with Down syndrome. The vocabulary and grammar are often described in relative detail in clinical reports of speaking children with language disorders, whereas the description of children's alternative language forms is usually kept at a minimum, without details about growth in vocabulary and utterance structure. It seems as though information about the changes in the vocabulary and the linguistic structure of signed utterances including manual signs in this group have not been regarded as significant, either by researchers or practitioners. The situation is the same for children acquiring graphic communication systems.

The lack of studies of children who acquire alternative language forms means that a critical knowledge base for intervention is missing. Knowledge about average development and the variation in the acquisition of alternative communication forms is necessary in order to form appropriate expectations about the children's development and for professionals to make decisions about intervention. Without this information interventionists cannot know how the acquisition of alternative communication systems may best be promoted in different groups of children or what kind of skills an optimal development would imply. This makes it difficult to plan and provide a language environment that truly supports development. Different alternative communication forms imply different forms of skills and knowledge. The relationships between the development of memory and other cognitive skills and children's acquisition of alternative means of communication have hardly been discussed or studied (see Light and Lindsay, 1991, 1992; Oxley, this volume). From a developmental perspective, it is critical that the natural course of alternative language acquisition is not known. The field of augmentative and alternative communication is coming of age, but the transactional processes underlying development (and intervention) are simply not known. Although the course of development is planned by professionals, it remains a fuzzy process characterized by ad hoc strategies without clearly defined milestones. Even the end point, mature adult competence, is obscure.

It is this lack of knowledge about the development of alternative communication forms that provides the background to the present volume. The aim of this book is to discuss the semantic, grammatical and pragmatic development of children using alternative language forms. However, the first significant finding of the present authors is that the empirical basis for such discussions is extremely meagre. One source of information comes from the small number of descriptions of actual language use by children developing alternative language forms at one point in time or over a short period (for example, Abrahamsen et al., 1990; Heim and Baker-Mills, 1996; Kouri, 1989; Light, 1985; van Balkom and Donker-Gimbrère, 1996; von Tetzchner and Martinsen, 1996). Most descriptions of the achievements of users of augmentative and alternative communication are based on intervention reports with few details about the non-speech language forms understood and produced by the children. In order to analyse developmental trends in the grammatical structure of utterances produced by children using various communication forms it would be necessary to have large language corpora produced by a representative sample of users. At present, such a corpus does not exist. There are no large-scale studies and studies with fewer subjects usually present little detail about utterance structure and changes in utterance structure over time. Even for children using Blissymbols, there are few publications including descriptions of the actual utterance structure used, as opposed to a description of the utterance structure that is taught. A few studies include information about utterances produced in a graphic or manual mode by autistic and intellectually impaired individuals (Bonvillian and Blackburn, 1991; Fulwiler and Fouts, 1976; Grove, Dockrell and Woll, 1996; Udwin and Yule, 1990; von Tetzchner et al., 1998; Wilkinson, Romski and Sevcik, 1994) but do not relate utterance structure to the communicative situation and what the child seemed to try to relay.

The chapters in this book may thus be regarded as a first attempt to look at the achievements of children using alternative language forms from a broad developmental perspective. The authors use small group data and excerpts from dialogues between children and adults for preliminary analyses of how the children use grammatical structures and strategies to convey meaning and solve communicative problems. The empirical base of these chapters has some of the same limitations as the field in general: the chapters contain mainly observations from educational settings and detailed descriptions of development are lacking. This does not reduce their importance. The developmental trends suggested here highlight the need for more studies and, in particular, studies that include children's communication with parents and other adults without an educational role in the children's life, as well as with both speaking peers and peers using alternative communication means. If this book serves as an inspiration for further investigation and contributes to a change in the approach of both research and clinical practice, it will have accomplished its overall aim. It is our belief that a shift towards a developmental understanding of augmentative and alternative communication will lead to new knowledge and a better basis for intervention practices, and thereby to improved social and societal participation for children using alternative means of communication (cf. Gerber and Kraat, 1992).

The primary focus of this book is not on disabilities, although the children described in this book have a variety of disabilities, some of which are the main reasons the children are following atypical developmental paths. Instead the focus is on the developmental achievements of the children as users of augmentative and alternative communication. Although the achievements of all the children are exceptional in the sense that they become able to communicate in ways that are not shared with many others in their environment, their achievements are not the result of uncommon or unique abilities. As McNaughton (this volume) points out: it is Kari's language and communication achievements, given her non-exceptional abilities, which make her story so valuable. The other case studies are similarly exemplary, describing ordinary children whose drive to communicate has been promoted through the creation of social environments that 'afforded' and 'scaffolded' language development. The term 'afford' is borrowed from Gibson (1979) who uses 'affordance' to describe how the actions of organisms are embedded in their perception of the world: newborn squirrels perceive branches of trees as 'climbable', young humans perceive floors as 'crawlable', and so forth. Affordance of language means that children perceive language as a target of communicative actions of a type that they are able to perform. For some children, this form is not speech. The term 'scaffold' was introduced by Wood, Bruner and Ross (1976) to describe adults' support and guidance of children's active contribution to their own language development. Scaffolding may comprise a variety of activities, including direct instruction and co-construction in conversation with vocal or non-vocal language. Within the framework of the present book, language development relates to the acquisition of language forms and structures through social interactions, both planned and incidental in nature, that take place in particular socio-cultural circumstances.

Development and language

It takes about 20 years from when a child is born to the time when it reaches adulthood. In these years there are enormous changes in social relations and in how the individual experiences the world, solves practical and intellectual problems, experiences and expresses emotions, and participates in different social and cultural activities. Development may be defined as time-bound changes in behaviour, knowledge and other attributes of humans (and other species) as a result of biological and environmental conditions. These changes may best be understood as a *process of adaptation*. According to the *orthogenetic principle* of Werner (1948), development always involves change in a positive direction, that is, change that implies a higher degree of differentiation, integration, organization, complexity, and so forth. In language development, the lexicon expands and differentiates, and sentences increase in length and complexity. In all species, development implies greater autonomy and independence from the parents. Developmental changes can only be reversed to a very limited extent. When a physical or mental structure has evolved, the organism will not return to earlier forms. When children have reached a certain height, they do not become smaller again. Complex skills and abilities do not return to simpler forms. When language is learned, it will normally not disappear. Even when skills and abilities are reduced through the ageing process, impairment or disease, they do not appear as immature forms (Thelen and Smith, 1994). Some aspects of development may be quantified, like children's height and the number of words they say. Other aspects cannot be easily quantified, like reasoning ability and social adaptation. They are qualitative in nature.

Not all change in children is considered development. A change is usually considered developmental when it appears at a certain time and in a certain order in a large number of individuals. Development is also usually related to biology. Learning is usually defined as a relatively permanent change in behaviour or knowledge related to the experience of the individual, not only to factors like maturation, illness, fatigue or impairment (Kimble, 1961). Unlike development, something that is learned may be unlearned or forgotten. To learn mathematics is not development, even if most children in the industrialized countries learn mathematics at about the same time and in a relatively stable pattern of achievements. When to learn, what to learn and in what sequence skills are taught, are determined by a society's opinion about how this best should be done. On the other hand, teachers' strategies will depend on their knowledge about children's cognitive abilities and skills at different age levels. The difference between learning and development is therefore not a clear-cut or simple one. Some theories will describe development as a process where new learning is based on former learning, independent of biological conditions, and that a general ability to learn is the only biological basis of development (for example, Bijou, 1993; Schlinger, 1995; Watson, 1928).

Development is thus the composite outcome of a number of processes that together lead to children accruing physical, cognitive and personal characteristics and establishing personal social relationships and their place in society. Development embraces all aspects of functioning in humans (and other species) and is the result of an interaction between biological and environmental factors. Culturalization – that is, how children acquire and adapt to the culture in which they grow up – is an important aspect of all forms of development.

Main effects and interactional effects

In describing developmental processes, it is usual to distinguish between main effects and interactional effects. A *main effect* means the influence of one factor is independent of other factors. For example, eye colour is only determined by a set of genes, and a motor impairment may be the result of a particular trauma. A skill or an ability may also be considered the result of *additive main effects*, that is, several independent factors influence development in an additive manner. Attempts by behavioural geneticists to assess the relative genetic and environmental influence on an ability – for example, intelligence – are based on an assumption that the influences of genes and the environment are independent and additive. A hypothetical example may illustrate this. One could imagine two groups of monozygotic twins (one of each pair of twins in each group) so that the groups were genetically identical, one growing up in a desert country where proteins are scarce, the other growing up in a country with abundant access to protein-rich food. If genes and environment have independent influences on height growth, the twin of the tallest child in the desert environment would be the tallest child in a protein-rich environment, but the second twin may be considerably taller than the first twin. The same would apply to the rest of the children. The heights of the twins within each pair would differ, but the rank of the twins would be the same in both groups.

Interaction means that the influence of one factor will depend on one or several other factors. Using the same illustrative example as above, if genes and environmental conditions interact, the rank order of the twins in the pairs will not be the same in both environments because the influence of high-protein and low-protein nourishment is not the same for all children, but depends on the genetic endowment of the children. Another example may illustrate the relevance of the interaction model for understanding alternative language development: an environment with a lot of communicative interaction involving speech and no manual signs may promote optimal language development in hearing children. The same environment may lead to non-optimal or even deviant development for profoundly deaf children, whereas development may be normal in an environment with manual signing (except for a less common language form than speech). Thus, in this case, what will result in an optimal development depends on the interaction between children's hearing and qualities of the environment. Similar interactions between child characteristics and language environment can be found in the development of alternative language forms.

Interaction effects do not always involve factors related to the organism's constitution and factors in the environment. There may be interactions between different constitutional factors, and between two or more environmental factors. For example, language acquisition in some children with autism is the result of both the provision of alternative means and a structured communicative environment (see, for example, Bonvillian and Nelson, 1978; Fulwiler and Fouts, 1976; Peterson et al., 1995; Schaeffer et al., 1977; Vaughn and Horner, 1995; von Tetzchner, 1984b).

Transaction

One of the most important theoretical insights into developmental processes comes from the transactional model that was introduced in the 1970s (Sameroff and Chandler, 1975). This changed the conceptualization of the relationship between the organism and the environment from being mainly a one-way influence, where children are influenced by events in the environment, such as parents' communication style, to the concept of a reciprocal relationship, where the child and the environment influence each other. At any point in a transactional chain, children will have certain abilities and attributes and the environment will have certain qualities. The environment will influence children and change their skills, abilities, knowledge, and the abilities and attributes of the children will influence the qualities of the environments, for example the way people act and react towards them. Active children evoke different reactions from other people than less active children. This occurs in ways that also reflect the styles of those who react to the children. One important contribution of this model is that it is possible to understand why parents behave differently towards their children. For example, an observed relationship between children's emotional reactivity and parents' behaviour does not imply that the child's emotionality is caused by the parents' style in any simple sense, as the parents' style may be influenced by how easy or difficult their child is to regulate. The child's ability to regulate its own emotional reaction will also depend on the help it has received from the parents in regulating itself.

The transactional model may be applied to most developmental phenomena. The influence of children on their caregivers is demonstrated by the simple fact that many parents with non-speaking children choose to use manual and graphic signs. The influences exerted by the child are crucial for the parents' choice. Without a non-speaking child in the family, or a child who is vulnerable with regard to language development, the parents would never have considered an alternative communication form. The reciprocal influences that constitute the transactional model may also be used to explain why communication partners of children using aided communication tend to be dominant and the children to be passive and lacking in communicative initiative and autonomy (see, for example, Basil, 1992; Harris, 1982; Light, 1997). The reason for this dominance is neither a general dominant trait in the parents nor a passive temperament in the children. The children have limited means of expression and their parents may take over in an attempt to manage communication and keep the conversation going (see Light, 1985; von Tetzchner and Martinsen, 1996). The parents' style of communication management may increase the children's passivity, for example by not giving the children the time they need to take initiative or a complex, non-responsive turn, which again will increase passivity, and so on.

The acquisition of alternative communication forms can thus be understood within a general developmental framework and the theories of language development in general may also be applied to these forms. In principle, it is only form and not function that distinguishes alternative communication forms from speech. However, vocal and non-vocal language forms may differ in both their underlying processes and the environmental conditions that together influence the paths children take to communication and language.

Theories of language development

Theories are different ways of reflecting upon phenomena in the world and theoretical terms are the tools of reflection. Theories of child development try to answer questions regarding *what* develops, *how* it develops and *why* it develops, and a number of theories attempt to explain the what, how and why of language development. Practitioners also need answers to these questions, and the answers will differ depending on the perspective of the major theories: nativism, behaviourism, emergentism and social constructivism.

Within the *nativist tradition*, the basis of language acquisition is assumed to be a species-specific neurological module that perceives certain experiences as linguistic and categorizes and structures what is perceived according to inborn linguistic rules and categories (Chomsky, 1968, 1988; Fodor, 1983). Petitto (1992) suggests that this 'linguistic structure-seeking module' is independent of modality but, except for sign language acquisition in deaf children, non-speech communication modes are rarely mentioned in discussions of language development. Within a nativist framework, the basis of language development is perception – that is, the recognition of linguistic forms and how they combine structurally – and the process is relatively automatic.

This tradition assumes that the acquisition of an alternative communication system would depend on the system being perceived as linguistic and on a certain amount of exposure. Even if the alternative form is perceived as linguistic, it may be difficult to establish a language environment that provides sufficient exposure to the alternative form (Martinsen and von Tetzchner, 1996). With some rare exceptions, the exposure to linguistic input in alternative modes is limited outside restricted training situations. For manual signs the quality of the linguistic input is typically extremely poor (Grove et al., 1996; Launonen, this volume; Light, 1997). This may severely limit a child's opportunity to set the parameters and 'calibrate' the language system 'naturally' as implied by Chomsky's (1988) theory and other nativist theories, and it is not known to what degree the effect of an impoverished language environment can be compensated by instructional activities.

One natural opponent to nativism is the *behaviour analytic tradition*, which maintains that learning language is similar to learning any form of behaviour. There is no distinction between language competence and performance and thus no need to explain language as a linguistic and meaning system (Schlinger, 1995; Skinner, 1957). Behaviour analytic researchers therefore tend to limit their efforts to attempts to demonstrate relationships between particular behaviours and schedules of reinforcing events (for example, Mirenda and Datillo, 1987; Reichle and Ward, 1985; Remington, 1994; Remington and Clarke, 1983). As a theoretical framework, behavioural analysis has little to offer to promote understanding of the cognitive, social and cultural processes underlying typical and atypical development of language and communication, and the behaviour analytic tradition has had negligible influence on discussions on language development since the discussion triggered by Chomsky's review of Skinner's book in 1959.

Despite the limited influence on general discussions of language development, there has been a considerable behavioural bias in the field of augmentative and alternative communication. Behavioural strategies may have some practical use in intervention with severely intellectually impaired individuals, along with other strategies, and reinforcing conditions may sometimes explain why individuals fail to use language skills that they have learned, but they do not explain how and why language develops. Language acquisition is not dependent on praise for 'good communicating' or other forms of metacomments about communicative acts, but on communicative success, on being understood and solving communicative problems that appear.

Within the theoretical framework of *emergentism*, or *connectionism*, there is both less dependence on detailed genetically specified mechanisms than in modern nativism and a clear biological foundation and a focus on social and cognitive processes not found in behavioural analysis. Language is regarded as the result of a dynamic process involving many underlying processes and the emerging function is more complex than a function obtained by a simple addition of these processes. Language is driven by organization of experience rather than pulled towards a pre-defined goal as implied by nativist theories (Elman et al., 1996; Plunkett et al., 1997).

According to the assumptions of emergentism, the acquisition of alternative communication in children with communication and language impairment may be understood as constituting distinct developmental paths. Impairments constrain the ordinary processes in such a way that typical language development is impossible or severely hindered, and the alternative language form must therefore emerge through a dynamic interplay of processes that is different from the foundation of typical language development. Speech perception and production, memory and other cognitive processes, and the communication partners' sensitivity and style and other environmental characteristics, may be processes in a dynamic model that contributes both to constraints and to the emergence of non-speech linguistic competence.

Within the *social constructivist tradition*, words and sentences are assumed to gain meaning through the social interchanges and activities in which children take part (Vygotsky, 1962). Language is made possible by both the human brain and human culture. Social constructivist theories do not deny the influence of biology, but maintain the limitation of biology as a sole explanation of the development of higher mental functions like language (Luria and Vygotsky, 1992; Vygotsky, 1978). The essence of language, from this perspective, is that language is an aspect of the children's cultural development and language acquisition consists in internalizing a 'cultural tool'. Language is learned, not because of pre-wired neurological structures or as a result of the reinforcement of certain behaviours, but through guidance from more competent language users (Bruner, 1975, 1983; Service, Lock and Chandler, 1989). Language competence is not primarily an individual skill, it is constructed jointly with others before it becomes an individual skill through internalization, and joint construction of meaning remains an integral part of language use throughout life.

The social constructivist conception of the acquisition process links the understanding of alternative communication to children's activities and social participation. The construction process of alternative language development will differ in important ways from typical language development (see Renner, this volume). One important question that this approach raises is how activities that involve alternative communication differ from activities with spoken communication. This answer will have implications for the design of intervention strategies. There is a strong focus on activities and participation in society and social constructivism has a strong position in educational discussions, but social constructivist approaches are only rarely applied in intervention or to explain characteristics of children's use of alternative communication means. This perspective has influenced several of the authors in the present volume, but with the exception of Renner's chapter on Vygotsky's developmental theory, they represent eclectic rather than pure social constructivist approaches.

The language environment

All theories of language development imply that there is an environment of language users and that the quality of the environment is related to the behaviour of these language users to a greater or lesser extent. Language intervention is based on the premise that it is possible to influence children's language development through environmental influence. The issues in question are what the critical influences are and how the environment may be adapted to influence the development of language in the best possible way for a child with particular characteristics.

There are significant differences between the language environments of children acquiring spoken language and children acquiring alternative communication forms. Children who acquire spoken language are surrounded by a community of speakers, even if there may be several languages spoken in a child's environment, and the influences are usually not planned. For children who use alternative communication, there is no natural language environment of competent users of the same expressive mode as themselves. Most of the input comes from direct instruction and participation in educational activities. For children who acquire manual signs, adults often sign 'key words' to support their spoken language, but the environment is very different from ordinary bilingual settings where the child in principle is equally well equipped to master both languages (Martinsen and von Tetzchner, 1996). The children hardly see the alternative language form used by competent users. Manual signs are rarely used by others even in special classrooms (Grove, 1995; Grove and McDougall, 1991). There is increasing recognition of the need for young alternative communication users to observe structures in the alternative mode, but a lack of evidence relating to the nature of the resultant transactions and the effects these may have on the acquisition of alternative language by the children concerned.

Outside the explicit teaching settings there is little information about the language environments of children using alternative communication. Grove and McDougall (1991) and Grove (1995) asked teachers who were familiar with the home circumstances to rate the extent to which manual signs were used at home. The teachers reported that manual sign use was very patchy outside the classroom, with primary carers (usually mothers) the most likely to sign. However, the home environment comprises many significant communicative partners and children spend more waking time there than in the pre-school and school. The strategies that evolve from the social interactions between children and their parents, siblings and other significant people may differ in important ways from the 'school language' (see Wells, 1987). A full understanding of the factors that influence the development of children using alternative means of language must therefore include information about all the environmental influences on their language acquisition (see Launonen, this volume; Smith, this volume).

The acquisition of alternative forms is therefore very unlike the implicit learning that is typical of spoken first-language acquisition, and many communicative activities will differ. This does not mean that the children acquiring alternative communication do not engage in typical interactions. There may be a whole variety of language experiences that are useful to children, even if they do not involve their primary communication system. There will be many aspects of communicative development that are not planned by professionals, and which will develop through implicit learning to greater or less effect. However, communicative interactions involving the alternative communication system are likely to be foregrounded by professionals. This is evident in the fact that there are very few detailed descriptions of alternative communication in the home, and child–professional interactions seem to have replaced the traditional parent–child interaction of the language development literature.

The scaffolding properties of the language environment depend on communicative acts and the explicit beliefs and strategic acts of professionals and other people in the environment (von Tetzchner, 1999a). An environment that supports the acquisition of alternative language forms does not seem to come naturally. There are several possible reasons for this. Firstly, the environmental strategies with children using alternative communication forms are very different from the ones usually employed by parents and familiar communication partners. For example, pointing to pictures and words is used as a supplementary strategy in typical interactions, but rarely as the primary means, and when it is used in this way it is underpinned by established competencies in spoken language. Secondly, the communication difficulties of children using alternative communication forms may skew the interactions so that regardless of what system they use, it is hard for parents to employ effective strategies that may feel counter-intuitive. Deaf parents are familiar with the visual mode and know how to gain and maintain the attention of their children, whereas parents of signing children with Down syndrome, for example, are likely to employ the same strategies they would use with speaking children (Clibbens, this volume). Finally, the very fact that the system of communication used is controlled and planned by professionals may disempower parents, and make it hard for them to adopt it as a natural form. The language environment therefore has to be planned, and explicit teaching, which plays little or no role in typical development, may be a major environmental influence for children who develop alternative communication. For example, the acquisition of new words and structures is assumed to take place primarily in the nursery or at school rather than at home.

An important quality of a language environment is how it relates to both the abilities and the limitations of children. In typically developing children, overinterpretation, that is, the tendency of parents and other significant adults to attribute more specific intentions to the child than it is reasonable to assume it has, is considered a driving force (Lock, 1980; Ryan, 1974). Children with motor impairment often have to prove themselves able before they are believed to have the ability to develop language. On the other hand, adults also often overestimate non-speaking children's language comprehension and thereby fail to provide a language environment that is adapted to the children's possibilities for learning. As the developmental opportunities of children using alternative communication are so dependent on planning, the beliefs and attitudes of the professionals (and parents) are crucial. One important question is whether the support usually given to young children using alternative communication is sufficient for promoting optimal development of their mode of communication. For example, the function of communicative abilities is to solve communicative challenges. Sometimes, but not always, such challenges are related to children's personal needs and activities, but such needs and activities seem to be emphasized in the provision of vocabularies and the communicative interactions planned at least throughout early childhood and often longer, even if the focus changes from the immediate setting to ordering hamburgers in restaurants (e.g., Fried-Oken and More, 1992; Mills and Higgins, 1984; Morris, 1981; Tavares and Peixoto, this volume). For example, McNaughton (this volume) reports that for Kari, who was considered to have good comprehension of spoken language, a brief attempt was made to introduce a picture board for choosing at snack time when she was five years old, but that it was soon discontinued because it did not make it easier for her to choose food at meal times where pointing worked equally well. Alternative communication means for other functions were not considered at this age.

Conversations about past and future events and issues not related to children's individual experience tend to be less prominent when alternative communication is planned. However, studies of conversational skills and narration suggest that the acquisition of alternative communication will gain from a greater focus on discourse skills, including discussion, narration and negotiation (see, for example, Brekke and von Tetzchner, this volume; Grove and Tucker, this volume; Waller and O'Mara, this volume). When only a restricted range of communicative functions are facilitated through professionals' planning of the environment, what is termed 'communicative opportunity' may imply only a situation where children can use what they have been taught and not an opportunity to expand the communicative repertoire by developing new vocabulary and skills.

The interplay between the planned and unplanned aspects of the development of children acquiring alternative communication also raises the question of whether a segregated or inclusive school environment best facilitates children's language development. There are no real comparisons of children's development of alternative communication in inclusive and segregated settings, and opinions about what constitutes an optimal language environment for these groups vary considerably – even in the chapters of the present volume. On the basis of clinical experience, McNaughton argues that early segregation and a gradual desegregation into mainstream school will give aided communicators the most optimal language environment. From the perspective of Vygotsky's cultural-historical theory, Renner argues for full inclusion. From a somewhat related perspective, Brekke and von Tetzchner and Soto and von Tetzchner argue that true inclusion requires that all the children in the class have some alternative communication competence and, to some extent, that they come to share this communication form. This implies that the alternative communication form is not used only for communication with the user but has general functions: Blissymbols, for example, may be written on the blackboard to record the date, the weather, mystery messages, daily activities and classroom projects (see Brekke and von Tetzchner, this volume; McNaughton, this volume). One concern, however, is that the communication patterns in schools reflect the communication patterns in society in general: when schools are segregated, society also tends to be (see also Woll and Barnett, 1998).

The attitudes and expectations of people in the environment may to some extent influence all children's language development, but they may be critical for children who use alternative communication forms because these children depend on the means and opportunities provided by professionals. It is common to hear professionals proudly report the achievements of children using alternative communication. Sometimes the pride arises from the successful introduction of new and creative strategies that helped the child overcome serious challenges to its communicative ability, but sometimes it may reflect low expectations and surprise over the children actually having the skills and abilities that they demonstrate. The fact that there are no established norms for children who acquire alternative modes of communication makes it difficult to determine the factors involved in failures and successes: the biological endowment of the child, the readiness or reluctance of the family, other significant people in the child's environment and educators to accept and use the system, the appropriateness of the alternative means of communication provided and the skills of the professionals responsible for the planning.

The onset of alternative language forms

The conditions that determine the onset of expressive language are very different in speaking children and children developing alternative means of communication. In speaking children, onset has been assumed to depend mainly on biological factors and the language environment has been assumed to have little or no influence (Lenneberg, 1967). For children who need alternative means of communication, it is the knowledge and attitudes of professionals that determine when and how a particular system of communication is implemented. Such children and their families will have developed forms of communication within their available repertoires – such as gestures, gaze direction, vocalizations and facial expressions – but they will depend on professionals for the introduction of linguistically structured communication.

With the exceptions of a small number of children with Down syndrome (Launonen, 1998; le Prevost, 1983), opportunities for linguistic expression in the form of manual and graphic signs are rarely introduced until after a child has shown a clear impairment in the development of spoken language (Calculator, 1997; Light, 1997; von Tetzchner, 1997). This means that the transition from pre-verbal communication (vocalization, gaze, pointing and gestures) to verbal expressive communication (manual and graphic signs) is not only much later than for typically developing children, but possibly also later than may be optimal for the child (see Launonen, 1998, this volume).

The language impairment of some children is not possible to predict, but delayed access to alternative language forms is the rule for children known to be vulnerable to of severe language delay or for not learning to speak at all. Even for children with known neurological impairment that may hinder the development of expressive spoken language, alternative communicative means may not be provided at an early age. One reason may be that both parents and professionals tend to focus on motor development in young children (Basil and Soro-Camats, 1996; McNaughton, this volume; von Tetzchner, 1997). However, for language development, communicative access is more important than physical access.

The late onset of expressive communication may influence children's processing of spoken and alternative language. Mature auditory discrimination and identification of speech sounds is the result of complex developmental processes involving both perceptual analysis and analysis of meaning (Eimas, 1985; Werker and Tees, 1984). It has also been demonstrated that the processing of manual signs among deaf individuals is influenced by the age at which sign language is introduced (Newport and Supalla, 1980). Developmental evidence thus suggests that a late onset may influence the emergence of expressive language in hearing children who acquire alternative language forms, but the nature of this influence has never been directly investigated and may be difficult to assess. It is, nevertheless, an argument for providing children with alternative means as soon as impairment or vulnerability is established.

Grammar and strategies

Together with the transition from pre-verbal to verbal communication, the transition from single-word utterances to utterances consisting of two or more words is the most important milestone in language development. The ability to combine words gives children a more versatile 'tool' for communicating. They can express more meanings with the same number of words and produce utterances with more complex and specific meanings. However, to fully use utterances with two or more words or signs, it is necessary to indicate the semantic relationship between the words or signs in the utterance. This may be done by presenting them in a regular order, for example to indicate who the actor and recipient of an action are. If the sign order is agent–action–patient, JOHN KISS MARY would mean 'John kisses Mary'. If the sign order is patient–action–agent, the same utterance would mean 'Mary kisses John'. Latin and many other languages have relatively free word order and provide the same information about the relationship between words by modifying (inflecting) the words. *Cecar necavit Brutus* means that Cecar killed Brutus, whatever order the words are presented in. Thus, inflections may relay the same information as word order, but they may also be used to give information about characteristics of the actors or patients, like number, gender, physical shape or entity (for example, individual or crowd) and time of the event. For example, the *-s* in *dogs* indicates that there are at least two dogs. Manual sign languages inflect for aspect rather than tense, have inflectional movements that indicate size and other qualities of the entity referred to, and sign order is relatively free (Klima and Bellugi, 1979).

Both word order and inflections thus add specificity and complexity and contribute the variety in meanings that can be expressed. The question is how children who use alternative language forms exploit the possibilities of their systems' creatively and productively as they acquire the use of the system, in similar ways to speaking children's increasing use of inflections and complex structure. The potential for combination and modification varies between the different manual and graphic systems. Manual sign systems will in principle have all the possibilities of sign languages, but whether these are realized may depend on exposure to linguistically governed input (see Grove and Dockrell, 2000). Blissymbols have some grammatical items that function as grammatical morphemes, like *PAST-TENSE, PLURAL* and *ACTION* (indicates verb), whereas the more pictographic systems usually do not have such markers and users would have to rely on presentation order to indicate the relation between the graphic representations in an utterance. However, presentation may also be used for strategic communicative purposes, for example to indicate topic and comment, or what is given and what is new (Lyons, 1968; Namir and Schlesinger, 1978; von Tetzchner and Martinsen, 1996, 2000).

Many children with autism and intellectual impairment who use an alternative communication system do not seem to make the transition from single signs to multi-sign utterances. One reason may be that the children lack relevant cognitive and linguistic skills. However, not all children who score low on tests of intellectual functioning have impairments that also constrain language development, and many use spoken sentences (Lenneberg, 1967; Rosenberg and Abbeduto, 1993). Thus, overall low intellectual functioning is not an explanation in itself.

Another reason may be that the children have not received appropriate input to learn a language structure, whether this is assumed to be based on modular knowledge or not (see Locke, 1994). Most intellectually impaired and autistic children who are taught manual signs are exposed to simultaneous speech and sign in the form of key word signing where only one or two signs accompany the spoken sentence. Even if two signed key words are accompanying the same sentence, they would rarely constitute a 'sentence' and key words are unlikely to provide sufficient cues to utterance structure (Grove et al., 1996). This leaves it to the children to create a grammar with minimal input support, a task that may surpass the productive powers of most severely communication-impaired children. That this may be a contributing factor is supported by the fact that structured input and help to form longer utterances seem to increase utterance length in general. In a case study where an autistic boy was provided with intervention that facilitated sentence knowledge, he both produced and understood graphic sentences with two to four items at the same time as he failed to demonstrate understanding of simple spoken sentences on the Reynell language test (von Tetzchner et al., 1998). The results support the assumption that insufficient environmental cues and scaffolding may imply a non-optimal development. Also the narratives produced by intellectually impaired children described by

Grove and Tucker (this volume) and the eloquent signing of a boy with Down syndrome (Launonen and Grove, this volume) suggest that some children may have unrealized developmental potential, and that intellectual impairment does not in itself explain a lack of multi-sign utterances.

A reason somewhat related to the limited environmental input may be that the lexicon is too small. Children typically start to produce sentences when they have an expressive vocabulary of between 15 and 50 words (Bates, Dale and Thal, 1995). Locke (1997) argues that a critical mass needs to be reached in the lexicon before analysis and segmentation of representation begin. It may be that the lack of structure is related to restriction on vocabulary size in children using alternative means of communication. Although intellectually impaired children who speak often have larger vocabularies before they start to make sentences than typically developing children (Rondal and Edwards, 1997; Rosenberg and Abbeduto, 1993), there is an example of severely intellectually impaired children with no speech and a vocabulary of 12 manual signs producing utterances with three signs (Bonvillian and Blackburn, 1991). Other children use a much larger number of graphic or manual signs without displaying any apparent understanding of sentence structure. It should also be noted that motor-impaired children with good comprehension of spoken language also tend to produce short graphic sentences (Brekke and von Tetzchner, this volume; Light, 1985; McNaughton, this volume; Udwin and Yule, 1990; von Tetzchner and Martinsen, 1996). This suggests that it is more difficult to produce graphic sentences than to produce spoken sentences, but also that the emergence of sentence structure may be more dependent on scaffolding strategies than the typical development of spoken language.

There are also studies that indicate that intellectually impaired children can use manual signs in a creative manner and apply untaught strategies in attempts to solve communicative problems. Grove and her associates (1996) demonstrate the use of sign modification to relay particular meanings. Similar findings are reported by Grove and Tucker (this volume) and Launonen and Grove (this volume). Very little is published about the self-made strategies of young aided communicators, but children using graphic communication also seem to explore their medium in untaught ways, for example by indicating parts of pictograms or using them in associative or metaphoric ways that far extend the literal meanings of their glosses (Brekke and von Tetzchner, this volume). The prevalence of taught and untaught strategies in children's communication is not known, or why some strategies are developed rather than others. This may be related to phonological and cognitive processing. For example, some motor impaired children actively use phonological similarity to relay meaning, like Yehonatan who indicated *HIDE AND SINK* to say 'hide and seek' (Soto and Seligman-Wine, this volume). Others rarely use this strategy to indicate a spoken word. This may reflect differences in phonological awareness and thus may be indicative of how difficult it is for a child to acquire the most advanced form of graphic communication, orthographic writing. Yehonatan started early to use this strategy and also seemed to learn to read and write with relative ease. Kari and Sander rarely used phonological similarities between words as communication strategies. Initially, Kari did not have the necessary orthographic skills for identifying unfamiliar written words and her progress in reading was mainly due to her learning to guess better when she attempted to identify unknown words on the basis of contextual cues (McNaughton, this volume). Sander also had significant problems in learning to read and write (Brekke and von Tetzchner, this volume). It is not known whether facilitating the use of phonological strategies with graphic communication systems will have a positive influence on the acquisition of orthographic reading, but this seemed to be the case with Sander (Brekke and von Tetzchner, this volume). It is also notable that Kari and Sander both seemed to acquire spelling skills only when they discovered letters as a communicative strategy for specifying meaning, while traditional reading instruction alone was unsuccessful. This demonstrates the double role of orthographic writing in the communicative development of this group: for literacy and for face-to-face communication.

Relationship between spoken and alternative language structure

It is a characteristic of children using alternative means of communication that they have little or no productive speech but their comprehension of spoken language differs widely – from no apparent understanding to comprehension that seems appropriate for their social and intellectual abilities. Consequently, relationships between the alternative language form and speech will also differ (Layton, 1988; Martinsen and von Tetzchner, 1996).

There seem to be two main developmental paths to alternative communication competence: one is based on the comprehension of speech, the other on the independent creation of a meaning system with other communicative forms (see also Sutton et al., 2000).

The first path is in some respects similar to second language learning. However, even for children who grow up with two or more spoken languages, or hearing children with deaf parents who grow up with one signed and one spoken language, the relationship between the two languages is not fully understood (Bialystok, 1999; Romaine, 1999). Similarly, there is little doubt that the comprehension of spoken language is an important foundation for the acquisition of alternative communication and that comprehension will influence development. However, there has been little investigation into the interaction between the two language forms (Romski and Sevcik, 1996; von Tetzchner et al., 1996).

The second developmental path is followed by children who have very limited or no comprehension of spoken language and acquire a communicative system without reference to speech, in some ways parallel to the sign acquisition of deaf children but usually dependent on more elaborated scaffolding. They must discover the functions of manual and graphic signs through joint activities with others where their independent or guided use of the system has communicative consequences of which they become aware. It is the scaffolding strategies of people in the environment that make it possible for those who follow the second path to learn language that they did not acquire through the use of spoken language in their environment, but it still needs to be understood why utterance structures tend to be so limited. One reason may be that most environmental adaptations are based on spoken instructions and thus mainly favour children who are attentive to, and have some comprehension of, spoken language. Bonvillian and Blackburn (1991) found a strong correlation between the size of the manual sign vocabulary and speech comprehension in children with autism. Romski and Sevcik (1996) found that children with higher comprehension scores tended to show better use of communication aids with Lexigrams and digitized speech output. An interpretation of these findings based on child characteristics would be that the use of manual signs and Lexigrams and speech comprehension all depend on a general symbolic ability. A scaffold-oriented interpretation of the same results could be that the scaffolding is based on spoken language comprehension and that the children's ability to comprehend spoken language therefore will determine the developmental result (see below).

Children with little or no comprehension of spoken language who follow the second developmental path will need scaffolding that is not based on comprehension of spoken language in order to fulfil their communicative potential. However, having acquired an alternative mode of communication, this may function as a basis for the acquisition of comprehension and use of spoken language, as in the case mentioned above of a four-year-old autistic boy who was taught the use of photographs and pictograms. He showed no evidence of speech comprehension at the time the intervention was initiated, but he later demonstrated both comprehension and production of speech (Tetzchner et al., 1998). Thus, for this boy, spoken language was acquired as a second language. Graphic communication was his primary communication mode and his language acquisition depended on appropriate opportunities for communicating with the graphic system. A probable explanation of this development is that the knowledge of the meaning system that the boy had developed through the use of graphic signs helped him to attribute meaning to the speech sounds that he heard and to start using them in a meaningful manner. Incidentally, the explanation may also apply to the failures of traditional language intervention that relies on imitation and other forms of non-functional instruction with children who do not understand the words they are trained to say. Their production of word forms is not related to meaning and hence not transferred to linguistic functioning.

One would expect that the manual or graphic sign utterances of children who understand spoken language show more influence from the spoken language structure than those of children with more limited comprehension of speech in particular, as they are not usually exposed to a competing structure. However, Grove (1995) found that the speech of such a group of children did not reflect spoken word order, suggesting that the alternative communication mode was dominant when it came to constructing output – or that the use of an alternative communication mode for output in some way affected the children's ability to apply what they heard around them.

There exist manual sign systems that follow the word order of the spoken language and have markers for all grammatical morphemes, like plural, gender and tense. It is also possible to construct graphic systems that can match the spoken language morpheme by morpheme. The alphabet is one such set of graphic representations, but it is based on phoneme-grapheme relations rather than on correspondences between graphic representations and morphemes. Blissymbolics contain some grammatical markers, but are not designed to follow speech in an absolute way and lack many of the morphemes used in various languages, such as the markers for the three grammatical genders in Norwegian.

It is also a question whether full correspondence to spoken morphemes is in fact the most efficient way to use a manual or graphic system. A French manual system based on morpheme correspondence was introduced by L'Épée in 1784 and since then similar systems have been introduced in many countries (see Loncke and Bos, 1997; Martinsen, Nordeng and von Tetzchner, 1985; Wilbur, 1979), but these were never adopted by the deaf community, mainly because they are inefficient as visual languages and involve incompatibility between the grammatical structures.

It is currently unclear whether the best approach to a manual or graphic language structure is to follow on the spoken language or to work within the constraints and affordances of the alternative mode. However, with regard to graphic communication, as aided communicators gain knowledge about orthography and their expressive communication approaches orthographic text (and spoken language), the word order may also come closer to this form. However, due to the time involved, children with relatively good motor co-ordination may be more likely to use grammatical markers than severely motor impaired children, and explicit instruction may be needed to facilitate this transition (see Brekke and von Tetzchner, this volume; Kaul, this volume; McNaughton, this volume).

Intervention as scaffolding

All intervention is based on the assumption that it is possible to influence children's development through environmental adaptation. In principle, traditional speech and language therapy and intervention with alternative communication systems try to establish the same communicative functions. When alternative communication systems are more successful than spoken language alone, it must be because child characteristics somehow interact with parameters of these systems to facilitate the emergence of communication and language skills. Moreover, it means that it is possible to circumvent the children's problems and establish improved, albeit not normal, communication.

One significant contribution of social constructivist theory to the understanding of language development is the notion of 'scaffolding'. This means that adults, rather than just presenting what needs to be learned, support children's own active striving to communicate. They do this by participating in activities with joint engagement, attributing communicative meaning to the children's actions (overinterpretation), guiding children in expressing themselves and negotiating meaning (Schaffer, 1989; Tomasello, 1999; Wood et al., 1976). The function of scaffolding is not only to help children communicate better in some situations, but to influence the processes underlying their language acquisition.

One of the main characteristics of effective scaffolding is the contingent relationship between the child's attention and the learning that takes place. Adults may follow the child's lead, using its immediate interests and preferences, or direct the child, which may promote the child's participation in activities deemed important for cultural learning. However, it has been shown that following children's attention may have a more positive effect on the very early acquisition of vocabulary than attempts to lead their attention (Grotnes and Urnes, 2000; Masur, 1997; Clibbens, this volume). Children who acquire alternative communication forms may have very few opportunities to take the lead, which may further delay their acquisition of systems for communicating meaning, and in turn, their participation in society.

Teaching and learning

Educational settings are an important part of all children's language environment. Their quality may both promote and constrain language development, and the educational environment may be critical for children developing alternative language forms. Many of the chapters in the present volume address the influences of this environment, including both direct instruction and the adaptations of the communicative environment made in nursery and school. Within a social constructivist perspective, children are considered to learn and develop their skills through a range of interactions, which will be characterized by different styles of interaction, depending on the goal.

According to social constructivist theory, co-operatively achieved success lies at the foundations of learning and development. Instruction and guidance, both formal and informal, in many social situations, performed by more knowledgeable peers or siblings, parents, grandparents, friends, acquaintances and teachers, are the main vehicle for the cultural transmission and acquisition of knowledge (Renner, this volume; Wood, 1998).

The type of scaffolding provided by adults and more competent peers will vary, from direct explanation and modelling to expansion and implicit direction of children's utterances (Snow, 1995; Wragg and Brown, 1993). In some cases and in some cultures, parents explicitly teach language structures to young children whereas in others children are expected to acquire language by exposure to child-specific registers or simply through exposure to language in general (Meisel, 1995; Schieffelin, 1979). This means that explicit instruction is not a necessary feature of ordinary language environments. In relation to alternative communication, scaffolding may be both more explicit and extended in age. It may be that linguistic and social competence is best acquired through more or less structured conversations in particular settings (see Hoff-Ginsberg, 1990), whereas strategic and operational competence may need more direct explanation and instruction (see Light, 1989). Wood (1998) found that in referential communication situations, explicit feedback by adults to children's ambiguous communications like 'I don't know if you want me to do x or y' seemed to help the children produce more explicit instructions, and thus supported their development of strategic competence. In narrative interchanges, an implicit style of feedback was more effective: teachers who paused, tolerated ambiguity and did not overload with questions were able to engage children in longer and more productive dialogues (compare Grove and Tucker, this volume).

We have argued that explicit teaching may be critical to children's acquisition of alternative means of communication. However, teaching alone is not enough to promote language comprehension and use, and the children's language development may not reflect the language skills taught in any simple manner (see Smith, 1996; Smith and Grove, 1999; von Tetzchner, 1985; Yoder and Kraat, 1983). An assessment of alternative language development that relates only to what the children have been taught therefore does not give a full impression of their language and communication skills. Word or sign order may serve to illustrate the difference between an educational and a developmental perspective on the structure of utterances produced with alternative means of communication. From an educational perspective, one might compare the word order of the children with the word order that has been taught, usually that of the spoken language in their environment, and deviations from that word order would be considered errors of learning. From a developmental perspective, one would search for patterns in the word orders the children are using and for changes in the word order pattern over time and try to assess the conditions that influence the word-order pattern and its development. For example, it has been suggested that children may use a topic–comment structure on their boards, first mentioning an event and then saying something about it (von Tetzchner, 1985). In order to qualify as a linguistic rule, it would have to be shown that there is a consistent marking of topics as distinct from comments, by word order or another marking.

Sutton and her associates (2000) suggest that users of pictorial systems may exploit order patterns that deviate from spoken syntax in order to clarify the relationships between the elements of the utterance and to avoid ambiguity. Adult English speakers used pictorial systems to communicate subject-relative clauses ('the girl who pushes the clown wears a hat') and object-relative clauses ('the girl pushes the clown who wears a hat'). Some of them used the same word order based on spoken English with both clause types *(GIRL PUSH CLOWN HAT)* and therefore confused the two structures. Others adopted a different strategy, based on proximity relations, and used *GIRL PUSH CLOWN HAT* for the object-relative clause and *GIRL HAT PUSH CLOWN* for the subject-relative clause. A similar proximity principle has been described for American sign language (Namir and Schlesinger, 1978). Sutton and her associates suggest that modality-specific strategies may help to disambiguate complex meanings. It is not clear at what point in development such consistent rules might be acquired and to what extent metalinguistic skills would be involved.

From both an educational and a developmental perspective, the relationship between spoken language and alternative language forms is of great interest. From an educational perspective, the comparison may be used to measure the success of the teaching and the errors would be used as a guide to understand the difficulties in teaching and learning word order. From a developmental perspective, the comparison may shed light on the reciprocal influence of the two language forms, and deviations from the spoken language would be a source of information about how children at that age try to solve communicative problems applying taught and untaught word-order strategies.

Scaffolding and non-scaffolding intervention

The planned language environment, intervention in a broad sense, may be considered either scaffolding or non-scaffolding. The difference between scaffolding and non-scaffolding intervention may be compared to the assistance given to developing countries. Some foreign help only aims to give people in the country food and shelter and help to overcome disease. When the aid is discontinued, the economic situation may be the same, or even worse. Other forms of foreign aid try to influence the economic processes in the country and sustain local economic growth in order to make the country independent of foreign aid in the future. Some forms of augmentative and alternative communication intervention may be of the first kind: they help disabled children cope in particular situations, but do not function to sustain and encourage the active role of the child as a learner and fail to influence the processes underlying language development.

Augmentative and alternative communication has changed over time. In the beginning, the use of manual signs along with speech, or the provision of a communication board with graphic representations, was regarded as a sufficient basis for the acquisition of alternative communication systems. There has also been a tendency to focus on physical assistance and on guiding children to a communication form that they can produce independently. For motor-impaired children, this part can be very difficult. It may take a long time to establish a system whereby children can select and indicate a reasonable number of graphic signs. However, even for this group, scaffolding is not only a matter of providing a technical aid. All aspects of the communication situation are affected, in particular by the child's problems in initiating joint attention and determining topic. Hence, the scaffolding of communication must also be adapted to these characteristics.

Similarly, it has become clear that the success of alternative communication systems for children with intellectual disability and autism is not only a matter of overcoming possible auditory problems or building on a preference for visual stimulation, as suggested by, for example, Peeters (1997). A failure to provide structured communicative situations for children in this group may hinder their acquisition of manual or graphic communication. Unlike typically developing deaf children, placement of autistic children in environments with manual signing does not lead to competent signing. More elaborated and adapted forms of scaffolding are needed. The use of sign sentences by people in the child's environment is important for supporting acquisition but it is not sufficient to trigger a development of sign language comparable to that of hearing children of deaf parents who use sign language. Neither do children in this group usually start to use graphic representations for communication by themselves, although there are no published reports of attempts at 'natural' stimulation of graphic communication development in children with severe communication impairment.

All young children need scaffolding to express themselves, provided by the people who are important to them and who are more competent than they are - parents and other relatives, siblings, friends and teachers. As the children grow older and gain better language competence, their communication also becomes increasingly autonomous. There are few restrictions on what they can say, and they are responsible for their own language productions. The ultimate goal of intervention is a similar *communicative autonomy*. Communicative autonomy is not the same as being able to formulate an utterance independently. Children using aided communication may need a lot of assistance in the physical formulation of their intended meaning. Autonomy refers to where the messages originate and whether the children have the means required to express themselves in accordance with their communicative intentions. Communicative autonomy means to have one's say, to be able to communicate one's own thoughts, ideas and emotions. The complementary dimension in the social environment is *communicative accessibility*, analogous to physical accessibility. Communicative accessibility means that there are people who understand the alternative communication form, who can scaffold it in the acquisition period, and who are able and willing to communicate in a manner that gives the individual maximal communicative autonomy.

The scaffolding strategies that optimally support the acquisition of various alternative communicative systems for different groups of children are not fully known yet, but it is evident that such strategies must build on knowledge about language development in a broad sense. By taking a developmental perspective on both instructional activities and other forms of adaptation of the environment of children using alternative means of communication, the authors in the present book contribute to this knowledge. Further innovation in this area is likely to lead to many children using alternative means of communication and acquiring more advanced communicative competence. The overriding issues that need to be investigated are how children's use of alternative means of communication to solve communicative challenges change over time, what principles guide the grammatical and pragmatic strategies children attempt at different points in the acquisition process, and what environmental conditions influence the developmental process.

CHAPTER 2

Joint attention and lexical development in typical and atypical communication

JOHN CLIBBENS AND GAYE POWELL

Successful communication, in whatever modality, requires communication partners to be aware of, and take account of, the information that each can access, and to make inferences about each other's current mental states, including intentions and desires. This shared framework for interaction has been described by Sperber and Wilson (1986) as the 'mutual cognitive environment' and it is important to note that it is distinct from the physical environment. Objects and actions (and other more abstract things) that are present in the immediate environment do not become part of the mutual cognitive environment unless both partners attend to them. Once given attention (and available as mental representations), they take their place alongside other pieces of information drawn from immediate and longer-term memory. In this way the physical and cognitive environments in which communication takes place can be seen to intersect, but they are not coterminous.

Joint attention within a shared environment is essential for many purposes but it has a particular role in communication and in the development of language. Managing joint attention to the environment is an important skill for communicators of all ages. When speaking to others, and drawing their attention to some object, for example, it is necessary to take account of their line of sight in order to ensure that they are able to see the referent. When the object of reference is a sound, or indeed when something is perceived through touch, smell or taste, this must be taken into consideration as well. Things become a little more complicated when using a form of communication other than speech. Deaf people using sign language must ensure that their interlocutor can perceive the signs addressed to them (including non-manual features of sign language, such as facial expression, as well as manual gestures) and what is being signed about. This is a consequence of the visual-gestural modality in which signing takes place. Signing as used by the deaf community is a natural form of communication, which has developed over an

28

extensive period of time, and skilled users of sign language have many resources available to them to manage joint attention (Clibbens, Powell and Grove, 1997). However, manual signs are frequently used as a form of augmentative or alternative communication by people who have failed to develop expressive speech (and sometimes as a way of boosting early communication in children who are also developing vocal expression). The same basic issues arise in these situations and with the use of any visually based communication system, including pictorial or graphic sign-based systems (Clibbens, 2001).

Joint attention and language development

The management of joint attention thus plays an important role in communication throughout life: however, it can be seen to play a particular role in early language development. It has become increasingly clear in recent years that the relationship between the language addressed to children and the focus of joint attention between children and adults can be a major influence on early language development. Studies published during the 1980s, by researchers working within a framework articulated by Bruner (1975, 1983) established that adults are responsive to their child's focus of attention (for example, Harris, Jones and Grant, 1983, 1984/85). Harris and her associates (1986) show that early vocabulary development, in particular, is affected by the opportunities provided by adults for children to make the connection between speech input and the objects and activities on which their attention is focused. Similarly, Tomasello and Farrar (1986) demonstrate that there is a positive correlation between mothers' references to toys to which the child was attending and the size of the child's vocabulary at 21 months. By contrast, references that tried to redirect children's attention to other objects were negatively related to vocabulary measures. One way to think of this is that talking about what the child's attention is already focused on is less demanding for children than trying to get them to look at something else, and allows them to focus their attention on the language input, leading to more rapid learning. This is supported by work by Bakeman and Adamson (1984), who also produced evidence that following the child's attentional lead (what they call 'passive' joint attention) minimizes attentional demand and frees resources for attention to the language input.

It does not follow, of course, that parents never seek to direct children's attention: it would be impossible for a parent to take an entirely passive role in interaction with a child, and it is hard to imagine anyone encouraging such an interactional style. However, it seems to be important that parents are aware of what their child is attending to during a crucial stage of early development. There is some evidence from research with both hearing and deaf children that there is an underlying factor of parental sensitivity – defined as the ability to read cues from their children and react appropriately, to resolve conflicts and misunderstanding, and to maintain a positive tone in interactions – which is associated with more effective interaction strategies and with more rapid language learning (Baumwell, Tamis-LeMonda and Bornstein, 1997; Pressman et al., 1999).

Discussions of the importance of joint attention for development are sometimes predicated on the assumption that vocabulary learning simply requires an association between a word and its referent. However, there is much more to language learning than this, even at the lexical level. In the first place, many words refer to abstract concepts, or to imaginary objects or beings. It is clear, therefore, that children are able to develop lexical representations in the absence of real, concrete referents. In addition, lexical representations are usually taken to include quite complex information, including specification of the syntactic category of a word and the type of grammatical structures it can enter into. Several recent accounts of lexical development propose that there are multiple influences on vocabulary learning, while differing as to exactly what these influences are. Thus Bloom (2000) argues that both cognitive and linguistic factors are involved, including the ability to acquire concepts, the use of syntactic cues to meaning and an understanding of the intentions and other mental states of other people. Other researchers argue that children also use specific lexical principles to aid word learning (for example, Golinkoff, Mervis and Hirsh-Pasek, 1994).

Bloom (2000) makes a strong case against a simple associationist account of word learning, but also plays down the role of joint attention in general. One reason for this is that strict spatial and temporal concurrence is not always required for word learning. As noted above, there is evidence that parents talk about what their children are attending to about 70% of the time (Harris, Jones and Grant, 1983), but this means that 30% of the time this relationship does not hold. It may be noted, however, that this '70% rule' appears to hold for sign language addressed to deaf children and to children with Down syndrome too. This is discussed further below.

More evidence against a simple associationist account comes from research by Baldwin (1991) who found that children needed to recognize that an act of naming was intentional in order for word learning to take place. A child who hears a novel word, whilst attending to an object for which they do not already have a name, will assume that the word is the name of the object. However, a child who hears a word spoken outside the room whilst they are attending to something, will not take that as an act of naming. This example shows the importance of understanding the referential intentions of others in word learning (an aspect of 'theory of mind' in the child).

Baldwin also found that children could learn in a 'discrepant looking' situation by 18 months of age – they would check that the adult was looking at the same object as them before assuming that a word was intended as a name for that object – but not at 16 months old. This and the evidence cited above do, as Bloom argues, militate against a simple associationist account of development, but they are perfectly consistent with evidence that naming in a context of joint attention plays an important role in the process. Children must initially make some connection between words and things and also need to recognize the channel, or modality through which language is transmitted. They can have no a priori means of knowing whether they have been born into a language community that uses speech or sign, for example, and studies have demonstrated that children have the ability to learn either type of language.

One argument put forward by Bloom (2000) against the general importance of joint attention in early language learning is the apparent difference between the learning of nouns and verbs. He points out that parents frequently name objects while children are attending to them, but rarely do this with actions – verbs tend to occur before an action with which they are associated takes place. Nevertheless, children are able to learn verbs. However, it must be recalled that the connection that needs to be established is not between a word and action per se, but between the respective mental representations of a word and action. As Bruner (1975) pointed out, much early word learning takes place in the context of highly familiar routines, in which the child may have a strong expectation about what is to happen next. In these circumstances the child may well have anticipated the action and therefore be able to associate it with the appropriate label in the input.

Bloom also argues that language learning takes place at a similar rate in all children, including deaf children learning sign language and children reared in environments where object naming is not emphasized. However, there is evidence that the rate of language development is variable, and correlated with the opportunities available to children to experience words in appropriate contexts, this evidence coming both from studies of typical development (for example, Harris et al., 1986) and of sign language development in deaf children (for example, Harris et al., 1989). Many of Bloom's points have force as an argument against the idea that all word learning depends on associations between words and physically present objects, however they are consistent with the idea that naming in the context of joint attention plays an important role in the early stages of language learning, and serves to kick-start the process. It may be that interaction of this type is particularly important for some groups of atypical language learners, and this possibility is discussed further below. Joint attention may also serve as a foundation for the more sophisticated use of shared context in older language users.

Atypical communication development

Most of the research discussed above was carried out with typically developing, hearing, children acquiring spoken English. There has been relatively little research with non-typical language learners (see Conti-Ramsden, 1994) and still less with children who rely on alternative means of communication. However, as noted above, the use of a communication system in a modality other than the auditory/vocal raises important issues for the establishment of joint attention and still more so when, as is often the case, multiple modalities are involved. A helpful starting point for thinking about joint attention and alternative communication is research carried out with deaf children learning sign language as their first language, as signing is a visually based system. This chapter will briefly review some research on this topic, then go on to consider some evidence on the use of manual signs as an augmentative communication system (especially with children with Down syndrome) and, finally, consider some implications for other atypical language users (such as children with autism) and other alternative communication forms (such as graphic sign and picture-based systems). It is worth noting again here that joint attention is not only important for early development, but provides a foundation for the use of a shared context (the mutual cognitive environment) in communication throughout life, and this point will also be discussed further below.

Harris and her associates (1989) carried out a study of early sign language input to deaf children learning British Sign Language as a first language from deaf, signing, parents. One purpose of this study was to test the claims deriving from work with hearing children that joint attention, and the recognition of referential intentions in others, were of crucial importance for early language learning. For a hearing child learning a spoken language it is possible for the child to attend to the speech input without directly looking at the adult with whom they are interacting. Joint attention is a triadic relationship between the child and adult and whatever they are jointly attending to in the environment, and much of the time the child can listen to what is being said whilst looking at a referent. Of course children will frequently 'check in' visually whilst engaged in a joint activity, but they do not need to be directly looking at the adult while attending to speech input. The situation for the deaf child is different because of the nature of the visual modality. Visual communication has to be in the direct line of sight to be of any use. Deaf adults who communicate using sign language use a strategy of switching attention between the activity in which they are engaged and a conversation partner (reinforcing the point made above that joint attention is of continuing importance for communication), but children must make the necessary connection between signing and communication before they can start to develop the ability to switch attention.

Harris and her associates (1989) focused on the strategies used by deaf mothers to enable their children to perceive both the signs which were addressed to them and the toys or other objects that were being signed about. The strategies that were found to be most effective (in that they were associated with more rapid language learning) were those that did not disrupt the children's attention. It was better, for example, to move the hands into the child's line of sight, than to try to redirect the child's attention. This is in line with the results reported by Tomasello and Farrar for hearing children, reported above. A particularly interesting strategy is that adopted by some mothers for signs that involve contact with the signer's face or body. A lot of signs that are of interest to young children (such as animal names) fall into this category and they are particularly difficult to produce in such a way that the child can see them unless the child is facing directly towards the signer. Deaf mothers in this study would often physically transfer the signs onto the child's face or body. This strategy, of course, meant that the way in which the sign was perceived was different, but Harris and her associates argue that adopting these special strategies for signing to children enabled the children to tune into the visual/manual modality, as the one on which important information was being transmitted. The children whose mothers made more use of these non-disruptive strategies learned quite rapidly to switch attention between the activity they were engaged in and their mothers. A consequence of this was that the mothers were able to revert to signing in the location that they would typically use when signing to another adult. All signs produced by these mothers were being produced in a typical manner by the time the children themselves started producing signs.

The finding that deaf mothers adopt special strategies for signing to their young children in the early stages of development has potential implications for other groups with whom signs are used and for the use of other systems that rely upon a visual or mixed modality. One group with whom signs are frequently used is children with Down syndrome (Clibbens, 2001). Harris, Kasari and Sigman (1996) found that receptive language gain in children with Down syndrome was positively associated with measures of joint attention. They also looked at the frequency with which adults maintained attention to toys that had been selected by the children and found that this was positively associated with receptive language. By contrast, there was a negative correlation between language measures and the frequency with which adults attempted to redirect children's attention especially away from toys that had been selected by the child. This indicates that joint attention is an important consideration for children with Down syndrome, and the findings reported above parallel many of those reported earlier for typically developing children.

Signing appears to have the potential to significantly boost the language development and communicative ability of children with Down syndrome

(Launonen, 1996; Miller, 1992; see Clibbens, 2001, for a review). Clibbens, Powell and Atkinson (2002) analysed the signs addressed to four children with Down syndrome by their mothers, using an extended version of the classification of signing strategies developed by Harris and her associates (1989) (discussed above). They found that the signs that were produced were generally perceived by the children and related to the focus of joint attention. However, the range of strategies used was very limited, and the mothers generally relied on taking advantage of occasions when the children were looking at them, or on trying to gain the children's attention before signing. The use of displaced signing strategies, where the hands are placed within the child's existing attentional field, was very limited, and the number of signs involving contact with the signer's face or body which were perceived by the children was also very limited.

The above study suggests that the strategies adopted by deaf mothers when signing to their children might fruitfully be adopted by parents of children with Down syndrome, and potentially with other groups who rely on manual signing. Some possible implications for intervention will be discussed in the final section of this chapter.

Joint attention and other alternative communication systems

A set of issues arises when other alternative communication systems are considered in the light of this research. Strategies that promote joint attention are likely to be fruitful for other children requiring visually based communication systems. However, signing, as a natural and unaided communication system, may lend itself to the adoption of such strategies more easily than some others (Clibbens et al., 1997). As has already been noted, joint attention is important for communication throughout life, and not just in early development: however, once a system has been acquired, it is possible to adopt attentional switching strategies that facilitate this. Graphic signs and pictorial systems that are fixed on a board or bound into a book do not lend themselves to the type of attentional strategies seen in signing parents, but if the pictures or symbols are produced on separate cards initially, then displacement strategies could more easily be adopted. There is a need for research on this issue with children using alternative communication systems.

Children with autism are one group of children who frequently have communication problems, and with whom the use of manual or graphic signs has often been found to be effective (von Tetzchner and Martinsen, 2000). A number of researchers have pointed out that these children do not follow a typical developmental path in terms of the development of joint attention (see, for example, Baron-Cohen, 1989). Leekam, López and Moore (2000) found that children with autism found difficulty in both dyadic (child–adult) and the more sophisticated triadic (child–adult–object) joint attention. The children were able to switch attention in response to an external stimulus, but had difficulty responding to attempts to gain their attention and in following attentional cues. This characteristic is likely to be related to the general problems children with autism have with 'theory of mind tasks', which involve understanding other people's beliefs, intentions, and so forth, and to underlie their communication difficulties (Baron-Cohen, 1995). As noted above, children need to be able to recognize the communicative intentions of an adult in order to take advantage of word-learning opportunities.

It is interesting that sign systems (manual or graphic) have been found to be effective with children with autism who have failed to acquire spoken language, or who have acquired it only to a very limited extent. Martinsen and von Tetzchner (1996) note that the establishment of eye contact is often seen as crucial for the communicative development of these children, but that there is no real evidence that this is a prerequisite for language. (Here, as always when dealing with atypical development, it is important to remember that what is 'normal' for typically developing children need not necessarily be so for all groups.) As Martinsen and von Tetzchner note, with alternative communication systems attention is often primarily focused on the signs themselves and their referents, and it may be difficult to combine this with eye contact. It is possible that, for children with autism, relaxing the require-ment to look into the eyes of the person with whom they are communicating may make it easier for them to learn. In view of the particular difficulties they experience with joint attention, and the apparent effectiveness of alternative communication intervention, children with autism will be a fruitful group for future research in this area.

Some implications for intervention

This chapter has considered the importance of joint attention for language development in typically developing children and in a number of other groups. Research on sign-language development in deaf children and its relevance for the use of signs with other groups (especially children with Down syndrome) has been discussed, and some of the implications of this work for children who rely on other alternative communication systems have been briefly addressed. A general issue in the field of augmentative and alter-native communication is that of the extent to which intervention programmes should be based on evidence about the interactional context of language development in typical learners (Calculator, 1997). In the case of children with Down syndrome, and others with intellectual disabilities, the use of signed input early on can confer significant benefits, and it would be possible to adapt many of the strategies adopted by deaf parents signing to their children for use with this group. There is anecdotal evidence that this is likely to be effective in giving the children access to more signs early on (Clibbens, Powell and Atkinson, 2002) but this needs to be tested in a more substantial, controlled research study. As noted in the brief discussion of autism above, however, it should not be assumed that what seems to facilitate learning in typically developing children can necessarily be applied straight-forwardly with atypical groups.

For many children using other alternative communication systems, lack of independent mobility and manipulative ability means that interaction with the environment is limited (Light, 1997). Consideration needs to be given to maximizing the opportunities these children have for interaction with the world around them, as well as strategies for establishing jointly attended reference in the context of such interaction. As noted by Romski, Sevcik and Adamson (1997), research findings from typical development may provide a useful perspective for the promotion of development in alternative commu-nication users, but they cannot always be readily used as a direct model.

One important issue for research on joint attention and alternative communication is that of the distinction between the systems used for recep-tive and productive communication by many children. Deaf children acquiring sign language are learning the same productive system used by their parents, but many children and adults who use alternative communica-tion systems normally rely on speech for input and use a manual or graphic signs system for production. This situation provides fewer opportunities for adults to model the use of the system. It may be noted here that Bloom (2000) argues that no one has ever tried to teach a child such an asymmetric language system and that it would be almost impossible. However, such asymmetry is characteristic of the relationship between speech and alterna-tive communication systems and raises important issues for intervention. It may be that where children rely on different systems for receptive and expressive communication, there is a case for modelling the use of the expression system by communication partners (Light, 1997). This has a number of possible benefits over and above modelling per se, in that it supports comprehension by pairing spoken words and manual or graphic signs, helps with the segmentation of the speech input and reinforces the effectiveness and acceptability of the alternative communication system (Romski and Sevcik, 1996).

The main purpose of this chapter has been to review evidence of the importance of joint attention for early language development in typical and atypical users. However, this discussion of implications for intervention suggests that a systematic research programme aimed at investigating strategies for promoting joint attention in children and adults communicating using alternative communication systems would be of great benefit, and might enable communication systems to be more effectively used.

CHAPTER 3

Memory and strategic demands of electronic speech-output communication aids

JUDITH D. OXLEY

The function of alternative communication is to enable children with severe speech and/or language impairments to develop and use language and communication skills that they need for success in society. Like all children, they require materials and support congruent with their linguistic and cognitive abilities. Social interactional and transactional models of development reflect a view that development can be facilitated when adults support the child by providing timely and developmentally appropriate situations for learning, and this holds true for children who use alternative communication (Vygotsky, 1978). Part of this facilitating role includes understanding what makes a task potentially difficult, because this knowledge guides when, where, and what support is needed. The purpose of this chapter is to present some of the possible challenges facing children who use alternative means of communication, with emphasis on the role of memory and strategy deployment in use of the alternative communication technology.

Alternative communication

Detailed reviews of alternative are readily available (for example, Beukelman and Mirenda, 1998; von Tetzchner and Martinsen, 2000). The following summary identifies features that are pertinent to the present discussion. Alternative communication methods may completely or partially replace oral speech as a primary mode of communication and, by convention, two methods are distinguished: unaided and aided.

Unaided methods include residual oral speech, manual sign language and gestures (for example, pointing, body orientation, use of gaze patterns). These methods are accomplished without the need for anything other than the communicator's own body, and are generally acquired with the help of a community who uses them as a primary means of communication (for example, a deaf community). The focus of this chapter is on aided communication so the complexities of hearing children acquiring manual sign language will not be addressed.

Aided communication requires additional materials, such as displays of graphic signs that constitute a selection set. The communicator touches or points to the choice through direct selection techniques (for example, using finger, fist, manual pointing tool or light beam), or indirect techniques (for example, controlling a scanning tool with a switch). Graphic sets may include orthographic signs (the alphabet) or pictographic signs (for example, coloured or black-and-white line drawings or photographs). Objects and partial objects can serve as tangible signs. A communication aid with speech output has multiple components, including a store of pre-programmed words and sentences, a graphical overlay (static or dynamic), a mechanism for speech output (digitized or synthesized) and capability for various input techniques (switch, joystick, use of body part to touch a key, and so forth). Many children, particularly those whose expressive communication is predominantly aided, must eventually come to understand and learn the roles served by these components and be able to execute this knowledge to communicate. Children acquiring language through aided means also lack the presence of competent users of the same communication form in the environment, thus reducing the naturalness of the language acquisition process (Smith and Grove, 1999).

Children who use alternative communication

Three main populations of users of augmentative and alternative communication have been identified (von Tetzchner and Martinsen, 2000). Members of the *expressive language group,* who have significant gaps between their comprehension of language and ability to express themselves, require alternative methods to replace severely impaired speech more or less permanently (these include, for example, some children with cerebral palsy or Down syndrome). Many of the expressive group have additional neuromotor impairments affecting use of arms and legs, balance, head control, and so forth. The *supportive language group* includes two subgroups: those requiring temporary support for language comprehension and expression (developmental group), and those requiring alternative communication methods in specific situations only (situational group). The *alternative language group* requires extensive support for both expression and comprehension. There is likely to be a range of strengths and weaknesses, including cognitive skills in all the three groups of children using alternative communication.

A discussion of the cognitive demands of learning the technology through which communication is achieved for aided communicators must consider how the tasks interact with the learner characteristics. A distinction must be made between products and processes. Two same-aged children may use the same communication device and similar overlays, but there can be large differences between the two children's understanding of their systems and their need for explicit understanding. One child may use the system automatically, without consciously knowing or caring how it works, whereas the other child may be able to organize the vocabulary and encode messages for future use.

Changing cognitive demands on language learning

Children begin developing language from birth and become increasingly masterful at co-ordinating verbal and non-verbal communication. Most of these tasks proceed with relative automaticity. Children progress from a phase of language learning, to a phase of language for learning, to a phase of advanced learning (Paul, 2000). Until the middle years of primary school, when children are approximately nine or 10 years old, they are still engaged in learning language but around this time the demands change and they must increasingly use language to learn about the world, particularly through literacy. The educational system assumes that, by this age, children have a strong command of their native language. Throughout adolescence, teenagers must refine their oral and written skills to be flexible in using and understanding many genres of spoken and written language to succeed socially, educationally and vocationally.

Language and cognitive development proceed in parallel paths, but there are synchronies and asynchronies in the paths (Bates, Bretherton and Snyder, 1988). Memory is a cognitive domain that is closely related to language, particularly vocabulary and conceptual development. When children use speech to communicate for everyday purposes, they do not think about whether they have the right words and morphology stored in their mental lexicons. Word retrieval is fairly automatic and success depends partially on how frequently they access particular words and related forms. Children typically learn new vocabulary incidentally when they hear people using it in everyday activities. Indeed, toddlers learning their first words benefit from a process known as 'fast mapping' to draw initial hypotheses about the meaning of a new word (Carey, 1978; Dollaghan, 1985). They infer the word's meaning (referent) from something salient in the immediate context, but only when the referent is simultaneously the focus of the speaker. Frequency of use seems to account for ease of learning and ease of retrieval of new vocabulary.

Learning a first language thus proceeds relatively automatically, whereas second-language learning is frequently much more taxing on conscious processes. Children using alternative communication probably learn words receptively in much the same way as children with intact speech, although ease of learning may be challenged by decreased expressive usage, which ordinarily helps cement vocabulary in memory, rendering retrieval easier over time. Empirical research suggests that fast mapping is apparent, although with limitations in children with intellectual impairment (Romski et al., 1995; Wilkinson and Albert, 2001; Wilkinson and Green, 1998). For example, Wilkinson and Green (1998) observed that non-linguistic factors, such as memory, could account for problems of language learning in the individuals they studied. Note that adequate language comprehension is critical to the success of fast mapping (Sevcik and Romski, 1997).

Once children enter formal schooling, they are increasingly required to memorize new material deliberately (for example, words in science class, and the names and faces of new classmates). Intentionally storing and retrieving this information can place heavy demands on attention and memory, and may suffer from interference from similar material in memory. Unlike adults, who automatically identify the need to recruit cognitive strategies to assist in storage and retrieval tasks, children must first be taught how and when to use certain strategies. Strategy competence is also required for the strategy user to be successful: strategies typically have sequenced steps or procedures collectively known as strategy mechanics. There are many types of mnemonic strategies that differ in terms of ease of use, cognitive demand and need for training. Simple rehearsal is first observed in three and four year-olds, who spontaneously rehearse by naming items, but just once (Baker-Ward, Ornstein and Holden, 1984). Repeated rehearsal emerges next, and in early elementary school, children may spontaneously learn cumulative rehearsal (Ornstein, Naus and Liberty, 1975). At school, children learn to use higher level strategies, such as visual and verbal imagery, key words, organization, acronyms made of the first letter of a series of words and paired-associate learning to assist studying (Bjorklund, Muir-Broaddus and Schneider, 1990). Eventually, many of the strategies become automated for use with mundane tasks. Communicating with communication aids will be shown to make considerable memory and strategy demands on the users that may be challenging, given this general developmental trend.

Challenges to aided language acquisition

Children's acquisition of aided communication can be challenging for numerous reasons. Challenges pertain to the child's particular impairments, to support systems surrounding the child and to the technology itself. The relative importance of each factor will differ according to the attributes of the learner. The following list includes some of the challenges:

- limited availability of intelligible, expressive means of communication to the child, particularly during the earliest years;
- impaired physical access to expressive means;
- reduced and/or impoverished opportunities for active participation in the full array of communication experiences;
- absent or limited peer and adult models of aided communication;
- high overall demands on the child's attention resources arising from need for conscious monitoring of typically routine activities.

Unlike typically developing speaking children, these children may not have access to intelligible methods of expression until formal schooling begins. Thus their expressive development is likely to be delayed. Severely delayed or impaired neuromotor development reduces the variety of alternative modes and available selection of items to be communicated and renders communication attempts more effortful. Even if they have had early intervention with simple forms of aided communication, they are likely to exhibit a grammar that is different from the spoken language in their environment. Tradeoffs are made between getting their idea across and using complex grammatical means to do so (Kraat, 1985). Unconventional communication methods that are effective within the family circle persist, making communication with strangers more difficult.

There are usually few, if any, role models in the environment to support the child's acquisition of aided communicative competence (Bruno and Dribben, 1998; Cirlot-New, Civils and Oxley, 2001). There has been a renewed interest in the role of imitation in social, cognitive and linguistic domains, such that they are now viewed as the foundation of social cultural learning (Tomasello, 1996; Tomasello, Kruger and Ratner, 1993). There are important implications in this theory for alternative communication. First, there are populations, such as individuals with autism, who lack the necessary social referencing skills upon which communication is premised (Tomasello, 1992). Second, without the presence of competent aided communicators as models, children cannot readily benefit from innate mimetic abilities that seem essential to the development of social cultural learning, such as communication (see Nelson, 1999).

In school, children may receive complex speech-output communication systems that require time and effort to master. Thus, the process of conveying ideas is complicated by the additional demands of the technology. An examination of the inherent operational demands of technology must consider how these demands compete or interact with existing demands on the developing child. The focus of this chapter is on two particular demands: memory and strategy use. Technology is moving ahead rapidly, opening new solutions to old problems, but it comes at a price. Compared with natural speech, aided communication places different demands on both the speaker and listener that are not yet well understood by the community, a situation that does not facilitate language development. This chapter will address the particular cognitive and linguistic demands of diverse aided communication modes and equipment, and how these special demands interact with various aspects of child development, including cognition and language.

Memory and strategies

Two cognitive skills are critical for successful mastery of aided communication, particularly electronic devices with speech output: memory and use of strategies. Memory is required for operating the device, for remembering the lexicon and means of accessing it. Strategies are required to facilitate communicative, linguistic, operational and social competence; and they are critical to support memory processes.

Researchers conventionally consider memory from several perspectives:

- how memory is structured;
- how information is processed as people try to store or retrieve it;
- how people exercise conscious control of memory processes.

Children differ significantly from adults, and children at different age levels differ significantly from one another across all three of these parameters of memory.

Short-term stores: sensory memory and working memory

Short-term memory includes a very brief sensory store, lasting just seconds, and working memory, often described as the mental desktop, having limited capacity, but one that increases with age. A digit span of two or three is typical for young children, but it increases steadily to adult levels (seven plus-or-minus two) through the years of formal schooling (Dempster, 1981).

Working memory can be defined as 'The dynamic part of the memory system that is responsible for maintaining temporary information during mental operations. It has limited capacity that constrains the performance of cognitive skills' (Hitch and Towse, 1995, p. 3). The development of working memory has been well researched, but there is not yet a universally accepted explanation of how it develops. Changes in working memory attributable to a combination of maturation and experiential factors have been proposed by Neo-Piagetians (see Case, 1995).

Efficiency-of-processing explanations draw mainly on the model proposed by Baddeley and Hitch (1974). In this model there are three components: a central executive and two modality-specific sensory storage buffers: the articulatory-phonatory loop system and the visual-spatial sketch pad. Speed of rehearsal, which is affected by the articulatory system, increases with age. It has been found that slower rates of rehearsal result in increased decay of memory traces in the peripheral store. Thus, children have more difficulty than adults in storing information through the loop because they effectively articulate more slowly.

Not all memory tasks are dependent on the phonological loop. Complex verbal tasks seem to be more dependent on the capacity for sharing workspace resources (Hitch and Towse, 1995). Guttentag (1984), for example, studied the ability of seven-, eight- and 11-year-old children to use cumulative rehearsal to memorize a list of words while also performing a secondary finger-tapping task. He found that across the age levels there was a decrease in the interference of the memory task on finger tapping. Thus, he concluded that over time, use of cumulative rehearsal required less and less processing capacity.

Use of special mnemonic strategies, a more elaborated knowledge base, and greater automation of mental operations can influence the apparent capacity of working memory as children develop. External and internal distractions and deficits in ability to process information through particular sensory modalities can effectively reduce this capacity.

Long-term memory stores: declarative and non-declarative memory

By convention, a first-order distinction is made between two types of long-term memory: declarative and non-declarative memory (Baddeley, 1986). Although a spatial metaphor of 'store' is invoked, this distinction does not imply particular sites in the brain. The declarative long-term memory store contains memory for factual or conceptual information, which is called semantic memory and includes world knowledge, language, rules and concepts. This semantic information can be thought of as conventional and may be quite abstract. Memory for events (temporal knowledge) is called episodic memory and includes individual, autobiographical knowledge and records of past experiences. Episodic memory is idiosyncratic and need not reflect conventions. Declarative memory is easily described as memory for 'knowing that' and reflects conscious, deliberate or explicit knowledge and processing. Knowing that Paris is the capital city of France (semantic knowledge) is not the same as knowing about Paris from one's visit there (episodic knowledge). Also in the declarative store is second-order knowledge called metacognition regarding both declarative knowledge (knowing that I know that) and procedural knowledge (knowing that I know how) (Kuhn, 1999).

Children organize information in a different way from adults. This influences how information is stored in memory and the relevance and reliability of cues that are helpful to children for retrieving it (Bjorklund, 2000). There is a developmental progression characterized by decreased reliance on perceptual features of objects and increased use of other types of categorization. Children aged two to three years use idiosyncratic classification (Bjorklund, 2000). They group items mainly in pairs, but either they cannot provide a rationale for their pairings or their reasons do not reflect logical organization. Three- to four-year-old children can use perceptual grouping, such as things that are pointed or red. By the time children are six to nine years old they organize items predominantly according to complementary relationships such as theme (for example, objects that go together during a familiar routine) or function, particularly as the child uses the objects (for example, spoon and spade because both are used for digging in the sand box). They also learn to sort objects by using more than one feature. Thematic organization is not stable: in one situation, a child pairs a spoon and spade, but in another the child may pair the spoon with a bowl. Complementary relationships include episodic relationships, which are relationships among objects made by the child according to his particular experiences using them, and may or may not reflect conventional association. So, while children may conventionally group toothpaste and toothbrush, they might also include coins, because the tooth fairy gives them money for nice teeth. Association stability is important for consistent use of pictographs, regardless of contextual interference, to elicit prestored vocabulary for a speech-output device.

More abstract organization develops slowly through school years and is influenced by academic demands. This developmental trend is known variously as the episodic-semantic shift or thematic-taxonomic shift. The developmental progression implied reflects decreased reliance on perceptions and personal experience (episodic memory) and increased reliance on abstract thought (semantic memory); and has implications for aided communication. Children's organizational ability is highly personalized and therefore likely to be idiosyncratic. The younger the child, the more the immediate setting is important, because rather than using it actively, children seem to be constrained by it. These organizational attributes influence how easily children who use communication aids will learn the way their vocabulary is arranged on a display, particularly how the 'invisible' selections are organized. Efficient word retrieval requires proficiency in navigating the device according to its organization, and not the transient organization supplied by the child.

Research specific to developmental patterns of association pertinent to pictographic encoding was conducted by Bruno (1991), who sought to establish a probabilistic hierarchy of serial associative responses to graphic and spoken words made by adults, six-year-old and four-year-old children. Her purpose was to determine how adults could best select semantically organized pictograph sequences for Minspeak applications to be used by young children (Minspeak is discussed later).

Four-year-olds used, in order, functional and then episodic associations to both words and pictures, typically in the form noun–verb. An example of a functional association to *book* would be *read* and reflects the use of some action, activity or use associated with the presented word; whereas an episodic association consisted of a narrative, such as: *You put it on a shelf.* Their use of abstract semantic associations was very low. Examples include rhyme – an auditory association – or use of a salient property of the word or picture presented, such as size, a visual association: ball-big.

Six-year-old children's first associations to both pictures and words were also predominantly functional, whereas the second associations were mainly nominal. According to Bruno, nominal associations fall within the grammatical class of the word and reflect different levels of relationship to it. For example, if *apple* is presented, an association could be *fruit* (superordinate), *pie* (subordinate), *banana* (co-ordinate) or *refrigerator* (location). This trend is consistent with other studies and reflects the general development of the semantic system (Nelson, 1999). The six-year-olds' second associations to pictures and words differed significantly from each other. They gave predominantly functional associations to pictures and nominal associations to words; and they made a greater variety of association categories to words than to pictures. Adults offered first nominal associations and second functional associations to both words and pictures, thus reversing the children's pattern. Goossens', Elder and Bray (1990) used the Semantic Compaction Competency Profile (Elder, Goossens' and Bray, 1990) to determine the ability of three- to five-year-old children to use previously learned pictograph sequences for communication. The children's recall of the sequences was very poor, even though the experimental settings were age appropriate. One conclusion is that whereas children may be able to associate certain pictographs or pictograph sequences with sentences, they may not necessarily be able to access or exploit this knowledge consistently over time because episodic organization is not stable in memory.

Thus, the episodic-semantic shift is relevant to representation itself, to ease of storage and retrieval processes and stability of memories over time. The role of context is very important in framing children's associate information. Without the right context, previously made associations may be meaningless to a child. Until approximately seven or eight years of age, the automatic knowledge base (perceptual knowledge) dominates causal behaviour. By nine or 10 years of age, metacognitive processes begin to dominate. For example, nine and 10 year-olds, but not seven and eight year-olds, actively use their knowledge of organization to direct memory strategy use (Hasselhorn, 1995). These issues will be taken up further under memory strategy development.

The *non-declarative long-term memory store* includes unconscious or implicit memory for skills. It includes procedural memory, emotional memory and priming (both classical and operant conditioning). Procedural memory can be thought of as 'knowing how'. Daily living requires that hundreds of simple and complex routines be executed automatically; indeed, focusing attention on them can actually impair performance (for example, handwriting). I know that I can write (declarative knowledge), but in order to write, I no longer think about how to grip a pen (procedural knowledge). If I injure my hand, I must readjust my grip; to do so, I would engage metastrategic information in declarative memory to self-instruct so that I could write again. Writing will no longer be effortless, will tax working memory, and will probably distract me from the information I am writing.

Basic memory processes: storage and retrieval

Information is moved from short-term to long-term stores and subsequently retrieved for use through basic processes of storage and retrieval, which can be conscious or unconscious. Procedural aspects of tasks are generally stored and retrieved unconsciously and are facilitated by repeated, motivated practice. Unconscious storage and retrieval of information occurs when the knowledge base is richly elaborated (Bjorklund et al., 1990). For example, new information storage can occur automatically in the course of completing an activity, but purposeful behaviours are often needed to achieve initial storage. These latter behaviours support prospective memorization (remembering something now for use later). Retrieval can occur automatically or may require the use of strategies.

Strategies

Conscious procedures designed to facilitate storage and retrieval processes are called mnemonic strategies. A standard definition of strategies states that they are cognitive operations in which the user does something special to achieve cognitive goals (for example, comprehending or remembering) (Pressley et al., 1985). The special behaviour may involve just one step or a sequence of steps. This mechanical knowledge is a form of procedural knowledge. It is generally agreed that strategies are potentially conscious, controllable activities, which may become automatic with practice. Strategy use progresses through a predictable developmental course that is characterized by growth in:

- the ability to use increasingly complex and sophisticated strategies across social, linguistic and cognitive domains;
- metastrategic knowledge concerning when and why to prefer one strategy to another according to the perceived goal.

According to the *overlapping waves theory* of Siegler (1996), use of a new strategy comes and goes in waves as the child repeats a task. Mastery of the procedural aspects of increasingly sophisticated strategies is just one part of development, and equally important in development is to relinquish less appropriate strategies when problem-solving calls for different strategies (Kuhn, 1999). Thus, metastrategic insights, although important in the long term, do not lead to immediate and permanent changes in strategic behaviour.

There is currently a well-established understanding of how children become competent users of various types of strategies, the errors they produce and benefits they accrue from strategy use (Miller, 1990). At a certain time for a given child, use of strategies with many steps can be challenging and can even detract from task performance. A consistent finding is that the more the strategy relies on use of symbols, the older the child must be to use it independently and reliably. Use of two distinct representation systems in aided communication (for example, pictographs and electronically stored speech) may complicate language production for children. Children may be required to use pictographs to represent pre-recorded sentences. Pictographs are thus transformed from simple representations to strategic shortcuts.

Efficient strategy development for storage and retrieval proceeds over the lifespan, probably occurring mostly during school years. While even two-year-old children demonstrate some limited awareness of the need to do something special to help them remember something for later (for example, location of toy or candy in an array of containers), their strategies are very limited. The younger children are, the greater is their reliance on non-specific, external cues for memorizing material for future use or remembering previously learned material. It is expected that there is a correlation between strategy use and improved recall (utilization efficiency or strategy effectiveness). Indeed from age eight, use of organizational behaviours is highly predictive of performance at any measurement point, and performance gains in strategy use itself are excellent predictors of performance gains in recall (Sodian and Schneider, 1999). The period spanning ages six to eight seems to be a transitional time for the use of organizational strategies. However, for younger children, neither use nor non-use of a strategy relates to recall. Because certain strategic behaviours are driven by an understanding of learning and remembering, it is not surprising that pre-schoolers can understand simple strategies (such as perceptual inspection and verbalization), whereas only children older than eight years begin to understand strategies requiring inferential processes (such as semantic organization or elaboration) (Sodian and Schneider, 1999).

Microgenetic studies suggest that simply knowing how to use a particular strategy, and even having a basic understanding of how it works and when it can be helpful (metastrategic knowledge), is initially insufficient to motivate its use. Children continue to recycle old strategies even if these are inefficient, and do not abandon them immediately. It may take a transition of many months or longer for children to develop consistent, preferential use of a previously learned strategy (Miller and Coyle, 1999).

Production difficulties occur when children 'forget' to use a known and understood strategy when it is needed. These lapses reflect the presence of too many competing demands on their attention and working memory. There are numerous examples in alternative communication: children try to use unintelligible speech repeatedly even when their alternative communication system is available, but happily use it when reminded; children use automatic procedural guidance to locate vocabulary instead of using a pictograph, and so forth. Children making these errors are capable of using a strategy that helps when it is used, but must be reminded to do so. Production difficulties occur in all age groups, but only when the strategy is relatively new to the user.

Utilization difficulties reflect a phenomenon that appears to be highly robust (Bjorklund and Coyle, 1995). They are observed in children of all ages, at a transitional phase of strategy use and in younger children attempting strategies that are cognitively too taxing, for example when four-year-olds are told to use strategies requiring higher level semantic organization. These difficulties reveal that strategy use represents only one way to enhance performance, and because of its cost in terms of mental effort, it may not even be the most efficient way. This is a finding that is very relevant to aided communication. Children's performance or non-performance of the many strategies that arise in aided communication should be considered in this developmental perspective.

Metacognition

Second-order knowledge residing in declarative memory, including metacognitive and metastrategic knowledge, may be important for mature use of aided communication. Second-order knowledge includes self-monitoring skills related to estimate of task difficulty and relevance of known strategies for the task. Using aided communication includes skills that are procedural and proceed automatically, without the need for conscious monitoring by the user. Task analysis suggests that as devices grow more complex, especially in terms of how information is organized, the demand on metastrategic knowledge and metacognitive knowledge increases. For example, a user would draw on declarative memory to recognize that the device does not contain a particular word or phrase, and on metastrategic knowledge from the metalinguistic domain to circumvent the problem. Similarly, the user would draw on declarative knowledge to know that the device has the word or phrase, but not 'where' it is located. Metastrategic knowledge includes the particular values inherent in specific strategies and their relationship to particular tasks.

It would guide strategy use in locating a word, such as application of knowledge of taxonomic organization or a paired-associate strategy (see below). Strategies may also be needed for initial learning, so that subsequent retrieval is facilitated (for instance, rehearsal). For example, children learn that the larger the set of information to be remembered, the harder they will have to try to remember it. They recognize that one type of rehearsal would be better than another. These insights may be learned automatically in the course of doing the task, or as a result of adults pointing out the relationship between improved memory performance and strategy use (Fabricius and Cavalier, 1989; Fletcher and Bray, 1996; McGilly and Siegler, 1989).

The relationship between metamemory, metastrategic knowledge and effective strategy use is still poorly understood (Pressley, Borkowski and O'Sullivan, 1985). Findings from microgenetic studies point to the likelihood of a bi-directional relationship. Kuhn (1999) suggests that the central goal of the metastrategic knowledge system is co-ordination of task goals and strategy components to attain an optimal intersection of the two. According to this view, understanding task goals and understanding strategies and their application to those goals follow distinct developmental tracks that interact to prompt effective, timely use of strategies. In terms of aided language acquisition, Kuhn's conjecture suggests that it is important that young aided communicators develop an understanding not just of the mechanics of the various strategies implicated in aided communication but the goals they serve to enhance rate, to locate vocabulary, and so forth. Children who develop this wider appreciation of the need for effortful steps or additional learning are likely to master these steps and become more proficient communicators than children who lack this insight.

Memory and strategy demands in aided communication

Numerous strategies, some nested within others, are implicated in aided communication. While some may eventually become automatic, others may always require attention, thus imposing demands on working memory. Strategy development is closely related to development of memory, problem solving, executive ability and motivation; and certain types of strategies may require quite sophisticated representation and organizational ability, which may be particularly demanding on children younger than eight or nine years, and on individuals with cognitive impairments.

Aided communication: status as a strategy

Aided communication is itself a strategy used to overcome problems in using speech or manual signing. A child must make a decision about when to use aided communication in preference to other communication strategies, such as speaking. This decision occurs in communicative situations, which itself imposes numerous demands on the communicator's attention to topic, setting, and so forth. There is ample anecdotal evidence that under various circumstances, children of all ages appear to 'forget' to use their aided communication strategies, even though they are operationally competent and can use them in other situations. This failure to use appropriate strategies may be predicted from the general knowledge of developmental strategy use. The younger the children, the more likely they are to be more interested in the ongoing discourse or activity than in consciously self-monitoring the need for aided communication. Children of all ages using aided communication are likely to experience great demands on working memory, particularly when they are just beginning to incorporate use of devices into their communication repertoire. Unlike speech, aided communication competes with ongoing activities, like play and storybook reading, many of which may be more compelling to children and thus better able to hold their attention. To use aided communication children must shift their focus of attention to the communication board and temporarily ignore the activity (Light, Binger and Kelford-Smith, 1994). The children most likely to be affected at this level are young children who have some functional use of speech, and children with cognitive delays.

Ellis (1997) noted that much of most studies of strategy development focus on improvements in speed and accuracy of performance by children of all ages completing problems in what she describes as 'socially decontextualized situations', for example experimental monitoring of strategies used to solve arithmetic problems. Unlike solving arithmetic problems, using aided communication depends greatly on social and cultural norms, which can shape cognitive performance (Goodnow, 1990; Nunes, Schlieman and Carraher, 1993). Thus, apart from strategy knowledge, children also take into account their understanding of what is expected of them and what is acceptable to others. Children's decisions to favour a particular mode of communication in some situations are likely to be consciously or unconsciously influenced by the positive and negative appraisals they have received previously (Borkowski and Muthukrishna, 1995). Their emotional memories of success and failure in particular situations could thus influence choices of aided communication strategies.

Evidence that children can have great difficulty co-ordinating social and task goals must also be considered (Schmidt, Ollendick and Stancowicz, 1988). Ability to regulate the focus of attention is one skill, but pragmatic development and strategic development also influence children's use or non-use of aided communication as a conversational repair strategy. Most children do not develop the pragmatic skills of monitoring themselves and using effective repair strategies during conversational breakdowns until ages nine or 10 (Brinton et al., 1986). Five-year-olds typically have few repair strategies other than simple repetition. This difficulty relates to lower ability to presuppose partner perspective, to co-ordinate communicator–partner perspectives and to complete metalinguistic analysis of the conversational breakdown.

Strategic demands for physically making selections from a grid on communication aids

To use aided communication, children may use either direct or indirect selection techniques, or both if needed. When physical and/or sensory impairment interferes with the ability to produce sufficiently accurate and reliable movements for functional direct selection, indirect methods are needed. For example, in partner-assisted scanning, a partner can read or name the available choices while allowing time for the child to choose one. The child is under minimal demand to perform motor tasks, but must rely on someone else to establish the topic and provide specific choices correctly. Children have greater independence if they use one or more switches to control an electronic scanner that highlights the choice, for example via adjacent lights, highlighter or cursor. The price of this independence is the need to learn individual procedures, including scanning and switch activation patterns and co-ordination and timing of these strategic operations. These procedures are initially physically and cognitively effortful for children, regardless of age (Ratcliff, 1994). Moreover, they serve as distractions to the act of communication. The younger and the more novice the aided communicator, the more likely it will be that these activities will tax working memory, rendering communication more challenging.

In the long term, procedural memory can guide spatial-kinaesthetic patterns driving switch use, scanning patterns and item selection from an array, thus reducing the cognitive load. However, children first need adequate practice of switch use in simple situations that are not complicated by additional demands. Similarly, children of all ages will automatically move their hands to the approximate location of a button or selection even without conscious attempts to memorize its location in an array if they have sufficient practice. Interacting with materials can be sufficient for remembering some aspects of the task or the items themselves (Ornstein et al., 1975). Identifying how much knowledge a child can acquire by using a system to accomplish a goal, such as locating a message from multilayered displays, and how much by the application of deliberate learning strategies, is an issue for aided communication. It is also important to determine the conditions that must hold for a procedure to become truly automated. In my experience, learning to use a switch, for example, initially requires attention, but even skilled seven-year-olds who have been given plenty of practice can guide scanning with apparently minimal attention to the scanning process. Children with severe neuromotor impairment may never be able to automate switch activation, attention to scanning and their co-ordination fully, and so must communicate with these as constant distractions.

Representational strategies for aided vocabulary development

Most typical four-year-olds already know several thousand words and use hundreds on a daily basis. Their lexicons also contain derivational and inflectional morphology that allows for modulation of meaning. They access the lexicon relatively automatically. To accommodate this growing lexicon, communication aids would have to contain a large number of pages of selections, but there are practical constraints on the size and complexity of the selection set available to the child directly, particularly for young children and children with cognitive impairments. Thus, although children's receptive vocabulary may be age appropriate, there is typically a huge gap between the words children know, compared with:

• what they can see directly on their displays;
• what is actually, but indirectly, available to them in organized books, eye-gaze charts or multiple virtual 'pages' or levels in speech output devices.

Representation strategies are critical for both guessing at available vocabulary and locating it. Clearly, children acquiring aided language must engage in extraneous tasks to support vocabulary development. Knowing which of their mental lexicons are available through the device is a metalinguistic skill, whereas knowing how to locate individual items, quickly and accurately during communication, includes strategic knowledge of representation and encoding systems and metastrategic knowledge about the strategies themselves. Each skill imposes separate cognitive demands on the child.

In devices with very small selection sets and simple representation, locating vocabulary may be procedural but, as a child's lexicon increases, a display can present only a small set of vocabulary for selection, necessitating multiple pages requiring logical organization. Procedural guidance is afforded by automatic use of spatial location on an array (for example, corner keys are easy to remember), colour codes, and kinaesthetic patterns. When an overlay has a large grid of keys, use of these strategies can narrow down the search, but may not fully specify which vocabulary is at which location (Oxley and Norris, 2000). These automatic methods for locating vocabulary may also be subject to conscious, metastrategic control; that is, children may strategically use the knowledge that some kind of vocabulary is in a certain quadrant to narrow their search. Without adequate understanding of pictographic representation, however, the child may not be able to complete accurate vocabulary retrieval. This child would have to search by trial and error.

Discovering the device's lexicon

There is not always an exact match between children's lexicon and the content of their communication devices, so children must learn which vocabulary is available. When presented with a new device, both children and adults engage in trial-and-error button pushing to establish what the device can say. They might or might not attend to the graphic representations on device buttons. If they do, they are relying on a representation strategy to guess at available vocabulary based on what the pictographs connote to them (see below). Depending on the child's cognitive abilities, the pictographs may be useful or entirely misleading. The device's vocabulary may be memorized in two ways: deliberately, through prospective memorization strategies, or incidentally, through procedural means.

Prospective storage strategies occur when children memorize available vocabulary intentionally and in advance of needing it, through some sort of rehearsal, for example pushing a key, listening to it and repeating the process as often as necessary for all keys. When three- to five-year-old children are told to 'try hard', they are able to remember information in the course of play (Baker-Ward et al., 1984). Investigations have determined that children's greater attention to materials is responsible for increased recall. Older children improve the quality of their rehearsal by using what is known as cumulative rehearsal; that is, instead of repeating each new item several times, they chain new items to previous items before they are rehearsed. Cumulative rehearsal is more effective for memorizing lists and helps with recall. Even five-year-olds can improve recall by using this strategy, although they exhibit problems with production unless they are prompted (Ornstein et al., 1975).

The most natural way children learn the vocabulary of their device is through everyday use, a process akin to second-language learning, in that children somehow come to know whether a word is available or not (metalinguistic knowledge). Vocabulary is learned incidentally, for example through trial and error, with or without adult support. Adult guidance to the messages can facilitate functional use of the available vocabulary. Learning of this type is automatic and therefore not strategic, that is, intentional.

Vocabulary organization and navigation

Even with adequate vocabulary in the device, there is the challenge of locating it. Individual items may be stored on different pages of a book or display; they may be encoded with sequences of keys on devices that have fixed displays; or they may be buried in complex nests of dynamically displayed pages. Young aided communicators must learn how to use these organizational systems to retrieve vocabulary.

Adults typically organize vocabulary in children's communication devices to make items easy to find, typically basing it on assumptions about the child's developmental 'level' (for example, Bruno, 1988). For novice users and children below the age of about eight, vocabulary is organized according to the environment in which it is most commonly used (in other words, thematically), with the exception of core vocabulary, which, by definition, includes items that are used across environments. This type of organization may be well suited to the organizational patterns used by young children. Later, vocabulary can be added using branching strategies based on conceptual organization more congruent with the cognitive abilities of older children.

There may also be special procedural strategies that provide the child with short cuts to producing multi-word utterances (for example, whole sentences programmed under one key, or short sequences of keys) and morphological markers. Some of the navigation and shortcut strategies required for retrieving vocabulary from a communication aid must be learned intentionally and may demand considerable understanding of how the lexicon is organized. For example, to locate an item of clothing, a school-aged child may use either taxonomic knowledge to determine that jeans are clothes, or thematic knowledge to determine that they are things to wear; and to know that these items can be found at one location, itself represented by a pictograph. While taxonomic organization may be appropriate for school-aged children, it may not make sense to a pre-schooler, whose associations are more perceptual or thematic. Thus, three- and four-year-olds might understand that pressing a button with a pictograph depicting a closet (thematic association) could lead them to a page of pictographs depicting specific items of clothing, such as jeans, but they also tend to react to perceptual associative features of the pictographs. More perceptually directed children might have difficulty using the dresser as a cue to the clothes category, and might instead select a button marked by any pictograph that bears some perceptual association to jeans. By contrast, one could argue that young aided communicators whose devices are taxonomically organized may still learn how to locate a 'hidden' item, stored at another location, without fully understanding why it is stored there. The difference here hinges on distinctions between deliberate and automatic memory access. The likelihood of both production and utilization difficulties is increased for younger children attempting to use these higher level strategies.

Representation

Perhaps the most complex developmental issue is how children come to understand how system designers relate pictographs to the stored vocabulary – how the stored lexicon is encoded or represented visually on a display.

This information must first be encoded before it can be stored in memory. Communication aid users are learning to represent language bimodally – they learn language in an auditory environment but express it, in part, through graphic signs. A problem for some aided communicators is that they might not understand speech and so, unless they have an adequate receptive understanding of the graphic signs, they will experience difficulty understanding the function of the communication aid.

Children using graphic signs to elicit speech from devices potentially face challenges arising from the need to co-ordinate graphic and auditory representations within working memory. Note that, when used on a speech output communication aid, a pictograph represents a pre-stored word or some other unit, and so it is part of a predetermined pair of associated items. Native users of either a spoken or signed language are believed to think using modality-specific representations. The question is what the equivalent modality is for children using bimodal language. Certainly, until they have formed strong associations between specific pictographs and related words or concepts it is hard to imagine anything other than a translation process in which the children first formulate the intended message through 'inner speech' and then translate this into pictographs that serve as a medium to generate an equivalent, but not necessarily identical, synthetically spoken utterance. Until it is automated, this translation process may be impaired by numerous distractions. First, children must retain the whole idea – presumably a whole utterance – in working memory while they complete the necessary operational procedures to retrieve individual words or a sentence from the aid. The phonological loop system would be activated for this task. There is mounting evidence that anarthria and dysarthria can impair efficient use of the phonatory loop system for rehearsal in working memory (Sandberg and Hjelmquist, 1996). Breaking down the utterance into chunks that correspond with stored units of language in the communication device constitutes another demand, suggesting that the visual-spatial sketchpad is activated. Thus, there may be multiple representations of multiple lengths of the planned utterance to be juggled in working memory. This situation lends itself to cross-modal interference such as the lexical selection errors observed in slips of the tongue. There is no empirical data on production errors of aided communicators to support these conjectures but adults using such systems report them (personal communication). It can safely be assumed that, however difficult the task is for adults, it will be more difficult and possibly overwhelming for children, particularly novice communication aid users. This may account for the fact that children use simpler expressive means at the cost of precise expression or even a more active participant role in conversation. Changes in technology may mitigate some of this demand, but even after automating as many procedural aspects of device operation as possible, children may find this form of communication very demanding. Working memory has limited capacity and the limitations are more obvious in children and populations with cognitive impairments.

A second representation issue is that visual-graphic representations (pictographs) require interpretation in a way that is not characteristic of spoken words. A single word can encapsulate the relationship among multiple arguments in a proposition. To achieve this task through pictographs on the display of a speech output communication device the designer must present the individual arguments on the same key and the observer must be able to infer the intended meaning as it relates to the stored utterance in a device. When shown a picture, both adults and children attempt first to name it, but they vary in their associations to words and pictures (Bruno, 1991). However, when the picture contains multiple arguments, it is not always possible for the beholder to know whether an individual argument is relevant, or whether the picture is to be interpreted as a whole.

Research has addressed the relevance of iconicity, which is 'the continuum that describes symbols by ease of recognition' to ease of learning of pictographic representation (Beukelman and Mirenda, 1992, p. 11). In some situations, it is argued, iconicity may be less important than 'the reinforcing value of an item' (Reichle, 1991, p. 54). Iconicity can also be exploited to hasten learning for some populations (Mirenda and Locke, 1989) but studies also suggest that iconicity can actually interfere with strategic use of pictographs as representations for children under the age of three years (DeLoache, 1987; DeLoache and Marzolf, 1992; Tomasello, Striano and Rochat, 1999). According to DeLoache, Uttal and Pierroutsakos (1998), 'no symbol system is fully transparent: it cannot be assumed that even the most iconic symbol will automatically be interpreted as a representation of something other than itself' (p. 326). *Dual representation theory* assumes that somewhere between ages 2;6 and 3;0 years, children develop representational insight, the ability to simultaneously treat the same object as an object in its own right and as a representation of something else (DeLoache, 2000). Before children develop this insight, iconicity and concreteness actually interfere with their use of objects as symbols to serve a goal. For example, only after 2;6 years old children were led to believe that a real room and its contents had been 'shrunk', were they able to use a miniature object to retrieve its life-sized counterpart in the original room (DeLoache, Miller and Rosengren, 1996). Similarly, use of pictures as markers for the objects they depicted interfered with children's ability to use the pictures to retrieve the matching objects hidden behind them (DeLoache and Burns, 1994). These findings have immediate relevance to aided communication. It is conventional to introduce pictographic systems to children as early as possible to facilitate expressive communication. The lack of representation insight can be observed when young children and cognitively impaired individuals treat pictures as the objects they depict. Experience seems to be a critical determinant of children's ability to distinguish a picture from its referent but it may be insufficient to allow children to co-ordinate both facts in service of a communicative goal.

Iconicity as a facilitator and a barrier

Electronic and non-electronic communication aids differ in terms of the helpfulness of iconicity. If a child can be primed reliably by context to establish meaning of specific signs or pictographs on non-electronic displays, their iconicity relative to the discriminative cue may be helpful. A child whose representation skills are perceptually driven may experience more success using a non-electronic picture display that lacks speech output than using a speech output device. For example, assume a child understands that a pictograph can represent some associated object or concept and has a partner who is willing to interpret a selection as a communicative attempt. Provided the child can associate an available pictograph with the idea to be communicated, the child can select that picture and it is likely that the co-operative partner will interpret the selection as it was intended. Indeed, different situations could render other pictographs more appropriate for conveying the same meaning. Thus, children using non-electronic picture boards can potentially use pictures flexibly to convey a variety of meanings, which may be metaphorical or literal, direct or indirect, depending on the situation. For example, a picture of the sun may mean 'sun' in one situation and 'hot', 'summer' or 'day time' in other situations. This metaphoric capability depends on the co-operation of the communication partner; that is, the partner's readiness to use context to interpret the intended message (Besio and Chinato, 1996; von Tetzchner and Martinsen, 1996). Sperber and Wilson (1995) define context as 'the set of premises used in interpreting an utterance', that is 'a psychological construct, a subset of the hearer's assumptions about the world . . . not limited to information in the immediate physical environment or the immediately preceding utterances' (p. 15). Contextual priming (unconscious) can help the child because the picture, which at that moment suggests the desired message, may be used to express that message.

By contrast, the same child with the same picture overlay attached to a computerized keyboard on a speech output communication device must eventually come to understand that apparent relevance of a pictograph may not always be a reliable cue for utterance elicitation because each pictograph maps precisely to one key and its pre-stored spoken vocabulary. Although two or more pictures may simultaneously suggest (connote) the same meaning to the child in one moment and in one context, only one of them will lead to the desired output from the device. Contextual priming can actually interfere with the child's selection (Brown and DeLoache, 1978). The child's ability to represent is not of itself the determining factor here; the child may well appreciate the content of the picture. Instead, the child should rely on memory for paired-associate information to resolve the dilemma (some relation between a specific pictograph and stored speech). Moreover, the contextual priming that assisted pictograph selection for the non-electronic board users might interfere with the selection process by leading children to 'forget' that a different strategy is required. Children's selection of an automatically primed pictograph, but not the one eliciting the desired word, would constitute a production difficulty. Thus, as children's vocabulary grows, part of the information to be learned may be a uniquely discriminating cue needed to resolve which of the competing pictographs actually signals the desired utterance. For example, a picture of the sun would be highly transparent as meaning 'hot' when a young picture-board user is outdoors sweating in a Louisiana July, but the same picture may be quite opaque as a symbol for 'hot' relative to a picture of a bowl of steaming porridge, when the child is using an overlay for retelling 'The Three Bears' story. A child using a picture-board overlay could use either picture to communicate 'hot', depending on the situation. Thus, contextual priming could actually help the non-electronic device user select a suitable pictograph for communication. However, it could induce a speech output device user to miscue and consequently suffer the penalty of miscommunication after inadvertently selecting the picture of the hot porridge and elicit *Who's been eating my porridge?* instead of *It's hot out here* (coded by a picture of the sun) (Oxley, 1995). A co-operative partner might ignore the spoken output and honour the 'sense' of the picture choice, but such co-operation cannot be assumed with unfamiliar communication partners who may not attend to the pictographic overlay – and even familiar partners might have difficulties disregarding the spoken utterance.

A hide-and-seek game is a useful metaphor for characterizing the search for vocabulary in a complex array. The spoken words cannot be seen, so users of communication aids with speech output must guess how to access them from available cues, which include pictographs. Clearly, children cannot always rely exclusively on the iconic properties of pictographs as guides to stored vocabulary during initial learning. In the case of communication aids with complicated encoding systems, children might need to learn that factors other than iconicity might govern the precise relationship between picture and utterance, regardless of the seeming appropriateness of a particular picture as the cue to the right place to push to speak the desired utterance.

Schneider and Pressley (1989) summarized the main findings from numerous controlled studies of pre-schoolers' use of pictures as retrieval cues for location in many everyday and naturalistic experimental tasks. The findings suggest that:

- children as young as two years can benefit from them;
- three-year-olds tend to use them only in very simple tasks;
- all pre-schoolers need prompting to use markers prospectively, to help locate a hidden object later.

Thus, with prompting, children may reflect on the need to do something special to memorize and remember which key to press from the array to produce a particular utterance and to search deliberately according to perceptual or spatial clues. But even if children can search deliberately, the search must be co-ordinated with the knowledge of which picture to search for, particularly when multiple pictures cue the utterance simultaneously.

Picture versus encoding strategies

For adults, the use of pictures as external reminders is an intuitive and obvious solution to remembering which key elicits which utterance. However, it is not an obvious solution for children aged five years and younger, and it is a skill they must be taught. Pictures and utterances can be interrelated transparently or opaquely relative to the user's understanding. For example, if on the overlay there is one simple line drawing depicting a dog and the utterance it elicits is *dog*, then it is clear that the picture represents the utterance transparently and at an association level accessible to a young child.

However, in order to locate vocabulary, aided communicators must sometimes employ a paired-associate strategy in which they use an invented relation between two pieces of information – for example, a picture or some element of the picture and an utterance. The relation is embedded in a spoken utterance or a visual image and memorized as a verbal mnemonic, for example via rehearsal. Later, either piece of information (the pictograph or the word) cues the relational mnemonic, which in turn serves as a mediator to determine which of several competing pictures marks the location of a certain stored utterance. For example, a pictograph depicting a dog with one ear up and one down could be used to produce, for example, *ear* or *listen* with the aid. An overlay may include the pictograph of the dog and other pictographs depicting a girl, a boy, a man or a woman (all of whom have ears and are capable of listening). Why should the dog, rather than one of the others, serve as the retrieval cue for *ear* or *listen*? The conflicting cues noted above occur because the decision to associate one and not the other pictures to *ear* or *listen* is obviously an arbitrary one from the perspective of the child user.

When children must choose from several pictures on an overlay that are all equally representative and suggestive of the stored spoken utterance they are seeking to communicate, the semantic relatedness of the picture to the stored utterance may constrain the search, but not complete it. To complete the search, the child must remember why one picture was used to encode the utterance. The 'why' of this process is really a memory strategy rather than a representation strategy. The 'why' accounts for the need for deliberate creation and memorization of paired associate information that effectively links a picture to an utterance or concept, and vice versa (Light and Lindsay, 1991; Oxley and Norris, 2000). An adult could remember to use the picture of the dog to elicit the utterance *listen* by recalling either a verbal mnemonic that relates the pair of associates (for example, 'Dogs prick up their ears when they listen'), or in an imaginal mnemonic (for example, a mental image of a dog moving its ears into a listening posture). Later, when the adult wants to say *listen* but cannot remember which of several potential pictographs actually marks that utterance, the adult could use an auditory image of the word *listen* to cue the mnemonic, and use the mnemonic to remember that the dog pictograph retrieves *listen*. An analogous procedure involving visual imagery could be used with the same outcome. Both of these examples use a verbal symbol (a word) as the starting point.

The strategically created sentence or visual image containing the relevant associations between the speech output device's bimodal representation of an idea serves as the real code in this situation, whereas the picture itself serves as a mediator for the code, rather than as a unique representation of the phonological referent stored in the device (Bray, 1990). Paired-associate mnemonic strategies do not typically develop spontaneously but must be taught. Studies suggest that it is not until late childhood or adolescence that they are used spontaneously to facilitate memory (Schneider and Pressley, 1989). To create and understand verbal or imaginal mnemonics of this type is just one part of the strategy. To retain them in memory, once created, they must also be rehearsed. The ability to co-ordinate simple and complex strategies can render access to utterances in speech output devices efficient for adults, because they can reflect on their use of strategies, while it may take time for young aided communicators to become capable of and efficient at exploiting these strategies. Until they learn the necessary strategy, they may continue to use simpler strategies that might yield inaccurate utterance retrieval.

With Minspeak and similar systems, it is important that children eventually learn how the code works in order to benefit from advanced software packages that exploit it. Minspeak exploits a coding procedure where up to three keys may be pressed in sequence to elicit utterances, thereby greatly expanding the number of utterances that can be produced from a single keyboard while retaining procedurally consistent access patterns. In communication aids with dynamic displays with multiple screens, it can be helpful if icons are situated in consistent locations to reduce visual search time.

Minspeak, with its potentially limited set of icons, can facilitate this automatization of searching.

The Minspeak system is essentially taxonomic: the first pictograph in the sequence encodes a global category high in a hierarchy, the second encodes a subordinate category and the third specifies a specific member of the subordinate category. A canonical example would be a sequence consisting of (first) an apple to represent food, (second) a lightning bolt to represent speed, and (third) another lightning bolt to represent French fries (based on visual similarity of icon to actual French fry). For young children using this system, initial training may include two-icon sequences: the first icon might be a rainbow (representing 'colour') and the second icon could be a red apple (specifying 'red'). When pressed in sequence, the two icons would elicit *red* from the device. Overlays are colourful so other red items could be potential sources of distraction. It is a completely arbitrary choice for the person programming the device whether one or another red item serves as the last key of the sequence, and so the child would have to learn to ignore distracters. To reduce the effort of recalling second and third pictographs in a coded sequence, visual prompting strategies have been incorporated into Minspeak hardware. After an initial key is selected, only keys that could be used as second items in the sequence are highlighted, thus narrowing the range available for selection. While providing support, the prediction strategy nevertheless adds another chore to retrieval.

Long-term efficiency with the Minspeak system would probably require children to develop understanding of taxonomic semantic organization, a skill that begins to develop during the pre-school years but is not the predominant classification strategy until adolescence (Denney, 1974), and the ability to co-ordinate two or more strategies, for example light cues and scanning. Minspeak is just one example of an encoding system that places demands on all aspects of the memory of the user. Dynamic systems also rely on some type of categorization to guide navigation through the network of virtual pages of stored, organized vocabulary. Moreover, unless individual pages are designed with attention to consistent placement of buttons, the memory demands of visually scanning pages for frequently used keys can be overwhelming even for adults.

Certain memory strategies are called 'encoding strategies' (for example, logical letter codes and iconic encoding). The relative efficiency of these for adults has been examined by Light (Light and Lindsay, 1992; Light et al., 1990), but there are few experimental studies on the developmental course of using pictures simultaneously as memory strategies and representations (Goossens', Elder and Bray, 1990).

As children are confronted with the need to learn more and more codes for vocabulary sets (for example, definitions for social studies class), declarative or explicit knowledge of paired-associate strategy use may be required first at the time of storage (when the child is learning the code needed to retrieve the word from the device), and then at the time of retrieval (when the code must be recalled to retrieve the word from the device). This knowledge goes beyond learning what the word means, itself a challenging task for children. The point is that it is one thing for children to be successful at procedural mastery of a limited set of icon sequences, but it is quite another to have the metacognitive appreciation of how the system works and can be expanded to apply to more utterances, including inflectional and derivational morphology. Procedural learning is unlikely to be adequate for fluent retrieval of low-frequency academic vocabulary, which may require intentional memorization. Children using aided communication may not have as many opportunities as speaking children to rehearse new vocabulary in natural situations, a factor that increasingly taxes general vocabulary development. Studies show that children with greater exposure to literate styles of communication, whether oral or written, are at an advantage when compared with children without this experience (Westby, 1998). Rate-enhancement strategies, such as using a small store of ready-made phrases, may also reduce practice opportunities.

Children of all ages must be highly motivated to exert the extra effort to memorize information purposefully (Guttentag, 1995). Motivation is typically present when children have sufficient insight to recognize that although memorizing information can be difficult, the effort will help them communicate quickly and accurately. In general, children are motivated to communicate, but even highly motivated children can become discouraged when the skills they need to communicate are too effortful. Similarly, children learning to ride a bicycle or hit a ball with a bat or practising numerous other skills they are eager to learn often temporarily abandon attempts when they are too frustrated. These skills, while important to many children, do not compare to communication. Yet, the same frustrations may apply. Cognitive insights into memory-related tasks reflect metamemory or metastrategic knowledge and typically develop with experience and adult support. As with other types of metacognition, metamemory exhibits a developmental progression (Schneider, 1985). Clinicians often hear complaints that a child is 'playing' with the communication device. Often, when adults observe a child pressing buttons and listening to feedback, they assume the child is engaging in inappropriate behaviour, an appraisal that may or may not be true of a particular child. One parent explained her observation thus: *He thinks it's just a pretty plaything.* She meant that while her son pressed buttons and listened to the device's feedback, he failed to recognize the communicative significance of the device. He had just received the device and had only just started to learn to use it. Clearly, coming to know what the aid can 'say' is part of learning its power. The importance of this kind of 'play' should not be underestimated. By exploring a device in this way, the child could be consciously and unconsciously learning the vocabulary it contains, the location and representation. Indeed, anecdotal parental reports suggest that some children consciously rehearse the content of their devices. Indeed, with older children, the need for practising icon sequences for specialty academic vocabulary is well established.

Implications for supporting aided language acquisition

Regardless of whether they use communication books, multiple-page eye-gaze charts or speech output communication aids, children acquiring aided language potentially face cognitive challenges that are not present in the typical acquisition of spoken language. It has been shown that many factors add cognitive complexity to aided communication by requiring more time and cognitive resources to locate and select individual items than in the production of speech or sign language, and with numerous competing demands on the young aided communicator's attention. External demands on aided communicators interact synergistically with intrinsic demands and limitations, such as cognitive abilities, overall experience with a particular communication system, degree of physical impairment, and so forth. Cognitive ability, skill and motivation can influence self-monitoring, memory skill, level of representation, susceptibility to distraction, tolerance of frustration, constraints of fatigue, and so forth. It is true that children can learn to perform many complex skills automatically and with little or no appreciation of how they learned them. Indeed, research findings may one day demonstrate that many aspects of communication aid use also develop automatically if given the right conditions. It is also likely, however, that there comes a point when the young aided communicators must bring new learning under conscious, explicit control in order to exploit the features of an aided communication system. Learning to read and write is a good analogy. Most children learn effective use of oral communication automatically, but they must be taught literacy. The conscious learning process forces children to consider language itself as an object of reflection, and so promotes metalinguistic development. Although many of the demands of aided communication appear quite daunting, evidence from second language learning suggests that even young children learning a second language face challenges and have enhanced opportunities to develop metalinguistic abilities that exceed their monolingual peers (Bialystok and Ryan, 1985). For example, being aware that one does not have the necessary words in one language can lead to greater awareness of language form, a metalinguistic process that is more characteristic of 10-year-olds than four-year-olds. Perhaps parallel challenges faced by children acquiring aided language also promote precocious metalinguistic development. Researchers caution reliance on typical developmental models for alternative communication development (Gerber and Kraat, 1992).

Efficient aided language acquisition may be further complicated for children younger than 10 years by premature introduction to packaged systems that include immense vocabulary choices accessible through logically determined sequences of pictographs or by dynamic pathways linking virtual pages on a dynamic screen. Game-like activities that lead children to rehearse and understand the organization may be helpful to children who are eight to nine years old or older and have the capacity to use the necessary strategies. Williams (1991), an experienced, adult user of Minspeak, argues forcefully for the need for intensive practice to memorize various aspects of that system. It seems important to maintain consistent placement of buttons on dynamic displays to facilitate automatic use of visual-spatial-kinaesthetic patterns, particularly for children with neuromotor or motor planning impairment, but probably also for cognitively impaired children.

Flavell and Wellman (1977) emphasized that metamemory is a form of social cognition or awareness that emerges through interaction with others. Thus, the need for adult guidance, particularly through use of a Vygotskian approach to memory training, appears to be as important to the strategic exploitation of the device as it does to language instruction (see Renner, this volume). Metamemory and metastrategic development should be taken into consideration when training is planned. Young children tend to focus on one aspect of a task at a time. This unidimensional processing leaves fewer resources available for applying strategies to the search for a desired message, particularly if the situation is urgent or the physical and sensory demands of the task are high (Bruner, 1964; Fletcher and Bray, 1996). Bruno (1988) noted that it is important for children to have mastered the ability to locate vocabulary in a communication aid automatically before using it in the classroom, because timing and accuracy are important in face-to-face communication. Specially created pages through which children could use speech output to rehearse codes might be helpful. Simple strategies, such as rehearsal, are suitable for four-year-olds discovering the lexicon of a device. Thus, allowing pre-schoolers to 'play' with their communication device by repeatedly pressing buttons may facilitate procedural memory for which utterance is elicited by which key. A child's own representational development and adult reminders regarding picture–utterance relationships influence how efficiently the child can learn a system.

Performance monitoring is a type of training in which children receive specific feedback during problem-solving tasks requiring strategy use.

Children learn to appraise several aspects of the task, including task difficulty, their own resources, knowledge of potential strategies and their suitability, and their success or failure during the task (Pressley, Borkowski and O'Sullivan, 1985). The more recent direction of microgenetic research suggests that such insights do not lead to immediate changes in strategic behaviour (Siegler, 2000). It is likely that children's attempts to use paired associate strategies, for example in vocabulary retrieval, may be inconsistent for months or years before stabilizing. It might be helpful to understand how adults best can support and guide the acquisition process. One way to support children is to recognize developmental error patterns that could signal why the child is having problems. Caregivers and educators should also be mindful of conditions that stress working memory. Extensive use of environmental support for children may help (Burkhart, 1994; Goossens', Elder and Crain, 1992).

CHAPTER 4

The development of communication with alternative means from Vygotsky's cultural-historical perspective

GREGOR RENNER

In order to develop effective approaches to intervention for children using non-speech systems of communication, it is important to consider several factors: the impact on development of missing or limited speech skills and the recruitment of alternative communication forms; how alternative means of communication should be designed, what criteria they have to meet; and in what ways such alternative routes to language can be facilitated and supported. The cultural-historical approach of Vygotsky (1962, 1978) may contribute to answering these questions.

Vygotsky's theory has a broad scope encompassing the historical development of cultures and children's development. This includes the construction of social structures by the individual, language development, the impact of impairment on development and dimensions of compensatory intervention. His discussion of development is not limited to language and cognition, but addresses what he calls the 'personality', that is, the personal attributes of children. These are areas that are of central importance for understanding the development of augmentative and alternative communication. The theory focuses on the significance of children's social interaction with people in the environment for their cognitive and language development, in contrast to Piaget (1950, 1959), who sees children's investigations of the physical world as the primary motivation of development. The aim of the present paper is to demonstrate how a focus on social interaction may contribute to the understanding of the development of children using alternative and augmentative communication.

The theory of development, impairment and compensation

According to Vygotsky, individual development is embedded in a cultural environment. Although a culture exists exclusively in the social structures of its members, it also persists beyond the lifespan of individuals and develops over many generations. Cultural achievements are continuously transmitted from one generation to the next and the culture evolves through this process. This is the basis of the cultural-historical perspective. As applied to psychological development, the theory assumes that the development of higher mental functions, such as memory, consciousness, thinking and language, is determined by the social environment, whose structures in turn are developing through the cultural-historical evolutionary process. This is the social constructivist perspective on the individual's development. Vygotsky's theory is underpinned by Marxist philosophy, holding that communication and language are related to the co-operative social structures embedded in the culture – that is, they function as means of co-operation.

From this theoretical viewpoint, the individual's development of language is a socially and culturally driven process, not purely a biologically driven one. This raises the question of what characteristics of the child and the social environment are crucial for the development of higher mental functions in the form that is determined by their culture. On the one hand, one may ask what underlying structures children need in order to develop the skills and abilities valued in the culture. On the other hand, one may ask how adults should interact with children at different cognitive and linguistic levels in order for them to develop such abilities, because children need to be guided towards culturally determined knowledge by more competent members of the culture.

Social developmental situations

Vygotsky applied the social constructivist approach to developmental psychology by evolving the concept of the 'social developmental situation'. This term refers to the relationship between the personal attributes and developing mental abilities of children and their relationships with significant others, and it is considered a major factor in development. For example, infants can hardly do anything on their own and their social situation is characterized by dependency on adults. They need help from more competent people in coping with both the social world of people and the physical world of objects. As children's motor abilities improve, they will no longer be content with adults doing things for them. They want to do them on their own. This brings about a transition into a quite different social developmental situation, where children have a new structure of personal attributes and a new form of consciousness. These situations are dynamic and continuously give way to the evolution of new mental structures. This means that the relationship between a set of personal attributes and a social environment changes with every developmental phase. This new social developmental situation is represented as a new mental structure in the child's consciousness and a new personality.

Primary and secondary developmental lines

It is a characteristic of development that different mental functions do not develop in parallel. The first to develop are those that are basic, and needed early in life. Each developmental phase or step has primary and secondary lines of development. A developmental line that is primary in one phase may become a secondary line in other phases and vice versa. For example, language is a secondary line for the babbling infant; a primary line in early and middle childhood and a secondary developmental line again in late childhood and adolescence. Each phase implies the transformation of the personality as a whole and thus a new structure of personal attributes. This transformation changes the nature of the child. The structure of personal attributes develop as an entity, with the development of attributes and subprocesses following. Hence, when the personal attributes of a child have changed at the end of a phase, the child's relationship to the environment and the developmental situation must change as well through a process of re-organization. This changing relationship between children and their environments is consistent with the reciprocal influences described in transactional models of development (see Sameroff, 1987).

Crises

Each re-organization of the social developmental situation leads to decisive turning points, or crisis phases. These are related to the transitions from one steady phase of development to another, and are necessary parts of development. They imply radical transformations and alterations in the personal attributes of children within a very short period where the main characteristics of the children change completely. There are three features that characterize the crisis phases:

- in contrast to steady phases, it is difficult to determine the beginning and the end, but easy to identify the peak of crisis phases;
- during crisis phases children may show considerable behaviour problems;
- the development during crisis phases may appear negative for people in the surroundings because earlier interests and activities are reduced before new ones take their place.

The reason for the crises is that each developmental achievement involves the dismantling or reorganization of an earlier achievement. An example is the transition from infancy to toddlerhood. Sensori-motor unity is a characteristic of development in infancy. Infants' actions are directly related to what infants perceive of the objects within their field of view. When language becomes a primary line of development in early childhood, the link between perception and action is increasingly constituted by language, in the sense that children gain mental access to things that are not present in the immediate environment, their here and now. Through language the sensori-motor unity, which is the basis of development of the infant, is dismantled. This facilitates the emergence of a new mental structure, a conception of the world that is not restricted to the representation of objects that are presently perceived by the child. According to Vygotsky, the use of language as mediator is an ability specific to the human species. He expands the scheme developed by Bühler (1930), where children pass through three stages of intelligence: *instinct, conditioning* and *intellect* by adding a fourth: *sign-mediated thinking.*

Zone of proximal development

An important aspect of the social developmental situation is the interaction children have with more competent members of the culture, who may be adults or older children. The developing abilities of children exist already in a mature form in the environment (Vygotsky's term is 'ideal' form). The social environment provides developing children with models of the mature forms of culturally valued skills and abilities. Vygotsky built the notion of modelled or guided learning into the concept of development of mental functions, by suggesting that this development always proceeds in two phases: *inter-mental* and *intra-mental.* The mastery of a specific task is preceded by a period where children can only solve the task in collaboration with adults or more competent children. The tasks children can master with support are the tasks the children will master next on their own. The tasks are within the children's 'zone of proximal development'. However, children of the same age may have different zones of proximal development, that is, be able to solve different kinds of tasks either independently or with the help of others (Vygotsky, 1987). The zone of proximal development should not be confounded with a general developmental level, the zone will vary between different areas of skills and knowledge (von Tetzchner, 2001a).

Impairment and compensation

Vygotsky rejects the position that development is limited to biological aspects and gives more prominence to social influences, so he regards the physical organs of perception and action mainly as social organs. The social environment always mediates between the human being and the physical environment. Therefore, an organic impairment is primarily an impairment of the social function. For example, motor impairment may contribute to the creation of a special environment, in that it typically involves behaviours that are labelled 'abnormal' in the social environment. Families may show particular concern towards their motor-impaired children. Also other people in the environment may react by giving motor-impaired children a special status and intervention, which may lead to segregation of these children from other children. According to Vygotsky, social segregation and special intervention may have far greater effects on these children's mental development than their organic impairment. For this reason, he considers it vital to their developmental progress that both the social contact with them and the treatment is as normal as possible. Vygotsky (1993) emphasizes the importance of placing the human individual before the impairment: the physical impairment is not a disease but a normal state for that person.

It follows that it is necessary to distinguish the reduction in function that follows directly from an impairment and the developmental consequences of the impairment – that is, the influence it may have on the children's social developmental situations. The social developmental situation, rather than the impairment in motor skills, is used to explain the resultant evolution of mental functions. The impact of a physical impairment on the psychological development of an individual is mainly on the process of enculturation. The development of culturally valued skills requires a set of capabilities from its members. For those who do not have these capabilities, the normal process of enculturation is constrained. The constraints affect mostly the higher mental functions, the mastery of cultural tools and cultural forms of behaviour (Vygotsky, 1987). Psychological development may take a different course from the norm, rather than just following a typical path at a slower pace. The set of capabilities that is required for enculturation will vary from one culture to another, depending both on its history and its concept of disability. This also implies that the consequences of impairments may be influenced by cultural attitudes and adaptations made by the social environment.

Vygotsky claims the same educational aims for disabled children at the same time as for other children. Special approaches to education may be necessary – for example, for teaching Braille or sign language, but above all disabled children need normal education and should have an ordinary life as far as possible. Vygotsky suggests that mankind will overcome disability in the future, but that this will happen earlier in the social and educational fields than in the medical and biological fields (Wygotski, 1975).

Sidetracks of cultural development

According to Vygotsky (1987), the way to overcome disability and optimize development is to create developmental 'sidetracks' of enculturation that may compensate for the consequences of a particular impairment. Vygotsky gives the tactile alphabet Braille and the sign language of deaf people as examples of how

> in the process of the cultural development of children there are substitutions of functions by other functions, a preparation of collateral ways, which open up totally new possibilities of development for the abnormal child. If this child cannot achieve something in the direct way, the development of collateral ways becomes the basis for compensation. By following these detours the child begins to achieve the same goal that it can not achieve directly. (Keiler, 1997, p. 300)

Braille is a good example of the substitution of one form by another. As an orthographic system it needs only to replace a limited number of letters, numbers and other characters. Braille is not an alternative language form. By contrast, sign language represents an alternative language to speech which mainly has developed naturally through a historical process (Lane, 1984), unlike the manual and graphic systems used as alternative means of communication, which have been developed artificially.

Central to this part of Vygotsky's theory is the idea that social functions have been established in specific manifestations, but that the implementation of a social function does not need to be achieved using these manifestations or forms. Children who learn social functions through the use of alternative forms of implementation follow a sidetrack in their cultural development, a course that may lead to normal or at least optimal abilities. The distinction between social *function* and *implementation form* offers a systematic approach for considering the use of alternative means for individuals who are unable to use the ordinary tools of the culture. Language plays a central role in the cultural development. It does not only provide critical access to the culture in general, in children's early development it facilitates the transition from the sensori-motor functioning to sign-mediated intelligence. The developmental steps of early and middle childhood are particularly important because it is during these periods that language is a primary line of the development.

For children with some kind of impairment, Vygotsky considers the effects on their enculturation as crucial and to be a primary line of compensation, mainly through the creation of sidetracks of cultural development. With regard to language impairments, this may involve the use of alternative language means.

Implications for development with alternative means of communication

Creating alternative communication means of communication

Vygotsky's notion of social function is related to the use of cultural tools, as when speaking and reading. They are the abilities that are used in the life of the society when people are living and working together. Social functions are closely related to the process of co-operation. Parents' caring for their infants is an example of early co-operation, where the signals of the infants, such as smiling and crying, lead to actions by the parents. This is a very broad concept of co-operation: the infants are not conscious of the co-operation and they are rarely actively involved. This construction of the social function may be contrasted with the concept of communicative function, which is typically applied in the literature on augmentative and alternative communication. 'Function' also includes aspects of co-operation (for example, requests for objects or actions) but focuses more on the intentions of the individual than on dialogues within dyads. Viewing the principle of co-operation as central to the development of social functioning means that communication and language become even more important to people with disabilities. As they will achieve more through co-operation than on their own, their development will depend on collaboration and interaction with others. The same is true for persons with intellectual disabilities, who typically need help for a longer period than typically developing peers, or even throughout life (see von Tetzchner, 1997).

Implementation form denotes the actual way of acting, the forms of actions through which social functions are realized, for example, a child speaking a sentence or indicating a sequence of graphic signs. The distinction between social function and implementation form is useful when designing alternative means of communication and language. The first step is to analyse the typical structures of communication and language within a culture with regard to their social functions and the way in which these functions are realized. The second step is to investigate the properties that an alternative form must have for a particular function to be implemented. Possible alternative forms may be analysed with regard to what functions may be implemented and what perceptual, cognitive, linguistic and motor skills are required for the individual to use these forms. A profile of skills needed for using a particular alternative form in various settings may be developed.

With regard to motor skills, this form of analysis is fairly well developed and there are different technical solutions for access to communication aids, like switches, special keyboards and scanning devices that may be used by people with limited motor skills. The linguistic analysis is only partly developed.

Linguistic analysis would involve consideration of semantic, morphosyntactic and pragmatic requirements for the functional use of an alternative language form. In the domain of semantics there has been a search for core or important vocabulary items to be implemented in a manual or graphic form (Balandin and Iacono, 1998; Beukelman, McGinnis and Morrow, 1991; Fried-Oken and More, 1992; Yorkston et al., 1989). Grammar and pragmatics are also increasingly regarded as central themes in the development of augmentative and alternative communication (for example, Grove, 1997; Smith, 1996; Sutton, 1997, Todman, Alm and File, 1999; von Tetzchner et al., 1998). Still, the real task is to create new language *systems* with alternative forms (manual, graphic and tangible) to encompass the whole world of the individual user – and not only small pieces of it. The communication systems are usually provided to the users by people who do not use such systems for communication themselves. An understanding of the structures of non-speech language forms based on general linguistic theories would contribute to solve the task. Research and debate is ongoing regarding the extent to which language structure can be optimally expressed through alternative forms (for example, Smith and Grove, 2001; Sutton, 1997), but there has been little analysis of the grammatical structures necessary for the achievement of social functions.

The distinction between social function and implementation form leads to the general question of what the social function of language and its structure is. Within the social constructivist tradition, communication and language are regarded as a means of co-operation. The social constructivist approach to language suggests that language has to represent all aspects of the world relevant for co-operation (Hildebrand-Nilshon, 1980). This notion of language is comparable to a structural approach to linguistics where language is not seen as a collection of names or labels for existing ideas or meanings. Rather the meanings of words are paradigmatic – that is, defined by the semantic relations that exist between each word and all other words within the language system (de Saussure, 1974). The meaning of, for example, the word *apple* is seen in relation to all other words of the language. If someone says something about apples, it is implied that in principle this person could also talk about pears, bananas, food in general, and so forth, but has chosen not to. This fact demarcates quite precisely what the person is referring to by the word *apple*. The situation is very different for users of communication boards with, for example, 100 or 1,000 graphic representations, where *APPLE* contrasts only to the other graphic representations on the board. Therefore the range of possible meanings intended by an aided communicator indicating *APPLE* might be much broader than the meanings intended by a person saying *apple*. From the structural point of view – language as a system representing the world – a graphic representation could symbolize anything that is not more closely related to one of the other graphic representations. In fact, the range of meanings symbolized by a graphic representation may be too broad to be useful for communication.

From this perspective, the critical question concerning artificial alternative language systems is how and to what degree they represent and differentiate the physical and social world. At present, most alternative communication systems consist of a small selection of manual or graphic signs that are related to the natural spoken language of the culture, which implies that the inherent systemic character of language is lost. It may not be possible to create a more differentiated and integrated language from a restricted number of signs derived from the language system of the environment. As the example with *APPLE,* the meanings would be different from the related meanings of the language system from which they were originally derived. This means that in the planned development of alternative communication, the vocabulary items provided to children will have different meanings and social functions than the meanings corresponding to their glosses. This is evident in the language productions of young aided communicators (see Brekke and von Tetzchner, this volume; Soto and Seligman-Wine, this volume). Because of the small number of items, the meanings have to be more general or multifaceted. The construction of more detailed meanings requires combinations of items. The combinations can either be sentences or the construction of a special (word-) meaning. The combination of *THINK* and *SLEEP* to say 'dream' is an example of the latter from McNaughton (this volume). If the elements of an alternative communication system are to evolve as a real alternative language, then grammatical structures need to evolve, especially to increase the number of meanings by using combinations of graphic signs.

This perspective also has implications for supporting alternative language development in children with severe cognitive disabilities. An important question is whether the vocabulary items provided for them will structure the world in a way that is appropriate for them and the social activities in which they participate, and whether the items they have give access to new social actions. The core question for alternative communication development is to what degree an individual's cognitive and linguistic impairments restrict the typical implementation form (speech) and language competence in general, independent of implementation form. If the impairments relate, for example, only to the processing of acoustic information, manual or graphic signs can be used as substitutes. But there might be also impairments in the underlying linguistic capabilities, as when the person does not understand the relationship between things and signs, or has not yet understood the temporal relationships of the present, the future and the past. The alternative communication may thus be different in both implementation form and content. The meanings of the graphic or manual signs might be different from the meanings of the spoken language of the environment.

The main criteria for alternative means of language and communication from a Vygotskian perspective are:

- the children are able to use them, that is, the alternative means meets the individual ability profile of each child within its cultural setting, for example in accordance with the three functional groups of children in need of augmentative and alternative communication described by von Tetzchner and Martinsen (2000);
- they can be used to implement the relevant social functions;
- the users can recognize the social functions (in a very basic sense) that are implemented by the alternative means.

As knowledge of the social functions of language is growing in the research community, the effects of the use of different alternative means can be better analysed, empirically examined and optimized.

Communication development with alternative means

An outstanding question relevant to compensatory interactions is how the social functions develop. The crying of a baby might be a starting point. It is a biologically determined signal of discomfort, which leads to caring reactions by people in the environment, and is possibly the first and most general social function. If a child cannot cry because of an impairment, this social function can be realized by the environment, by ascertaining the specific signals of discomfort of this child, and react accordingly.

Next it is important to find out if the child is awake and interested in interacting. Interaction games provide a frame for repetition and variation (Bruner, 1983). If children react with smiling and laughing, adults may interpret this as wish for 'more' or 'again'. Their reaction to this could be seen as the realization of the function 'do-it-again'. The children still do not need to be aware of this function. For children with impairment these expressions might have a different meaning. Papousek and Papousek (1989) point out the vulnerability of children whose impairment may restrict their signals and by this the interaction with adults, so that the 'innate didactics' may not work. This can be circumvented by people in the environment searching for a child's specific signals of early social functions.

The 'do-it-again' function might be an example of the development from an inter-mental to an intra-mental ability. First, the child watches what the adult is doing. The adult pauses for a short while and the child smiles, which is only an expression of its emotional state. The adult repeats the action that the child has been watching and the child shows even greater joy. Over time the child comes to realize that there is a connection between its own actions and the reaction of the environment: it experiences its own social efficacy. At this point, the game or event may become the object of the child's intention and lead to its initiation of interaction games. Other early functions that are important for communication are the focus of interest of the child, gestures and triangulation, and the ability of the child to switch the focus of attention between an object and a person (see Bates, 1979).

To use alternative means as a compensation for impairment in early development means to recognize the signals of the child and react according to them in a way that the child can come to understand. Gestures are possibly the first means that are not determined solely by biological functions. Children learn them from models provided in the environment and they can be substituted by other forms if children cannot perceive or produce the ones that are usually used in its culture. It is not necessary that the children know the social functions of the alternative means before they can use them. On the contrary, children learn what can be achieved by these means, through the reactions of people in the environment. Described as a transactional chain: people in the environment interpret children's actions and reactions, determine how far they succeed in meeting the intentions and expectations of the children, and moderate their own actions and reactions accordingly. It is a cyclical process of mutual reactions that leads to a process of co-construction of shared meanings.

Thus, from the Vygotskian perspective, the provision of means for more social functions than the child actually masters is important. For example, when an adult in dialogue with a child communicates about people, objects and events outside the immediate situation and the child's contribution to the dialogue and construction of meaning gradually increases, this indicates that the child is developing more advanced language skills and a broader and more stable conception of the world, less dependent on immediate perception.

The dependence on an adapted language environment will be quite different for the three functional groups described by von Tetzchner and Martinsen (2000). For the alternative language group, which is characterized by no or very limited comprehension of spoken language, a language environment that contains the mature form of the children's own language form – or at least an approximation of this – is absolutely necessary because children in this group do not understand what adults say. In order to enhance their understanding of other people, their ability to express themselves, and their enculturation in general, co-construction must take place through the children's communication form.

However, even for the expressive language group, which is characterized by a large gap between comprehension and use of spoken language, a language environment that comprises the mature form would be helpful. The language development of these children is complex and they need significant cognitive and linguistic resources if translations between the different modes have to be done continuously by each child. On the other hand, if children have full mastery of the relationship between speech and the alternative communication means, it may not be necessary that adults in the environment use the alternative form. However, this relationship does not seem to be a simple one and the available evidence indicates that it may take time to understand it fully (see Grove et al., 1996; Smith, 1997; Smith and Grove, 1999; Woll and Barnett, 1998).

The scaffolding function of the environment

In the view presented here, communication development with alternative means is supported by the environment by 'joint' realization of social functions, starting with the environment having the major part, which is reduced concurrent with the increasing active part of the child. This also includes functions that the child is not aware of in the beginning. Children are searching for connections between events in their environment and especially between their own actions and reactions in the environment (Nelson, 1996; Papousek, 1969). With the support of the environment children can experience social efficacy, which then can become the goal of their intentions, that is, the children can try intentionally to achieve the reactions they experienced. At this point children have some insights into the function and the way to realize it, but still need help from more competent interactive partners. The ability is now within the zone of proximal development.

The process whereby more competent interactive partners support the development of abilities in children has been termed 'scaffolding' by Wood, Bruner and Ross (1976). Adults are not solving the problem for children but guiding the children's own problem solving. A child can only try to solve a task and use help with a basic understanding of the nature of the problem, of what needs to be solved (von Tetzchner, 2001b). Through development the independence of the child will increase and help from the people environment will be reduced until the child masters the task without any help. This also applies to language comprehension and production. Children must have a basic understanding of what communication is about in order to understand the utterances of others and try to communicate something. For example, children with severe intellectual disability or autism may not have this understanding. Language comprehension tends to precede language production. For example, even very young children with a limited expressive vocabulary and grammatical knowledge are able to understand some of the language produced in the environment, and this comprehension will influence their zone of proximal development for expressive language.

An example of scaffolding is the way in which adults use situational cues and follow children's attention and interests when they name objects and events, direct the children to culturally significant objects and events, and help them to construct utterances that are relevant for these objects and events (Harris, 1992; Schaffer, 1989; Tomasello, 1999; von Tetzchner, 1996). The finding that adults' naming of objects within children's attentional focus is more efficient for children's early word learning than directing children towards objects and then naming them, lends support to a social constructivist framework (see Carpenter, Nagell and Tomasello, 1998; Masur, 1997). Both children's comprehension of spoken and non-vocal language forms and the meanings relayed by their utterances will differ in many ways from those of adults. Hence, co-constructing messages is important for the children to relay meaning and for the people in the environment to understand the meanings of their child. Through co-constructive learning and enculturation children's language comprehension and use gradually approaches the mature adult form.

One implication of this perspective is that the adults who plan and adapt the language environment of children who use alternative means of communication should be providing models of language use in their own form. Moreover, these should be used for genuine communicative purposes, not only for restricted educational purposes, in all types of everyday settings and when the children are a very young. One advantage for adults using a child's alternative language forms is that they may be able to identify shortcomings of the system and suggest ways and means to overcome them, as well as demonstrating to the child how the system may be best used. It is a major problem for the development of children who develop alternative language forms that the adults in the environment are unlikely to have personal experience with the use of such language forms and sufficient mastery of them to be able to provide their mature form (for an exception, see Launonen and Grove, this volume).

Steps into society

So far in this discussion, the social environment has mainly been related to the family. The family provides the most important environment for young children's development. A systematic integration of alternative communication means into the social environment implies that children with severe speech and language impairments will be provided with alternative language forms that they can use and a communicative environment that promotes and supports these means. This requires considerable efforts from the members of the children's families (see Launonen, this volume).

As long as most of a child's life is within the family setting, the number of communication partners is limited. As they grow older, children become part of an increasing social environment, including pre-school, school and the society at large. Outside the home environment, communication with alternative communication forms is not likely to function without intervention directed at this part of the social environment. Compared to other people in the environment, the children use an alien language form. With the transition into other environments, more and more persons must be able to at least comprehend alternative language forms, people who also tend to have less time and be less devoted to understanding it.

The situation within the German-speaking area in Europe varies considerably. In German discussion groups (via electronic mail), there is currently an intense exchange between parents about the considerable difficulties they have in establishing the alternative communication form of their children in kindergarten. The attitudes of professionals seem to be a major participation barrier for young children using alternative communication in Germany. A more positive example may be found in a Swiss intervention study, where alternative communication was established in a big institution for persons with disabilities by training the staff of all departments, including those involved in administration, cleaning and catering (Lage and Antener, 2000). The residents using alternative communication could communicate everywhere within the institution, but unfortunately not in the local environment outside the institution. In Somerset (UK) there is a district-wide adoption of graphic representations to convey information across the whole community (Jones, 2000).

The challenges that arise from children's expanding social environment are only partly solved through translation of alternative language forms into a common language form, like orthographic written language or communication devices with artificial speech output. Such translations may to some extent work for children belonging to the expressive language group. However, for children in the alternative language group there is also a need for translation in the opposite direction and at present there is no technical solution besides using interpreters who translate spoken language into the alternative language form and vice versa. Von Tetzchner and Martinsen (2000) report the use of a sign language interpreter in a group of intellectually disabled people where one young woman with Down syndrome used manual signs, but at present, this form of potential adaptation of the environment does not appear to have been investigated.

The situation is easier for the expressive language group because they have at least some understanding of spoken language. Still, the process that underlies this learning is not well researched. Except for the fact that different implementation forms seem to support each other, knowledge about the developmental processes in such cases is limited. In one sense, the children develop within a bilingual environment (Martinsen and von Tetzchner, 1996). The situation of alternative language development may contribute to the wider discussion of language development within a bilingual context, and vice versa (see von Tetzchner et al., 1996; Woll and Barnett, 1998).

The historical development of culture and society

It is generally acknowledged that it is often difficult for users of alternative language forms to engage in spontaneous conversations with unfamiliar persons. If an environment consists of the same people living under relatively stable conditions over time, it will be easier to establish a community of users of multiple language forms, a language environment that includes a bilingual or supplementary use of alternative language forms, a society where children without the ability to speak grow up as ordinary members (Singleton, Goldin-Meadow and McNeill, 1995). One related example is the general application of sign language among deaf and hearing people in Martha's Vineyard in the US (Groce, 1985).

Vygotsky's theory encompasses not only the development of children but also the development of the structures of culture and society. This accords with the general aim in the field of augmentative and alternative communication to establish communication with alternative language forms as different but known and accepted ways of communication. In such a situation, an alternative means of communication would become 'normal' – which would in fact imply that it would not be 'alternative' in the same sense any more.

It is the responsibility of society to find and implement the relevant sidetracks of cultural development that are needed for its members with disabilities to achieve effective participation. This responsibility is also in accordance with the International Classification of Functions (World Health Organization, 2001). In contrast to the former International Classification of Impairments, Disabilities and Handicap (World Health Organization, 1980), this classification focuses on functioning and distinguishes the physical, psychological and social aspects of disability. It emphasizes the importance of social participation for reducing disability. Within the field of augmentative and alternative communication, the participation model suggested by Beukelman and Mirenda (1998) is an example of a strategy for identifying and reducing barriers to social activities. Participation implies that all people of the society have (active) social roles. An example of the inclusion of the development of social roles is the concept of the 'individual habilitation plan', which is part of the Norwegian support system for children with disabilities (von Tetzchner 2001c, 2001d). Whereas the provision of treatments for children tended to be the main focus when planning various forms of intervention (and still is in Germany), the first focus of the habilitation plan group is to develop a vision of the child's personality, interests and activities five years into the future. The different interventions and methodologies are then directed towards this joint vision. A similar approach, with emphasis on the active involvement of persons with disabilities, has been raised for discussion in Germany by Hömberg and her associates (2001).

Conclusions

Vygotsky's theory and later elaboration of his approach offer both a broad and a differentiated view on typical and atypical language development by embedding the social constructivist view in a cultural-historical perspective. It is a developmental theory that not only comprises the individual but also includes the social environment. Concepts of particular importance for language development are what Vygotsky calls the 'ideal form' of language, that is, the shared cultural tool of a society; and the 'zone of proximal development', where children develop language by solving communicative challenges with the help of more competent members of their language environment.

The theory also has explicit implications for the understanding of the role of impairment, compensation and intervention in developmental processes. The distinction between social function and implementation form is central to the theory. Both this distinction and the idea of creating sidetracks of cultural development may be directly applied in theoretical work and empirical studies of alternative communication development, and when designing intervention for children.

All cultures are constantly changing. From a cultural-historical perspective Vygotsky suggests that disability will be overcome by society. In order for this to happen, society has to afford the realization of social functions by alternative means. This is what augmentative and alternative communication represents in the field of communication and language. Moreover, establishing a culturally shared use of alternative language forms may be advantageous for other members of the culture because it also expands their possibilities of expression.

Acknowledgement

The author wants to thank Stephen von Tetzchner and Nicola Grove for their comments on earlier drafts of this chapter. Funding to write the chapter was provided by the Hans-Böckler-Foundation, Düsseldorf, Germany.

Note

All translations from German to English are by the author.

CHAPTER 5

Manual signing as a tool of communicative interaction and language: the development of children with Down syndrome and their parents

KAISA LAUNONEN

This chapter describes the communication development of 12 children with Down syndrome from the age of six months to eight years. As part of an early intervention programme, the parents were taught manual signs to augment the children's early communication and language development, and to provide a shared communication system for the whole family. All of the families used manual signs when the children were young, and most of the children learned later to speak. All of them had effective communication skills at the age of eight. The longitudinal study of this group of children with their individual paths to communication, illustrates the transactional nature of communication development. Intervention may be seen as an environmental influence on the developmental process, and its outcome is the shared achievement of the children and their families.

Interaction is the basis for communication and language development

In whatever form language is used, its purpose is to function as a tool for human interaction, that is, sharing of experiences, information and emotions. The earliest forms of interaction seem to have few other functions than creating and maintaining interpersonal contacts. The routines that are co-constructed in the early interactions of children and their caregivers provide the foundation of the children's emerging model of the world and later language content (Nelson, 1996). Early communication, developing along with interpersonal tuning, turn taking and joint attention, forms a basis for the subsequent development of language (Bates, Camaioni and Volterra, 1975; Mundy et al., 1995; Wetherby, Yonclas and Bryan, 1989). Each individual child has its biological prerequisites for language development, but language acquisition is a result of social construction, interaction between an individual and its social environment (see, for example, Nelson, 1996; Tomasello, 1999). Adults 'scaffold' children's contributions by interpreting and overinterpreting their actions and by encouraging them to be active partners by means of their existing skills. In the mutually regulated interaction, people in the environment provide developing children with a shared form of communication system that will enable them to adopt the life form of their society and to become members of the society (see also Vygotsky, 1978). Spoken language has a pivotal role for typically developing children. Children with severe communication disabilities and their communication partners may use alternative means of communication for the same purposes, such as directing the other's attention to 'objects' of interest and sharing experiences.

Successful communication and language development is the result of a transactional process. The vulnerabilities of children and environmental risks that may hamper development are not simple cause-and-effect chains. Children with congenital or early acquired impairments may be more vulnerable to the development of language disorders than other children, but the effects of biological vulnerability depend on the presence of relevant risk or protective factors in the environment (see Horowitz, 1987; von Tetzchner, 2001a). The young developing organism may thus be influenced positively or negatively, depending on the quality of the environment.

Intellectual impairment will always imply vulnerability for language disorders. Down syndrome is a chromosome deviance implying an intellectual level that varies from low normal intelligence to profound impairment, and a specific vulnerability for communication and language disorders, as demonstrated in a number of studies (Jones, 1980; Kasari et al., 1990; Smith and von Tetzchner, 1986). Down syndrome is usually recognized at birth and diagnosed soon after, and therefore it may be possible to establish an environment with protective rather than risky qualities for this group of children.

Interaction is a reciprocal process, in which both partners have their role. Due to low muscle tone, infants with Down syndrome often give their parents few opportunities for interpreting their behaviour as communicative and give weak reactions to their parents' communicative attempts (Ryan, 1977; Smith and von Tetzchner, 1986), and parents often find them more passive than other children (Fischer, 1987; Kasari et al., 1990; Levy-Shiff,

1986). Parents may find it difficult both to attract their children's attention and to maintain eye contact, and to interpret their early expressions (Jones, 1980). This uncertainty in interpretation may, in turn, cause problems in turn taking and inefficiency in interactions. In this situation, it may be difficult to create activities with joint engagement and mutual play, which would encourage the child to be an active communicator.

Most children with Down syndrome develop speech but have a later onset and a slower progress than typically developing children (Chapman, 1995; Miller, 1988). Their expressive vocabulary growth starts to fall behind at a time when vocabulary normally starts to develop quickly (Chapman, 1995; Dykens, Hodapp and Evans, 1994; Miller, 1988) – that is, at the time when children's expressive vocabulary has grown to about 20 to 40 words (Barrett, 1995; Kunnari, 2000). However, although the expressive vocabulary of children with Down syndrome falls behind their cognitive development and their language comprehension, it still develops faster than utterance length and syntactic skills (Miller, 1988).

Many studies of people with Down syndrome suggest that their difficulties in communication and language are first and foremost in the development of expressive speech (for example, Bray and Woolnough, 1988; Dodd, McCormack and Woodyatt, 1994; Dykens et al., 1994). Both children and adults with Down syndrome tend to have many phonological and phonetic errors, both on phonemic, morphemic and word level. Primitive patterns are persistent and speech is often very dysprosodic, even to the extent that it may be very difficult to understand without situational cues (Bray and Woolnough, 1988). A number of explanations has been suggested for the special impairment in speech development in this group of children, including deviant learning strategies (Morss, 1985; Wishart, 1987), disorders of auditory perception and processing (Lincoln et al., 1985; Pueschel et al., 1987; Varnhagen, Das and Varnhagen, 1987) and primitive or deviant motor control of speech (Brown-Sweeney and Smith, 1997; Devenny and Silverman, 1990). The marked slowness of phonological development may have effects also on the development of language and communication skills (Smith and Stoel-Gammon, 1983), in interaction with disorders of speech rhythm, dysfluencies and dysprosodic features that are found to be common with people with Down syndrome (Bray and Woolnough, 1988; Devenny and Silverman, 1990).

Whatever the reason, or combination of reasons, for the development leading to deviant communication is, it is clear that this developmental path starts very early. New developments must always build on the results of earlier developments, so the longer that one waits before intervention, the more established an aberrant developmental course may be (see, for example, Casto, 1987). Traditional language intervention with direct speech training has not proved to be successful with children with Down syndrome, while many authors report of good results with early use of alternative communication, particularly manual signs (Launonen, 1996; Launonen and Grove, this volume; le Prevost, 1983; Remington and Clarke, 1996; Spiker and Hopmann, 1997). The evidence also suggests that the use of manual and graphic signs may facilitate acquisition and use of spoken language (Launonen, 1996; Romski and Sevcik, 1996).

At present, there is limited knowledge about the actual developmental course of communication and language in children who use alternative communication forms (Bara, Bosco and Bucciarelli, 1999; Oxley and von Tetzchner, 1999; von Tetzchner et al., 1996), about how the bimodal situation and other environmental factors in early communication affect language learning (Smith and Grove, 1999), and about the structure and functionality of alternative language forms in people with learning disabilities (Grove et al., 1996). Parent practices have rarely been described in the literature, even though parents provide the most important communication environment for very young children. There is a need for studies that can provide an empirical basis for understanding the developmental consequences of qualitatively different early communicative environments, including both planned interventions and the natural communication taking place in homes and in nurseries.

The aim of the present study is to describe children with Down syndrome who are exposed to manual signs early in life, their language acquisition and changes in their language environment. The early intervention programme, including manual signs, is regarded as a scaffold for supporting the children's acquisition of communication and language skills, both signed and spoken. The main aim of scaffold-oriented language intervention is to influence the forces that have effects on children's acquisition process, including the language environment (von Tetzchner and Grove, this volume).

Method

The children

Twelve families took part in an early intervention programme from the time their children with Down syndrome (trisomy 21) were six months old to when they were three years old. The children were born to Finnish-speaking families in Helsinki between May 1987 and January 1989. There were six girls and six boys in the group. None of them had other known disabilities that were likely to affect their communication and language development. At the age of five years, psychological assessments suggested that one of the children had borderline intelligence (IQ 70-85), three had intellectual impairments from borderline to mild, another three had mild impairment (IQ 50-69), and two had moderate intellectual impairment (IQ 35-49). According to an audiologist's examinations and routine child clinic examinations, none of the children had hearing impairments. Five of them had congenital heart defects – a common condition in Down syndrome – which were operated on at an early age.

Seven of the children were first born. By the age of eight, two were in single-child families, the others had between one and three siblings. Before school age, which for children with disabilities in Finland is six years (for other children seven years), all of them attended mainstream nurseries: seven children from one year of age, four children from the age of three, and one child from age 4;6 years. When starting school, all of the children attended special classes in mainstream schools. The family of one child moved to an English-speaking country when she was five years old. She attended an English-speaking school while the family continued to speak Finnish at home.

When it was initiated, early intervention with manual signing was offered to all families who had a child with Down syndrome living in the Helsinki area. The development of the 12 children was therefore compared with 12 children with Down syndrome who were born in the period immediately prior to the introduction of the manual sign intervention (for more detailed information about the comparison study, see Launonen, 1996). There were nine girls and three boys in the comparison group. One child had translocation trisomy, the others trisomy 21. None of them had other impairments that were likely to affect their language development. Four children had a congenital heart defect, and three had surgery at an early age. The child who did not receive surgery developed well, but tended to get easily physically tired. Three of the children were first born. At eight years of age, they had between one and four siblings. The families were Finnish speaking, with the exception of one family that spoke Finnish and Swedish (Finland is an officially bilingual country with a Swedish-speaking minority of 7% in the Helsinki area).

In the comparison group, there were one-year assessments for five children and two-year assessments for seven children (before they were part of the present study). All the children in the comparison group were assessed annually from when they were three to when they were five years old, and at eight years, but the number of children who were available varied somewhat. There were 12 children at the three-year and four-year assessment, 10 children at the five-year assessment and 11 children at the eight-year assessment. Only the Portage assessments were made at the first two age levels, at the other age levels, the assessments were the same as for the early signing group.

Intervention

The families were referred to a clinic for people with learning disabilities soon after the children were born. All the families of the signing group were visited in their home during the first months after the children's births, and offered an opportunity to take part in an early intervention where manual signs would be used to support and enhance their child's communication development. All of the families decided to take part in the intervention and parents were also willing to take notes on their children's communication development.

The intervention was initiated when the children were six months old. The focus of the intervention was to change the communication and language environment of the children by promoting family interaction and increasing parent competence and confidence. In the advice given to parents, it was particularly emphasized that they should try to:

- support the active communicative role of their child;
- follow the child's attention in interaction;
- use manual signing in everyday activities (for more detailed description of the intervention programme, see Launonen, 1996).

When the children turned three, the experimental intervention was terminated and most of the children continued with language intervention on an individual basis. One child finished individual speech therapy at the age of four, another at five, and two children at the age of six. For the remaining eight children, individual speech therapy continued at least until the age of eight years.

The language environment of the children in the comparison group did not include manual signs at an early age. Otherwise, early support and services were the same for the families in both groups.

Assessment and follow-up

The parents in the signing group recorded the children's communication and language on a pre-prepared form on a daily basis in the children's second year of life, and monthly in their third year. There was space for comments on the forms and some parents wrote fairly extensive observations. These informal comments are used here to illustrate the development of the children's communication environment.

Every six months, the parents filled in a form describing the communication in the family and the child's comprehension and use of language. They also estimated the number of manual signs and spoken words the child used, and possible combinations of manual signs and spoken words. These forms were used until the four-year assessment. By then many of the parents had great difficulty in estimating these numbers because their child's vocabulary was too large. When the children were eight years old, the parents were interviewed about the children's communication environment and interactive behaviour.

The author made notes on the children's communication during her bi-weekly sessions from the time the children were one to when they were three years old. Twice a year, these sessions were videotaped.

Formal assessments were made twice a year from one to three years of age, and after that when the children were four years, five years and eight years old. Parent interviews were used in the assessment with the Portage Assessment Scale which gives a developmental profile of children's skills in five different areas: *social, language, self-help, cognitive* and *motor* (Tiilikka and Hautamäki, 1986). The scoring was adapted so that the children who signed were given two scores: one with and one without signing. The Portage Scale was used up to the age of five.

The eight-year assessment included the Reynell Developmental Language Scales (Reynell and Huntley, 1987), conversation and descriptions of event pictures. The assessment was videotaped and the analysis of the children's communicative behaviour and language use was based on the researcher's written notes and transcribed conversations from the videos. The children's teachers filled out a questionnaire about the children's social adaptation, academic skills and communication and language skills in the classroom. The questionnaire consisted of 21 statements concerning four areas: *sociability, academic work, communication and language*, and *reading and writing*. The teachers indicated degree of agreement from 1 (disagree) to 5 (agree).

The emergence of communication

According to the parents' notes, the children seemed to live quite an ordinary infant life during their first year of life. Following the advice given to them, the parents tried to create and maintain interpersonal contact and encourage their children to be active. Many of these activities were traditional games like 'See saw Margery Daw', 'Round and round the garden', and 'This little piggy'. Most of the parents said that they and their children also created their own, individual variations of these games. Also in accordance with advice they received, the parents introduced activities where the focus was on the use of hands.

In the second half of the children's first year of life, the parents started to learn conventional manual signs and to use simultaneous signing with speech in everyday situations with the children. Many parents found that using manual signs in games, play and singing was easier for them than using signs in other everyday situations where the children did not yet appear to be so attentive to the signs.

By the age of 12 months, all the parents said that their child communicated actively, even if skills were limited. Most of the parents felt that their child managed to express wants and needs, but four parents were worried that they might not always understand what the child wanted. Most mentioned hunger, thirst, tiredness and wet nappies, but many parents listed also a variety of requests that their child was able to express: to be picked up, to be moved to another place, and to be given ice cream, toys and company. However, the parents had been advised to interpret their children's behaviour in social situations as communicative acts and many of these attributions may have been a result of overinterpretations. According to the observations from the videotapes, some of the children seemed to be able to establish joint attention whereas others were more dependent on the adult's support for maintaining interaction.

Formal assessments at 12 months showed that the children's Portage scores for cognition and language were lower than their social scores. Language was at the level of 5.0 months, cognitive skills at 5.1 months and social skills at 11.4 months. However, these scores probably do not reflect the children's development accurately as the Portage scales have very few items related to pre-linguistic communication. According to the parents' descriptions of the children's communicative means at the age of one, many were significantly more advanced than typically developing five-month-olds. Most of the children would hold their hands up to be picked up and clap their hands when the parent did, and six children waved bye-bye (see Table 5.1).

The forming of the early communication environment

All of the children made notable progress in the development of communicative skills in the second year of life. Their communication environment

Table 5.1. Age in months at the appearance of early communicative skills of the early signing group

	Mean	Range	Median	Information missing
Clapping	11	10–12	11	7
Waving	13.6	9–21	13	4
Pointing	16.7	14–22	16.5	0
First manual sign	17.8	14–21	17.5	0
>20 manual signs	26.3	17–48	21.5	0
First spoken word	19.3	14–30	18	0

changed as the parents started to use manual signs consistently around the time of their first birthday. However, there were significant differences with regard to how much the parents signed. In the very beginning, most parents expressed motivation for signing and curiosity about what would come. Some of them seemed to expect a fast development, and after a couple of months without the children yet having started to use signs, some parents felt disappointed, frustrated and lacking in motivation to continue signing. They said that it was because of the child they were using the signs, and if the child did not use signs, they did not see why they should do so. Some parents commented later that without the engagement and support from the other families in the group and the speech therapists, they might not have continued signing.

The parents started with fewer than 10 signs, which they were taught when the children were 10 months old and after the children's first birthday, the parents' signing vocabulary grew with about 10 signs per month. The first signs were selected to be useful both in play (for example, BALL, CAR and BABY) and in routine situations (for example, COME, EAT and SLEEP). Thus, the number of signed words that the children were exposed to in communication with their parents, increased with their parents' growing signing skills.

The parents were speaking normally when they signed with their children. They signed the key words of the spoken sentences according to their interpretation of their child's receptive skills and their own signing skills. Those parents who started to use more than one sign in an utterance – which some parents never did – always followed the sign order of spoken Finnish. When parents were signing along with songs, which they did a lot, the children saw combinations of signs, and the signing followed the song. This means that the children were exposed to both individual signs and spoken words, but structure was evident in the spoken language only. This pattern is usual with hearing children acquiring alternative language forms (Grove et al., 1996).

Differences in parenting style appeared gradually. In the beginning, most of the parents used manual signs in two main ways: in everyday situations, parallel with their spoken utterances, and in more direct instructions where they guided the child's hands to making the sign. Direct guidance was usually given in situations where the parents tried to anticipate what their child might want to express, but they also modelled for the child how it could express a particular wish with the help of signs. Many parents said that they expected the child to learn signs mainly from imitation in everyday situations. They said that because their hands were occupied by a variety of activities, it was often difficult for them to find a way to use the hands even for their own signing, let alone to help the child as well. Some parents reported that their children did not like to be guided by hand but threw their hands back when the parents tried to take hold of them.

Mothers and fathers also used signs when they were together in home 'sessions' with the child. They had been advised to have these kind of activities in the beginning of their sign learning, both to become familiar with signing and to provide their child with signing experience in shared activities, often in the form of contact games and songs. One of the parents would sit opposite to the child and model a sign while the other parent was sitting behind the child, guiding its hand to make the signs. If only one parent took part in the sessions, the parent and the child often sat together in front of a mirror. However, some parents did not find this kind of an instructional session a natural way of being with the child, and they soon abandoned such sessions. Other parents said they found it a good way of becoming acquainted with signing. One mother wrote: 'Particularly in the beginning, the signing sessions were happy, shared singing sessions for the whole family.' Several families continued having such sessions until their children had learned their first signs and had started both to imitate and use them for communicative purposes. From this point on, imitation was generally considered the child's main way of learning new signs.

Whilst, in the children's first year of life, signing had been mainly part of contact games and songs, during the second year it became a part of the families' general communication. In families with more than one child the siblings were often the fastest to learn new signs. The parents commented that taking the siblings along in the sessions where manual signs were taught to the families increased their own engagement: they did not want to look unreliable in the eyes of their own children. The parents felt that the monthly sessions of the family group were also important in providing their own family with a wider community with a shared communication system.

Expanding the physical and social world

During the children's second year of life, their physical and social world expanded in many ways. All of them could sit without support and move around, and some of them started to walk before their second birthday. When they did not have to support sitting with their hands any more, the children could use them more easily both for signing and for exploring objects. Their mobility gave them even better possibilities for exploring the world (see Prechtl, 1993). Many parents wrote in their diaries that their children had become more active in communication and demonstrated increased understanding when mobility increased. Improved mobility also made it possible for the children to choose their company. One parent wrote: 'Lisa goes now straight to find her sister and brother, and she wants to be in the centre of children's group.'

As their skills were growing, the children also contributed more to the development of their own communication environment. In the records from both the parents and the speech therapists it is evident that when the parents became able to interpret more of the children's behaviour as communicative, they also treated the children more as real communication partners. The more successful the communication became, the more motivated the parents seemed to be to support its development. When the children had learned their first signs and started to use them spontaneously, the parents also began to use signs more consistently in their everyday communication with their children. At the same time, there seemed to be a general increase in the parents' awareness of communication. They commented on the children's use of signs and other forms of communication more than before and asked more questions concerning both their own child and language development in general. They wanted to know what they could expect and whether their child followed the usual course of language acquisition.

An important change in language environment took place when seven of the 12 children started to attend a nursery during their second year. This expanded their social world from family and close relatives to comprising a greater variety of people, particularly of their own age. All of the children were the only one in their nursery group who used alternative communication. The staff was informed about the rationale for the sign use and taught the same manual signs as the families. However, the staff's use of manual signs varied a lot. In some of the nurseries, the staff went to sign language courses and made a great effort to make manual signs part of everyday life, not only for the children with Down syndrome but for all the children in the group. For the children with Down syndrome in these groups, their two major language environments were relatively consistent. In other nurseries, manual signs were never really used in spite of the good will expressed by the staff. The children in these nurseries had a genuinely shared communication form only at home.

The first signs and words

Most of the children had started to point before they were 18 months old (mean 16.7 months) and all of them did so before their second birthday (Table 5.1). Lisa was the first to start signing, producing TIRED and LAMP at the age of 14 months. Most of the other children were not far behind: nine of the 12 children had used their first sign before the age of 18 months. The slowest developing children learned their first sign at the age of 21 months. At 48 months, all the children used 20 or more signs, and seven children used more than 20 spoken words.

In most of the first signs, the signing hand touched or patted the body, like EAT, TELEPHONE, DOG and HAT, or had symmetrical movement of both hands, like SHOE, BIRD and CAR. Also a one-handed sign, LAMP, was among the first signs for many of the children (Figure 5.1).

Most of the parents reported their child's *first spoken word* around 1.5 months after the appearance of the first sign, at an average age of 19.3 months. However, the number of spoken words did not increase notably during the second year of life. By the age of two, the children used 3.9 spoken words on the average, and even the most advanced child used only ten words.

Formal assessment at two years showed that the language scores on the Portage scales still were lower than the social skills scores, which were 27.8 months when signing was taken into account. However, the manual signs made a notable difference in the language scores, with means of 14.9 months without and 17.9 months with signing. The social and cognitive age scores were about one month higher with than without signing skills included.

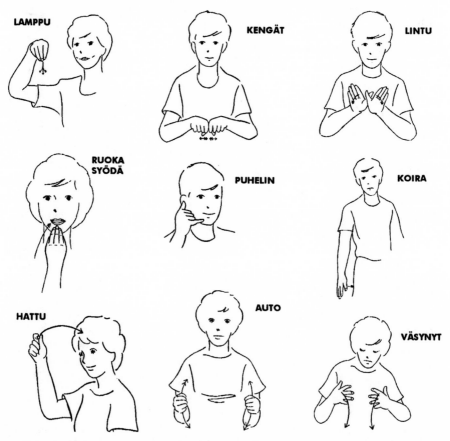

Figure 5.1. Finnish manual signs: LAMP, SHOE, BIRD, EAT, TELEPHONE, DOG, HAT, CAR, TIRED.

Early use of signs in interaction

With one exception, all families reported that their children used manual signs communicatively at the age of two. However, most of the parents listed a variety of early communicative means, including vocalizations, gestures, mime and actions, and manual signs seemed to be only a part of this rich, but rather undifferentiated, communication. The focus of the children's communications were mainly things they wanted to get or to do, like toys, juice, ice cream, playing, listening to music, reading books, eating, drinking, going out, being picked up and bathing. Expressions of resistance were also mentioned by many parents. The parents said that their family generally understood their children's communication, but most of the parents mentioned occasional difficulties in understanding their child.

According to the parents, all the family members were signing as part of their everyday communication with their child with Down syndrome. However, spoken language was the dominant form. One family said that it was '80% speech and 20% sign'.

Early growth of shared communication in child and family

The time from the children's second to their third birthdays was the flowering in sign use for most of the children. Only a couple of months after the children had started to use their first manual signs, their manual sign vocabulary started to grow rather rapidly. At the time of their second birthday, the children used an average of 34.2 manual signs, with a range from 10 to 74 signs (Figure 5.2). The growth in sign vocabulary was at its strongest from the age of 2;0 to 2;6 with an average monthly increase of 6.7 signs, and significant also from 2;6 to 3;0 years, with an average monthly increase of 4.8 signs. Thus, at 3;0 years, the average number of manual signs was 93. Three children had 25 signs or less at this age, while seven children had 100 or more manual signs and one girl, Mary, was reported by her parents to use more than 200 signs.

The acquisition of spoken words proceeded more slowly than that of manual signs, although there were large individual differences. The number of spoken words used increased with only four from the age 2;0 to 2;6 years and with nine from 2;6 to 3;0 years, to 17 words, an average of 1.1 word per month (Figure 5.2). Two children used more than 50 words and one child between 20 and 50 words. Six children used less than ten words, three of them only one to two words.

Thus, during the third year of life, the children on the average learned 69 manual signs and 13 spoken words, but individual differences were becoming more evident. Some children began to include spoken words in

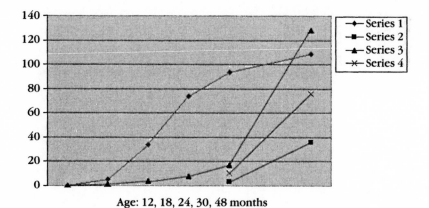

Age: 12, 18, 24, 30, 48 months

Figure 5.2. Early vocabulary growth in sign and speech in the early signing group and the comparison group; (1) signs, early signing group, (2) signs, comparison group, (3) words, early signing group, (4) words, comparison group.

their utterances towards the end of their third year, while others did not speak at all and were still in an initial phase of sign use. After the children were three years old, the growth in manual signs diminished and the vocabulary of spoken words started to grow for most of the children.

First sentences

The children used mainly single-sign utterances. However, with the exception of one child, Jake, they also started to use combinations before their third birthday (Table 5.2). These were combinations of manual signs, spoken words, or both. Combinations of manual signs and pointing were most common according to the parents' and the speech therapists' observations, but the age of their emergence was not recorded.

Many of the early sign combinations were of the type WANT + OBJECT and WANT + ACTION. In describing the content of pictures, combinations like BABY CRY, CAT SLEEP, THROW BALL, EAT BREAD and CAR GRANDMA were common. The three most advanced sign users frequently used longer combinations and sometimes put together several combinations, like in this narrative from Lisa at age 3;0 years:

    CAR DRIVE-FAST.
    DANGER PLAY ROAD.
    HURT *Lisa* CAR UNDER.

Combinations of manual signs and spoken words were of two main types. One type consisted of sentence-like structures, like *actor* + ACTION or *actor*

Table 5.2. Number of children who made different combinations of symbols at the ages of 36, 48, and 60 months in the early signing group (ESG, 12 children) and in the comparison group (CG, 11 children). W = combinations of spoken words, W+S = combinations of spoken words and manual signs, S = combinations of manual signs

	36 months		48 months		60 months	
	ESG	CG	ESG	CG	ESG	CG
W		3	4	6	6	5
W, W+S				1	1	
W, W+S, S	2		1		1	1
W, S	2					
W+S, S	1	1	3			
S	6	1	4		4	
No combinations	1	7		5		4

+ OBJECT, where the actor was the child's own name or the name of another person, as in *Dave* EAT, *Susan* SWIM and *Daddy* CAR.

The other way to combine spoken and signed words was to use them simultaneously, with the same referent, like {EAT *eat*}. In the beginning, the spoken words that started to accompany the corresponding signs were often incompletely articulated. When Kate was 2;9 years old, her parents wrote: 'We think that in addition to signs, Kate has tried to speak more and more words lately. She will often say the first syllable of the word, in parallel with the sign.'

Nick's parents also reported that he combined signs with syllables, but he would say the last syllable of the word. It seems that the parallel signing and speaking may have been a sort of transitional strategy that the children continued to use only as long as the spoken word would not be understood by itself. Some children seemed even to be aware of this option. When Kate was 3;0 years old, her mother said: 'Sometimes she notices that she can use a sign to make others understand – the words get less mixed.'

The examples of first spoken word combinations mentioned by the parents were of the same type as the other combinations, like *Lisa juice*, *Grandpa travel*, *Want milk*, *Mary sleep* and *Mummy take*. Because of poor intelligibility, it was often difficult to determine the morphological form which the child might have been attempting to realize. The Finnish language is exceptionally rich in inflectional endings and the adding of an ending often implies a change to the stem (see, Launonen and Grove, in this volume).

At the formal assessment at three years, the children still obtained relatively low language and cognition scores on the Portage scales, but at this age, their signing skills made the biggest difference in the Portage language scores: they obtained an average age score of 24.3 months without signing and of 29.8 months when signing skills were taken into account, a difference of 5.3 months. Signing also increased the age score for social skills with 1.9 months and cognitive skills with 1.3 months on the Portage scale.

Communicative functions

All the families reported that their children used manual signs for everyday communication by the age of three, and seven children had signing as their main form of communication. All the families except one said that they accompanied their spoken language with manual signs when communicating with their intellectually impaired child. One family said that they used speech and gestures.

The children were now communicating more varied topics of conversation. The parents still mentioned lots of wants, but some of the children were also reported to use signs to talk about emotions and events, like Mary (age 3;0) in the example given by her parents:

> Mary has started to tell us, for example, about what has happened during the day. One evening, after she had been on a day-trip with the nursery group, we asked how it had been. She signed BOAT WATER EAT. They had gone to an island by a boat and eaten their lunch bag there. When we discussed the same trip with her sister, the most important events during the trip had been exactly the same for Mary: going by boat and eating the packed lunch.

The parents maintained that the family understood what the children expressed most of the time, but half of the families said that their children had more to tell than they could understand:

> We don't always understand her. She keeps on repeating the same sign and she has become more impatient. Depending on the importance of her message, she will take it to the end by pointing or action.

The parents of two children mentioned negative reaction when the children were not understood: 'She gets hurt and offended when we don't understand. Her chin starts to tremble.'

As the children's expressive skills were growing, the parents' examples of communicative behaviours in the children became more versatile. Many of the parents said they found it difficult to imagine how the children could have expressed the same variety of communicative functions if manual signs had not been available to them. However, the situation was not the same in all families. The parents of the slow learners frequently expressed frustration and doubt about their children's development, and many of them found it difficult both to keep on signing and to make written notes because the note writing made it clear for them how little had happened since their last notes. These parents often expressed a need for strong professional support. However, the strongest motivation seemed to appear when there was some progress, even a small step, in the expressive communication of their children.

Changes in the communication environment

Despite the fact that the children continued in the same nursery as before, the communication environment was changing significantly. The early intervention programme was terminated when the children were three years old and after that communication support was arranged individually. The goals of the communication intervention varied according to the children's communication environment and their individual skills, but also with the working styles of the professionals. If the parents and the child's speech therapist continued to emphasize signing, the nursery staff tended to continue using signs.

With the speaking children, manual signs were gradually abandoned by people in the environment. However, little attention was also given to signing for some children with limited speech. Although a shared form of communication had been developed, for some of the children the use of manual signs by their everyday communication partners decreased. For others, manual signs continued to be an essential part of their daily communication environment and intervention. This was the case with Oliver, whose manual signing was good and who had severe problems in speech production, caused, as it seemed, by oral dyspraxia. When his speech started to emerge he was four to five years old and it remained unintelligible for a long time. The words were fragmented and consisted mostly of end syllables. In order to make himself understood, Oliver used augmentative signing for many years and the parents and nursery continued to sign too (see also Launonen and Grove, this volume).

Modality changes

After the children's third birthday, the differences in expressive skills became even more apparent than before. Some children were quickly changing from manual signs to spoken language whereas others were only starting to use signs actively for different communicative purposes. The average number of manual signs still increased between the ages of three and four, but more slowly than before. For five of the children, the number of manual signs used,

as estimated by their parents, started to decrease between their third and
fourth birthday. For three children it remained on the same level and for four
children it increased. Three children had a 'spurt' in their manual sign growth
during their fourth year of life.

Their average number of spoken words slightly surpassed the average
number of manual signs by the age of four. Five children had a 'spurt' in the
growth of spoken words at this age, and the vocabulary was growing so fast
that the parents were unable to estimate the number of spoken words when
the children were four years old. Among the four children who used 10 to 50
spoken words at the age of four, one showed a rapid increase in the spoken
vocabulary between four and five years. For the other three, speech vocabulary developed slowly during the late pre-school years. Three children were
practically non-speaking when they started school at the age of six years,
even though all of them were reported to say occasional single words.

All the children had started to combine words, signs or both by the age of
four (Table 5.2). The spoken utterance length increased with vocabulary size
and at the age of four, four children used spoken sentences or sentence-like
structures. At five years, six children did that. At four years, one child used all
three forms of combinations whereas three children combined only manual
signs or signs and words. Four children only combined manual signs at five
years, whereas the others combined both words and signs, or used combinations with spoken words only at the age of five.

The formal assessment at four years revealed that the advantage of signing
on the Portage scores decreased when the children began to speak more. At
four years, the average difference in language score with and without signing
was 4.1 months (34.4 versus 38.3 months in average age score). At the five-
year assessment, the difference was 3.6 months (44.7 versus 41.1 months). A
small advantage of signing was also evident in social and cognitive scores,
due to the six children who used at least some manual signs at the age of five.
The language and cognitive scores continued to be relatively lower than the
social scores on the Portage scales.

Continued benefit from manual signing

The parents consistently reported that their intellectually impaired children
were active communicators, including the parents of the children who were
slow to acquire signed and spoken language. For example, when Paul was 3;3
years old, his parents' comments indicated that his communicative skills had
increased faster than his expressive vocabulary: 'The number of manual signs
hasn't increased very much, but he uses them actively.'

High activity and persistency were mentioned by most parents, but also
creativity and emerging metalinguistic skills in the children's use of manual
sign. Many of the children started to create their own signs which were

adopted as 'home signs' (see Lane, 1984), as in these examples with Mary (3;9 years) and Oliver (4;0 years):

> She wants to find new signs, and she will suggest a self-created one if we are not able to tell her the 'right' sign. When she has made her own sign, she will always use it consistently.

> He signs his message persistently, many times. He has developed lots of his own signs; even mother doesn't always understand them.

Although they were encouraged to continue signing until the spoken language had truly become the main form, when a child started to speak, many of the parents seemed to take this as a signal to abandon manual signs:

> You make those decisions, that from now on you go back to using the signs, and the next moment you find yourself not doing it. It is so much easier just to talk, and when you know that the child will understand it anyway, you are just not bothered using your hands.

For the children who were mainly speaking, the role of manual signs decreased correspondingly. However, they would use signs when their spoken message was not understood or was not effective enough. They thus showed developing metacommunicative awareness, like Mary at 4;0 years:

> Mary signs 'difficult' words if others don't seem to understand her speech. For example, if she has tried a couple of times to ask for juice, and has not succeeded, she may draw the partner's attention to her: *Mum, look at me!* And then she signs JUICE.

Several parents of children who were mainly speaking reported that the children would use manual signs when they were angry or wanted to emphasize something. The speaking children also continued to sign along with songs, particularly with songs they had learned with manual signs early in life. They also used signs with new songs, possibly because it was the way they had first been acquainted with singing, or because it was easier for them to follow songs with signs than with spoken words.

The slow learners also showed both persistence and creativity, but also frustration if not understood. For example Jake, who at five years used between 50 and 100 manual signs and less than 20 spoken words, would use actions in addition to manual signs and words. He was usually able to make himself understood with the help of his total communication, although with some trouble. His parents wrote: 'Sometimes he gets carried away if we don't understand him. He is persistent, however, and gets his message through.'

The school years

School attendance offers new challenges and opportunities for the use of language and the development of communication. The children started school in the autumn of the year when they turned six years. They all attended a special class in a mainstream school, where the students had mild to moderate intellectual impairments. The children were assessed at eight years, but not followed up in detail in the period between the five-year and the eight-year assessment.

Manual signing

Manual signs were the main expressive communication form of three of the children: Jake, Mike and Peter. However, none of them seemed to use the signs they knew in an optimal manner. In the eight-year assessment situation they used manual signs when they named pictures and described events in pictures but during conversation they used mainly other strategies. Mike and Peter would listen carefully and answer *yes* or *no*. In addition, they both used pointing a lot. Peter, who was one of the boys with oral dyspraxia, showed a strong interest in reading and the staff at his school were pondering whether written language might later become his main communication form, and whether learning to read might gradually lead him to spoken language. The third non-speaking boy, Jake, was very persistent in making himself understood through vocalizations, actions, gestures and touching, patting, pushing and pulling the partner. He used manual signs occasionally, particularly if encouraged to do so.

Four of the speaking children used manual signs alongside speech (see Table 5.3). Paul and Oliver quite consistently combined manual signs and spoken words. Paul used them both in parallel, for example {*Play* PLAY-VIOLIN}, and in sentence-like structures, for example *Daddy and* BABY. Oliver used manual signs mainly in parallel with spoken words, similar to key word signing, like in: *Evening.* {*Evening at home* EVENING HOME}. *Evening. This is home.*

Six of the nine speaking children started to use manual signs in the eight-year assessment when asked to explain the meaning of words in the expressive part of Reynell. Only two of the children, Kate and Lisa, did not use manual signs at all at eight years. Mary spoke as fluently as Kate and Lisa, but occasionally used signs together with speech, without any obvious problems in speaking, as well as at school where she had a friend who used manual signs.

Spoken language

The formal eight-year assessment showed that the children's average age score on the *expressive* part of the Reynell scales was 2;7 years. The average

Table 5.3. Details of language skills in the children in the early signing group at the age of eight years

Child	Spoken language use	Manual sign use	Reynell (raw scores)
Mary	Sentences with good syntax. Substitutes /s/ with /h/. Strong interactive use of language.	Occasional signs along with speech, and at school with schoolmates.	Expressive 50 Comprehension 55
Oliver	Sentences with simple syntax. Articulation not very well developed, dyspraxic. Intelligibility varies. Strong interactive use of language.	Signs along with speech. Explains words in Reynell vocabulary by manual signs.	Expressive 47 + signed explanations Comprehension 50
Paul	Mostly one-word expressions (or short sentences). Articulation simple; intelligibility very poor without situational cues. Strong interactive use of language.	Uses manual signs if partners use them. Sentences often combinations of manual signs and spoken words. Explains words in Reynell vocabulary by manual signs.	Expressive 31 + signed explanations Comprehension 53
Ann	One-word expressions and short combinations; unintelligible 'private speech', Intelligibility occasionally very poor; contextual cues or augmentative means are needed. Interactive use varies.	Knows many signs, uses some along with speech but does not take full advantage of them.	Expressive 28 Comprehension 45

(contd)

Table 5.3. (contd)

Child	Spoken language use	Manual sign use	Reynell (raw scores)
Susan	One-word expressions and short sentences. Stutters some. Intelligibility poor and situational cues and/or augmentative means are needed. Interactive use varies	Uses some manual signs to augment her speech (mostly in songs and rhymes). Explains words in Reynell vocabulary by manual signs (and repeats the spoken word).	Expressive 35 + signed explanations Comprehension 39
Kate	Uses sentences with good syntax. Speaks also English fluently. Articulation mostly good, some minor immature forms. Occasionally some stuttering. Intelligibility mostly good. Strong interactive use of language.	Does not use manual signs.	Expressive 50 Comprehension 50
Mike	Does not speak. Vocalizations very undifferentiated	Main communication form. Does not use signs spontaneously and actively. Names pictures in Reynell vocabulary by manual signs; does not explain words.	Expressive 7 + signs object names Comprehension 32
Peter	Some spoken words.	Main communication form. Does not make full use of signs. Names pictures and explains words in Reynell vocabulary by manual signs.	Expressive 12 + signs object names. Comprehension 44

Name			
Rose	One-word expressions and short sentences. Articulation and syntax display some immature forms. Intelligibility mostly good, but situational cues help. Good interactive use of language.	Uses manual signs occasionally. Explains words in Reynell vocabulary by manual signs.	Expressive 37 + signed explanations Comprehension 52
Lisa	Uses sentences with good syntax. Articulation mostly good, some minor immature forms. Stutters occasionally. Intelligibility mostly good. Strong interactive use of language.	Does not use manual signs.	Expressive 51 Comprehension 54
Jake	Does not speak. Uses strong, affective and expressive vocalizations.	Knows many manual signs but does not use them very much. Names pictures and explains words in Reynell vocabulary by manual signs.	Expressive 8 + signed explanations Comprehension 31
Nick	Uses sentences with good syntax. Articulation generally good, some minor immature forms. Intelligibility mostly good. Stutters occasionally. Interactive use varies.	Knows manual signs but does not use them. Explains words in Reynell by speech and signs.	Expressive 39 Comprehension 35

age score of the nine speaking children was 3;3 years. Five of these nine children were fluent speakers with a reasonably good sentence structure. The other four speaking children used single-word utterances and short sentences (Table 5.3). According to the teachers, one of the four consistently signed along with his speech and the three others signed to augment their spoken utterances.

All of the speaking children showed varying degrees of deviant and imperfect morpho-syntax and many phonological and phonemic errors. Two of the speaking boys and one non-speaking boy showed evidence of oral dyspraxia. The speech of one of these boys, Paul, was highly unintelligible without situational cues or manual signs, while the intelligibility of the other speaking boy with oral dyspraxia, Oliver, varied. He also stuttered occasionally.

The average age score on the *receptive* part of Reynell was 3;6 years for the whole group. The average age score was 3;10 for the five fluent speakers, 3;8 for the four less fluent speakers, and 2;10 for the three non-speaking children. This means that the receptive scores were higher than the expressive scores for all of the children. The teacher evaluations showed the same tendency. When indicating on a scale from one (disagree) to five (agree), the teachers agreed strongly with the statement that the child was understanding well in the classroom. The average scores were 4.5 for the nine speaking children and 4.0 for the three non-speaking. The teachers also indicated moderate agreement with the statement that adults understand the child well for the fluent speakers (3.6), and lower agreement for less fluent speakers (2.8) and the non-speaking children (3.0). The difference in favour of speaking children was particularly large for the statement that children understand the child well: 3.4 for fluent speakers, 2.3 for less fluent speakers and 1.7 for non-speaking children. This indicates the other children in the children's special classes had poor comprehension of signs. The statement 'her/his means of communication seem to meet her/his needs' received an agreement score of 3.8 for the children who spoke fluently, 2.3 for less fluent speakers, and 1.3 for the non-speaking children, which may indicate poor general communication skills in the non-speaking group and/or poor understanding of signs among the people in the schools.

Kate had an unusual career: when she was five years old, she moved from Finland to an English-speaking country. Her family kept speaking Finnish at home, while she went to an English-speaking school for students with learning disabilities. For the five first years she had been one of the most advanced children of the group in both signed and spoken language. At the time of the eight-year assessment she was fluent in both Finnish and English.

The language environment

The information from the parents showed that the families had mostly stopped signing, including the families of the non-speaking boys. The parents of Jake and Mike said that most of the time there was no need for signing at home and that their son used signs if he needed them. Peter's mother said that she did not believe that signs would be good for her son any more. She expected him to learn spoken or written language and use these forms for everyday communication.

Paul's speech was highly unintelligible, and his mother said that she knew it would have been good for Paul if they signed at home. However, because Paul understood spoken language well and they thought that he had very good communication skills, they were unable to continue signing even if the mother admitted that she sometimes felt guilty about it. Paul was happy and sociable, and she was not worried that he might not be able to express everything he wanted to.

Oliver was one of the late speakers. He started to speak after his fifth birthday. His oral dyspraxia had been so obvious from an early age that his parents were aware of his not-very-promising speech prognosis. They used signs at home as long as it was needed, as did the pre-school teachers in the nursery with strong support from his speech therapist.

Manual signs were used in the classrooms of all the children, at least to some extent, because there were students in each class who needed manual signs. The frequency of use and the quality of the signing probably differed considerably, but details about this are lacking.

Social function

Regardless of communication form, all the children were regarded as having good contact skills at the age of eight years. The teachers generally indicated high agreement with the statements that 'the child has functional contact with adults' (4.3) and 'the child has one or more friends at school' (4.1), and more moderate agreement with the statement that the child has 'functional contact with children' (3.4). They indicated moderate agreement with the statements that 'the child is active in communication' (3.9), that 'interaction is reciprocal' (4.0) and that 'the child is active in the classroom' (3.5).

According to the researcher's evaluation, the children generally showed good contact skills at the eight-year assessment and appeared focused and motivated to do the tasks they were given. This assessments did not simply mirror the children's ability to speak: the three non-speaking boys were assessed as equally focused and motivated in their interactions as the speaking children. However, Jake's persistent expressive communication, mentioned above, made his attention to the partner's utterances somewhat variable, but maintaining contact still seemed to be important to him.

The comparison group

The communication environment

The main difference between the early communication environments of the signing group and comparison group was in manual signing and the fact that guidance of the parents of the children in the comparison group was mainly based on typical communicative development. The parents in both of the groups were advised to support their child's early interaction and to encourage an active communicative role. The parents in the comparison group were not asked to make regular notes on their child's development and thus missed the awareness such detailed note taking tends to imply.

Also the children in the comparison group attended different mainstream nurseries and each was the only child with learning disabilities in the nursery. Prior to the onset of ordinary language intervention, the nursery staff was not advised about adaptation of the environment to facilitate communication. In the comparison group, individual language intervention started on the average when the children were 3;6 years old, with a range from 2;3 to 5;0 years. One girl started with manual signs when she was 2;3 years old because her parents wanted to use signs with her. Manual signs were also included in the intervention of some of the other children at a later stage if they showed special difficulties in speech development.

Development of communication and language

There was large variety in communication development in the comparison group. On the average, the children's expressive language started to emerge around the age of three years. At that age, their mean spoken vocabulary was 10.3 words, with a range from 0 to 40 spoken words. The girl whose parents started with signing when she was 2;3 years used 17 signs at the age of three. Most of the other children had not been exposed to manual signs, and the group as a whole used an average of 3.3 signs.

As in the signing group, the vocabulary started to grow more rapidly between the third and fourth birthday. At the age of four, the children in the comparison group used an average of 75.8 spoken words, ranging from 0 to 300 words. Their manual sign vocabulary was increasing as well, with an average of 35.7 signs at four years. However, this growth in vocabulary was mainly caused by the one girl mentioned above who used 300 manual signs at the age of four. Thus, on the average, the expressive vocabulary was considerably smaller than in the signing group.

Three of the children in the comparison group had started to combine spoken words by the age of three, two combined manual signs, whereas seven children did not use any combinations at this age (Table 5.2). The number of children who combined spoken words increased to six by the age of four, according to the parents' information. However, at the five-year assessment, only five parents said their child combined spoken words. One child combined words and signs at the ages of four and five. This means that five children had no combinations at the age of four, and four children had no combinations at the age of five. This contrasts with the signing group, where both the speaking children and the non-speaking children used combinations.

The differences between the two groups were apparent in the formal assessment also. The average Portage scores in the comparison group were clearly below those of the signing group at all assessments from two to five years, even if signing was not taken into account. The differences were particularly evident in the areas of language and cognitive development (for more detailed comparison, see Launonen, 1996).

At the eight-year assessment, the variation within the group was even greater, and there were two main subgroups: six speaking children and five non-speaking children with limited expressive language in any form (Table 5.4). Within these two subgroups, too, there was large variation, particularly among the non-speaking children. Four children spoke fluently with a reasonably good sentence structure. However, one of them used language in an idiosyncratic way. Her speech was most fluent when she was talking to herself, and she was often reluctant to share her interests with others. At the eight-year assessment, she refused to co-operate most of the time.

Two children used single-word utterances and short sentences. One of them used manual signs to augment her speech, while the other one knew some manual signs but did not use them very much. As in the signing group, the speaking children in the comparison group had different degrees of deviant and imperfect morpho-syntax and many phonological and phonemic errors. The girl whose parents had started with manual signs before she began to speak was the only one at all who mastered all Finnish phonemes,

Table 5.4. The number of children using different forms of expressive language in the early signing group (ESG; 12 children) and the comparison group (CG, 11 children) at the age of eight years

	Spoken sentences	Spoken one-word utterances and short combinations	Spoken words and manual signs language	Signs and gestures	Limited expressive
ESG	5	3	1	3	0
CG	4	2	0	0	5

but even she showed some immature phonological processes in her sponta-neous speech.

The five children without functional expressive means differed signifi-cantly, but all of them had poor interaction skills. Two of the children were generally lower functioning than the others. One of them displayed autistic features and was very passive in interactions. He had been taught some manual signs and some pictograms (Pictogram Ideogram Communication, Maharaj, 1980) but did not use them spontaneously. The other low-functioning child seemed more interested in social interaction but would mainly participate actively in simple contact games. For another child in this subgroup, it was assumed that written language would become his main communication form in the future. He could write his own name and showed interest in drawing and copying letters. He had been taught some manual signs and pictograms. He could use them appropriately when prompted to do so, but did not use them spontaneously for communication when he was eight years old. He was, however, attentive in social situations and occasionally participated voluntarily in shared activities. For example, after the assessment, in which he was very passive most of the time, he was asked to help with collecting the video equipment. He was eager to do so and followed spoken instructions willingly.

Another child in this subgroup was very passive during the assessment but participated occasionally in reciprocal activities, like tapping the surface of the table in turns. Her teacher said that she was active and had good self-help and motor skills, but that she rarely reacted to the efforts of other people to direct her attention towards something. She knew some manual signs, but rarely used them and when she did, it was always so unexpected that people usually failed to catch them. When asked to, she never repeated her signs. Sometimes she seemed to use spoken words in the same manner. She lived in a bilingual family and according to her parents, unexpected spoken words appeared both in Finnish and Swedish.

The fifth child of the subgroup without functional expressive language used spoken utterances both when she was playing alone and when she actively resisted interaction initiatives from other people. Her speech consisted mainly of fluent jargon with lively intonation, in which it was sometimes possible to recognize some words and phrases. The phrases would always contain *no*, as in *no hold* and *no want*. Both the information from her teacher and the author's observations indicate that she did not use her speech in reciprocal communication. This girl was active and had good self-help skills when left to her own. When presented with some dolls during the language assessment with Reynell she started a pretend play where the dolls seemed to have appropriate roles.

The eight-year assessments could be completed only with six of the 11 children in the comparison group. The five others were selective in their interactions or totally refused to co-operate. The six speaking children obtained an average age score of 3;1 years on the expressive part and of 3;0 years on the receptive part of Reynell, somewhat lower than the speaking children and only marginally higher than the non-speaking children in the signing group. Most of the non-speaking children in the comparison group were not testable.

The teachers of the children in the comparison group indicated moderate agreement with the statement that the children understood spoken language in the classroom. The agreements were 4.0 for the fluent speakers (four children), 2.5 for the two less fluent speakers and 2.8 for the non-speaking children (significantly lower than for the signing group). The teachers also agreed moderately with the statements 'adults of the school understand his/her expressions well': 2.8 for the fluent speakers, 3.0 for the less fluent speakers and 3.0 for the non-speaking children. For the statement 'other children of the school understand his/her utterances well' the teachers indicated 3.8 for the fluent speakers, 3.0 for the two less fluent speakers and 1.6 for the non-speaking children. For the statement 'his/her means of communication seem to meet his/her needs' the teachers indicated 4.0 for the fluent speakers, 3.0 for the less fluent speakers and 3.0 for the non-speaking children. Somewhat surprisingly, this is higher than for the signing group, especially for the non-speaking group although the non-speaking children in the signing group had better expressive skills than the non-speaking children in the comparison group. It is possible that the teachers of the non-speaking children in the comparison group did not think the non-speaking children had a high need to communicate.

Discussion

This chapter described the communication and language development of children with Down syndrome, with and without the influence of early communicative intervention with manual signs. The focus is not the direct instruction given to the children and their parents by speech therapists and other professionals, but the way this advice – together with the children's development – influenced the parents' perception of their child, their interactions with the child and the children's everyday language environment. Signing was introduced at a very early age, so implementation was directed mainly at parents. When the children started to attend nursery this became the children's second major language environment and the staff played a significant role in the children's development. The language and communication development of the children who are described in this chapter demonstrates well the transactional nature of communication development (see Sameroff and Fiese, 2000).

The home environment

Parents' interactive behaviour, a result of their skills and attitudes, forms an essential part of the early communication environment of children. Manual signs were introduced to the families in the signing group so early that the children were not yet assumed to develop language. The parents were advised to use manual signs in early contact games, songs and other common forms of early interaction. In families with more than one child, siblings play an important role in passing the family's communicative means on to younger sisters and brothers (Dunn, 1988, 1999). When the siblings in many families also took part in these shared play sessions, this setting seems to have formed a sound basis for the children's early development of communication skills. The main difference between the communication environments of the two groups of children in this chapter was related to their parents' communication during the children's first three years of life, to whether they used manual signs or not. The use of signs modified the interaction between the children and their parents and may have made it easier for parents to focus on achievements rather than deficits (see Dunst, 1985).

The communication environment was also different in their nurseries. The environmental changes there were not followed systematically but it is likely that the attitudes of the staff also had an influence on the parents' behaviour. From the time children were three years old, new differences in the children's communication environment appeared as a result of individually planned intervention and the effects the children's communicative behaviours had on their environment.

When intervention starts early, parents are still processing the unexpected situation of having a child with learning disability. The intervention may have a positive effect on parents in this process, because despite the stress they may feel after having heard that their new-born child is intellectually impaired, they are usually willing to do all they can to support their child's development. Many studies confirm that parents of children with Down syndrome adjust their communication style according to their child's skills, especially if they are given guidance and support in this process (for example, Fischer, 1987; Murray and Trevarthen, 1986; von Tetzchner and Smith, 1986). As Mary's mother formulated it: 'When you get a child like this, you are ready to do everything for it, but you don't know what that everything could and should be, and therefore you need somebody to tell it to you.' It may be that when parents get support and guidance in coping with the situation, they feel more confident in their parental role, which in turn facilitates building up the relationship with the baby. A number of authors have pointed out the important role of parent empowerment in early intervention (Dunst, Trivette and Deal, 1988; Turnbull, Turbiville and Turnbull, 2000).

When early intervention focuses on interaction in particular, it is more probable that the children's environment provides opportunities for developing an active communicative role from early on. The signing allowed parents to look for communicative expressions in the children before they had intelligible speech and may have made them more sensitive to the children's expressions. When children can contribute to their communication environment they enable their parents to interpret their behaviour and see them earlier as competent communicators (Martinsen, 1980). Through the signing introduced in the present study, both the children and their parents experienced successful communication with a shared communication form. When the children used manual signs, they were able to take an active role in the interaction. It is probable that when the parents believe that their child can be given the lead, this will lead to a more reciprocal communication on shared topics (see Kelly and Barnard, 2000; Ryan, 1977).

Early positive communication experiences in the family are likely to influence children's later development of interaction and social skills (Guralnick, 1998). The children in the early signing group would communicate with an unfamiliar adult (the researcher) at the age of eight years, while many of the children in the comparison group seemed to have problems not only in taking instructions from an unfamiliar adult but more generally in joining in social interaction. According to the teachers' ratings, the children in the early signing group interacted better with both peers and adults than the children in the comparison group.

Planned development

When alternative communication forms are introduced to children with disabilities, an intervention plan is usually emphasized as a starting point. This starting point may lead to the teaching of manual or graphic signs to children in selected settings where the child is assumed to have certain expressive communication needs. When the child has learned to use signs in these settings, the teaching may be expanded to other situations. This developmental path is very different from the way typically developing children acquire their first expressive language, and typically developing children do not learn different expressive and receptive language forms. However, when people use key-word signing, they tend to speak more slowly, use shorter sentences and put stress on the words they both speak and sign (Whitehead et al., 1997; Windsor and Fristoe, 1989). This, together with the bimodal information, may make it easier for the children to be attentive to the most important aspects of the speech input.

Although the introduction of manual signs may have resembled the language learning situation of typically developing children more than for many other children acquiring alternative communication forms, the signing group still had an exceptional early communication environment. Manual signs were 'taught' to the children and their parents knew that it was their responsibility to provide the 'communication tool'. This teaching is very different from the 'teaching' that may be part of early parent–child interactions, for example in joint engagement with picture books (see Snow and Goldfield, 1983). For typically developing children, speech serves mainly the purposes of the play and games chosen. For the signing parents and children, the case may have been the opposite: certain games and plays were explicitly introduced to serve the purpose of using the hands and making signs. In many of the families, signing was particularly strongly related to instructional situations, and this may have led to activity-specific learning (see von Tetzchner, 2001a). The fact that most of the children in the signing group at the eight-year assessment tended to make the corresponding sign when solving problems of word descriptions may be a late reflection of the teaching approach used in the children's ordinary language environment (see also Smith, this volume).

To some extent, the parents were also advised to assist their child in making signs by moulding the handshape and guiding the movements, a practice that has no equivalent in parents' encouragement of infant speech. Hand guiding was recommended to the parents in the beginning because imitating signs was considered too cognitively demanding for children with Down syndrome at this early age. As it turned out, some parents did not do this, either because they did not find it natural or because they thought their child did not want or need it. All the children used some signs, and hand guiding can therefore not be necessary for early manual sign acquisition. Hand guidance is not usual in interactions where children learn signs naturally from a deaf parent, but it may facilitate signing in children with intellectual disability who show little or no imitation (see Iacono and Parsons, 1987; Mogford et al., 1980). This emphasizes the need for future research that compares the efficiency and efficacy of different approaches to promoting early manual signing in different groups of children. It is, however, possible that using different means to make signs explicit for children who are in the process of learning them will raise their awareness of signing and promote later metalinguistic skills.

Maintenance of signing

Despite the successful communication development of the children in the early signing group, observations in the present study indicate two critical phases in the maintenance of a signing environment. The first crisis appeared some time after the parents had started to sign and before the child had begun to produce signs. Many parents said it was difficult for them to go on using signs when their child did not seem to be responding, or even to be interested in the signs they were using. This crisis was particularly salient among parents of slow learners. They compared their child with the more advanced children and may have attributed the signing difference to intellectual level of the children. In these families motivation increased rapidly when the child finally used its first signs. This means that the children to some extent had to prove for the parents that signing worked. It is probable that in these cases, the parents' expectations were higher than the growth of their children's skills. To avoid the risk of an unbalanced situation of this kind, it may be necessary to guide parents in seeing their children's strengths, the need to accept their developmental tempo and maintaining the best possible communication environment.

The second developmental crisis appeared when the children started to speak. As soon as the children seemed to acquire a growing vocabulary of spoken words, most parents reduced their use of manual signs or abandoned signing totally. By this time, the children's comprehension of spoken language had usually reached a level where the parents felt that their child understood everything that was said in most everyday situations. They found it difficult to maintain motivation for signing when they believed the child could understand what they said without signs. However, at the same time the parents would tell that their child had started to create its own idiosyncratic signs. This is probably partly due to the limited number of signs used in the environment, but also typically developing children make new words to 'fill semantic gaps' (Clark, 1995). However, it is notable that the children who had early sign language produced new vocabulary in sign rather than speech after they had started to speak. This indicates that sign was still their best mode for communicative creativity and extending language and that speech alone was less efficient for expressing what they wanted to say.

It thus seems that the growth of signed vocabulary started to level out when the children were around four years of age, not only because the children started to speak but also because their environments did not contain enough signs and it was not thought necessary to provide them. Some of the parents with speaking children estimated the manual sign vocabulary of their child to have decreased from age three to four, at the time when the spoken vocabulary started to grow quickly. It is not plausible that the children had forgotten their signs that fast and the parents may have estimated only the number of signs their child used actively. In addition, they may have underestimated their child's manual sign use because they have paid less attention to the signs the child used, and some signs may not have been noticed because the spoken words were understood (see Launonen and Grove, this volume).

At the eight-year assessment, most of the parents said that their child did not use manual signs in any setting, but during assessment, most of the children used signs to describe words and occasionally also in other situations.

One reason signing was quickly abandoned may have been the reduction in family support of signing. At the time when the early intervention was terminated, most of the families were still in the most active phase of manual sign use – and some were just approaching it. The follow-up showed a fast degradation of the children's language environment. After the termination of the early intervention many families abandoned signing, some quite fast, others more gradually. In some families, this was a consequence of the child's speech, but the parents of non-speaking children also seemed to have difficulties in maintaining a signing environment for their child. This is somewhat surprising considering that the parents for several years had shown awareness of their child's need for a non-speech communication form.

Whatever reason, or combination of reasons, there was for the fast abandonment of manual signs in some families, it may indicate that manual signing was not seen as a real communication form but rather as an early intervention method, restricted to a certain age period. There also seemed to be a conceptual change from early intervention directed at parents to 'speech therapy' performed by a professional. In the early phase, intervention took place mainly in the home, the role of the parents was emphasized and the parents believed it was their responsibility to create an optimal communication environment for their child. When the early intervention programme was terminated, intervention sessions took place in the nursery or at the speech therapist's office. The parents seemed to believe that the professionals should take responsibility for the education of the child. A similar transfer of responsibility has been seen in other studies of family-oriented early intervention. When the early intervention is terminated, parents want to be relieved of the burden of training. Professionals are supposed to take over all instruction or training and the task of the parents is to provide the best possible family environment for the child to use its new abilities (McConachie, 1986).

The case of Peter demonstrates how difficult it may be to maintain an optimal language environment. When he was three or four years old, Peter knew more than a hundred manual signs and used them in combinations. Although the early communication development with manual signs had been successful, his parents said they did not believe in manual signs as a permanent communication form. Manual signing was more or less abandoned on the basis of the belief that he would start to speak or learn to read and write in the future. However, at the age of eight years he was still without expressive means that corresponded to his apparently good intellectual skills.

Two other families maintained a signing environment and thereby demonstrated the positive long-term effects this may have for some children. From an early age, Oliver appeared to have severe difficulties in speaking intelligibly. Eric, described by Launonen and Grove (this volume), had a poor prognosis for developing speech. The people around these two boys treated manual signs as a genuine language form that the children needed for communication and language development. The families did not have the necessary knowledge and skills and were dependent on strong support from the professionals. This demonstrates that, in order to maintain signing as long as a child benefits from it, parents may need sustained guidance and support, in particular in order to increase their own competence to be ahead of the child.

The parents' need for support and guidance and the transfer of responsibility for intervention imply that the knowledge and attitudes of the speech therapists who took over the responsibility for the intervention of each child would be critical for the use of signs. They all obtained information about the child's communication history and present skills but it was up to them to decide further measures. They may not have been totally aware of the situation of the children and the families or for some other reason did not continue intervention with manual signing. As the field of augmentative and alternative communication was still rather new at this time, many professionals did not have enough experience or an understanding of alternative communication forms as genuine communication. If individual speech therapists did not follow-up the early intervention, the parents and the nursery staff were left without proper supervision and were therefore unable to maintain signing. There is no basis for estimating how many of the speaking children would have benefited from continuous use of manual signs. It seems evident that the three non-speaking boys would have benefited from an environment with more active sign use, but the speaking children's use of signs in some situations suggests some of them would have gained from augmented use of signing.

Communication, signs and speech

All the children with an early signing environment learned signs, but there were large individual differences and their vocabularies were much smaller than those of normally speaking children (see Barrett, 1995; Clark, 1995). For many of them signing was a temporary phase on their way to spoken language. The children who, at the age of eight years, still had little speech continued to show benefit from the early signing period even if people in their environment did not maintain or enhance this communication form later. They had better language skills and were more competent communication partners than the non-speaking children who had not used manual signs at an early age. Long-term effects of the early guidance of parents were most notable when the slow learners of the two groups of children are compared, but even the best speaking children in the two groups differed somewhat. The children in the early signing group showed better comprehension of spoken language and social skills (see also Harris et al., 1996; von Tetzchner, 1984c). The children in the early signing group also had significantly higher cognitive scores on Portage. This suggests that the early signers had better opportunities for gaining knowledge about the environment and building up understanding of the world than the children without early signing.

The observations demonstrate that, in initial language development, signing was easier for the children than speaking. For all of them, the expressive sign vocabulary grew earlier and faster than their vocabulary of spoken words. There may be several reasons for this, connected both to input from others and to the children's sensori-motor skills (see von Tetzchner, 1984b). It may be easier for the children to attend to than the auditory forms of spoken words. Signs are often produced slowly by new learners, and the parents were learning signs together with the children (see Whitehead et al., 1997; Windsor and Fristoe, 1989). Spoken words cannot be articulated very slowly without loosing intelligibility. If children are more likely to attend to manual signs than to spoken words, they are also more likely to model them from other people. The possibility of hand guiding makes it possible for parents to assist their children in making signs in a way that is not possible with speech. The first signs of the children were usually easy to help the children to do by guiding their own hands: clapping and patting own body parts, but not all parents used hand guidance (see above).

The signing seemed to have a positive influence on spoken language, as has been demonstrated in other studies (Abrahamsen, Cavallo and McCluer, 1985; Casey, 1978; Creedon, 1973; Kouri, 1989; Romski, Sevcik and Pate, 1988; Rostad, 1989). In their early development, the signing children also used more spoken words than the comparison group. Simultaneous signing and speaking may also have made it easier for the children to comprehend what others were saying and to separate the elements in the flow of speech. However, possible long-term effects of early signing on the children's later speech development are less clear. At the eight-year assessment, some children in both groups spoke in sentences, whereas others had no or very limited speech. There were more children without speech in the group without early signing. Thus, although signing seems to have a positive effect on speech development and possibly increase the probability that a child with Down syndrome will start to speak, signing does not guarantee speech. Many children with Down syndrome will start to speak even without early signing. However, they tend to start to speak later and possibly have more negative experiences related to poor communication skills early in life than signing children do.

The results of this and other studies indicate that although signing may not be necessary for children with Down syndrome and other forms of intellectual impairment to speak, signing seems to have developmental benefits. However, in spite of the fact that many studies have demonstrated positive influences of signing on the development of spoken language (for example, Abrahamsen et al., 1985; Kouri, 1989; Launonen, 1996, 1998; Rostad, 1989), some researchers still warn that manual signs should not automatically be used with this group of children (Miller, Leddy and Leavitt 1999; Spiker and Hopmann, 1997). Miller and associates (1999) are particularly worried about the fact that children who use manual signs seldom live in a language community where manual signing is in common use. The present study shows that difficulties often exist in maintaining an optimal language environment that includes manual signs. More important, however, is that it also shows that the result would be even worse without an environment with manual signs. A language environment with speech only would hinder the children from developing in accordance with their possibilities and leave them with poorer communicative means than necessary. The results show the importance of supporting and guiding parents and professionals in giving children with intellectual impairment better possibilities for developing the communication means within their reach, including increasing the signing competence of people in the environment and their knowledge about how to use signs to enhance both spoken and signed language.

The transitional stage where intellectually impaired children using manual signs gradually change to speech has not been well described in the literature on augmentative and alternative communication. When the children in the signing group started to use spoken words, some of their early words corresponded to manual signs they already were using, and thus represented mainly a change in form (see Abrahamsen et al., 1990; Kouri, 1989). Other words referred to new categories and expanded the children's vocabulary. In their early word attempts, many of the children would articulate either the first or the last syllable of the word. Many of these would not have been understood and the simultaneous sign was often needed for the communication partner to recognize the spoken word fragment, and this may partly explain why the signing children had larger spoken vocabularies in the early phases of speech development. Many of the children seemed also to be aware that they could use manual signs to augment their speech. Even when they were mainly speaking, they would use signs if their spoken utterance was not understood. Using language in this manner may have contributed to their development of metalinguistic skills.

The development of syntax

Typically developing children begin to combine words when their expressive vocabulary is around 15 to 50 words (Bates, Dale and Thal, 1995). All the children in the present study who used more than 20 signs began to combine manual signs with other signs, spoken words or pointing. It is a general finding that multi-sign combinations are relatively rare among children with severe learning disabilities who use manual signs (Grove et al., 1996; Grove and McDougall, 1991; Udwin and Yule, 1990). The high frequency of combinations in this study indicates that the usual lack of structure may be linked with the signing produced in the environment. The parents in the present study were advised to use sign combinations from the very beginning, and particularly signing with songs may have facilitated the use of multi-sign utterances and thus given the children more complex linguistic input in the manual mode. However, also for these children, the early combinations consisted mainly of 'sign + point' and 'sign + spoken word'. The most advanced signers occasionally used sentences with three or more signs. The period with sign combinations was, however, quite short for most of the children because it took place during their transition from mainly signing to mainly speaking.

There was not a clear structural pattern in the first combinations. The utterances were telegraphic and included main words only (for an exception, see Launonen and Grove, this volume). Many of the early sentence-like structures of the children's spoken utterances seemed 'formulaic' rather than productive – that is, ready-made structures learned from adults, which are gradually used with different words (Braine, 1963; Kauppinen, 1998, Peters, 1983; Pine and Lieven, 1993). As with formulaic speech of other children learning Finnish (Kauppinen, 1998), many of the spoken words in the first combinations of the children in the signing group were correctly inflected (this cannot be seen in the English translations), even though the children had not yet mastered the corresponding grammatical rule. At least in this respect their adoption of spoken language seemed to follow the processes of normally developing children learning Finnish.

Implications for intervention

A comparison of the two groups suggests that early manual signing enhances later development of interaction and language in children with Down syndrome. The case reported by Launonen and Grove (this volume) indicates, however, that manual signing may develop as a genuine language form for an individual and its communication partners even if this communication form is not introduced until the child is four years old. Another example of a successful late start was the most advanced child in the comparison group, who was introduced to manual signs at the age of 2;6 years and quickly learned several hundred signs before she started to speak and then changed to spoken language as her main form of communication. On the

Children with Down Syndrome and their Parents 121

other hand, Peter's family started signing early. He learned several hundred signs but, although signing was his main means of expression, it never became a mature language form, possibly because his family abandoned signing when the early intervention period was over. Nor did early speech guarantee functional communication later in life: the girl with the largest vocabulary of spoken words in the comparison group at the age of four had substantial difficulties in communication at eight years.

Together, these findings demonstrate the complex interplay between biology and environment, the transactional nature of communication development and the importance of children's everyday communication environment. For children who are vulnerable to difficulties in learning to speak, an alternative communication may best ensure an optimal language development, either as transitional means or as a lasting expressive communicative form. If one waits until language problems are manifest, the developmental path has already taken a non-optimal direction and has to be turned through environmental influence. This is not the way normally developing children learn their first expressive language. For them, their future communication form, vocal speech, forms an integral part of their interaction with their parents from very early on. Even though the multimodal nature of alternative communication learning is not yet properly understood, it seems a warranted conclusion that whatever a child's future communication forms will be, they should be at the child's disposal from early on, so that each child can use them in accordance with his or her own individual developmental tempo.

Down syndrome is usually recognized and diagnosed soon after birth. Most of these children spend an ordinary infant life in their own home, and therefore the establishment of an optimal early communication environment may be easier for this group than for children with other developmental disabilities. Many conditions that may cause vulnerability for difficulties in learning to speak are recognized much later in development. On the other hand, in the most obvious cases of early developmental disabilities new-born infants may be so ill or otherwise physically so weak that they spend long periods in hospital, or even if they live in their own home, their parents' main concern may be their physical care. It is a challenge for professionals to develop methods both for the early identification of risk conditions and for different ways of promoting early interaction of individual children and their parents who are in need of early support.

Another challenge for intervention, implied by the observations presented in this chapter, is in making the people involved consider alternative communication as real communication forms and not as intervention methods. In addition to keeping up the motivation of the families and other communities to use alternative communication forms as long as they are needed, professionals should develop methods for evaluating total communication, instead of concentrating mainly on spoken language skills. Methods for evaluating communication in its rich variety, both of form and function, would enable professionals to obtain a better picture of individual skills and needs. This, in turn, would guarantee the people in need of alternative communication forms the best individual choices in communication form and intervention practices.

Acknowledgement

The author wants to thank the families for their participation and friendly collaboration in the present study.

CHAPTER 6

A longitudinal study of sign and speech development in a boy with Down syndrome

KAISA LAUNONEN AND NICOLA GROVE

A growing body of literature has shown that not all children follow the same path to language and that the linguistic tool that transmits cultural knowledge from one generation to the next does not need to be based on spoken language (Meier and Newport, 1990). For some children, language intervention may have a significant influence on the developmental path they take. Within the social-pragmatic framework of language development (see, for example, Bruner, 1975; Nelson, 1996; Tomasello, 1999), communication intervention can be defined as a means of creating opportunities for interaction between children with language and communication problems and people in their environments. The role of interventionists is to guide children's acquisition of culturally shared means of communication and facilitate their use of these means in a wide range of communicative settings, a process von Tetzchner (1996) calls recontextualization. Parents and other significant adults and children form an essential part of the supportive communication environment for children with developmental communication disabilities, and a primary goal of intervention is to influence how they interact with the children.

Traditional language intervention is based on a large number of studies of typical language development, including detailed diary studies of individual children. However, there is hardly any language-oriented description of children who acquire alternative modes of communication, which means that a significant knowledge base for language intervention with this group is missing. This chapter discusses the development of sign and speech in a boy with Down syndrome over a period of 17 years. Manual signs were introduced to Eric and his family when Eric was 3;6 years old and had not yet started to speak. He started signing at the age of four, and manual signs and gestures were his main means of communication for the following eight years. He started to speak when he was 12 years old and at the age of 17, speech had become his main form of communication although he still needed to support it with manual signs and gestures. Using the framework developed by von Tetzchner and Martinsen (2000), he initially seemed to belong to the expressive language group, which consists of people who have a large gap between their comprehension and use of spoken language, and who will have an alternative language system as their main form of expressive communication throughout life. Eric's later development showed, however, that he in fact belonged to the supportive language group, comprising individuals who use alternative communication systems only in a limited phase of development, and to support their speech in situations where they need it. Even if Eric's ability to speak developed very slowly, speech eventually became his main communication form and manual signs were used only to make unintelligible spoken utterances more comprehensible to the communication partners. Eric's development illustrates some features that appear to be critical to the effective use of other communication modes than speech, and offers insights into the dynamic relationship between different modes of communication.

The development of children who need alternative communication forms is usually very different from that of normally developing children, and individual developmental paths are often unique. Case study designs make it possible to collect rich contextual information and to discuss the transactional effects of various developmental factors (see also von Tetzchner, Rogne and Lilleeng, 1997). Case study methodology was therefore chosen for the present study. Eric's development has been strongly influenced by the various interventions provided and the written reports of professionals are also the main source of information about his development, in particular reports from speech therapists. Although these have been supplemented with information from the parents and videotaped material, it has been difficult to obtain a large body of detailed information about his language. However, Eric's case study is unusual in offering a long-term perspective, over 17 years of development. This makes it possible to look at processes of development and not only at specific phenomena at different ages.

Method

The description of Eric's development is based on clinical reports, speech therapists' notes and statements, information from Eric's parents, and videotaped sessions. The clinical reports cover the period from 10 months to 16 years. During the pre-school years, Eric was observed once or twice a year by a multidisciplinary team in a clinic for people with learning disabilities, and each member of the team made notes for Eric's clinical records. Information used in the case history comes mainly from the notes of the speech therapist, with supplementary information from a paediatrician and a psychologist. There are annual reports from speech therapists when Eric was four to nine years old, and again from when he was 12 to 16 years old. There are detailed notes, including information given by Eric's parents, during monthly sessions at home and occasional follow-up discussions, from the time when Eric was 4;7 to 7;1 years old.

Speech therapists are thus the main informants in addition to the parents. Eric had four speech therapists, whose views to a large extent determined the focus of his communication intervention. Until the age 3;8, when his speech therapy started, the family came to the children's clinic, and the first author and a colleague saw him and his family. The next speech therapist worked with him between the ages of 3;8 and 4;7. The first author worked with him in the period from 4;7 to 7;1. Two more speech therapists supervised his language intervention in school from the age of seven to 16 years. The first author became involved with the family again when Eric's signing was reassessed when he was 12 years old, and visited the family when Eric was 17 years old with the purpose of collecting more information for this chapter. Eric's development was also discussed in some detail with the parents when he was 12;10 and 17;6 years old. The audiologist who has followed up Eric's ear problems since the time he started school, has provided information on his hearing history and the results of hearing assessment when Eric was 18 years old.

Eric was videotaped on four occasions. In the first two videos, at the ages of 5;2 and 6;3, Eric is discussing the pictures in a children's book with the speech therapist. The second two videos, made when Eric was 12;10 and 17;6 years old, consist of picture naming, descriptions of event pictures and conversation. In the last of these two sessions, Eric also viewed and retold one of the 'Mr Bean' stories.

A broad phonemic transcription was made of the signs, gestures and speech Eric produced in each video. The Stokoe Notation System (Stokoe, Casterline and Cronenburg, 1965) was used to identify meaningful modifications to handshape, location, movement or orientation of manual signs and errors in the articulation of signs. Eric did not speak in the first three videos. In the final video, spoken words were transcribed phonemically.

Eric

Eric had Down syndrome (trisomy 21). He was born after a normal pregnancy in 1983 to Finnish parents living in Helsinki. He lived at home with both of his parents, an older brother and a younger sister. Psychological assessments when he was five years old suggested that he had mild to moderate intellectual impairment. He has had a continuing problem with secretory otitis media, causing a fluctuating hearing impairment. A mild conductive hearing loss was discovered in his left ear when he was four years old, associated with glue ear, and he had grommets in both ears from when he was four until he was 16 years old. At the age of 17, Eric's hearing in his left ear was, even at its best, slightly impaired (25–30 dB). At 18 years of age, he was again given a grommet in his left ear. The difference between the ears influenced sound localization and made it slightly difficult for him to hear in noise conditions. His vision was within normal limits and he was predominantly right handed. He attended a mainstream nursery until he was six years old, a special class in a mainstream school until he was 12, and finished his education in a special secondary school at the age of 17.

Early communication development

Eric's condition was diagnosed when he was born. The family had their first visit to a special clinic for children with learning disabilities when Eric was 10 months old. According to the reports of the multidisciplinary team, he was developing well. The parents were given general advice about how to support this development, and were told to pay special attention to Eric's active role in interaction. When Eric was 14 months old, the report said he had good interaction skills and vocalized a lot. The vocalizations were undifferentiated, with no canonical babbling, but were clearly social and used in interactions.

Good early interaction skills are mentioned repeatedly in the records from Eric's first years of life. The parents were encouraged to continue supporting his non-verbal communication in their customary way. When Eric was 3;6 years old, the team found that his speech development was delayed compared to other areas. At this age, manual signs were mentioned in the clinical reports for the first time as a possibility for enhancing Eric's communication and language development.

Individual language intervention was initiated when Eric was 3;8 years old. Manual signs were included from the very beginning but only in the individual sessions held in the nursery once a week. The significant people in Eric's environment were not considered active partners in the intervention at this point. His family and the nursery staff continued to speak with Eric and according to the reports, speech was the focus of intervention.

Information from the first period of intervention is somewhat contradictory. After three months of intervention, the report of the speech therapist indicates that Eric imitated actions and performed simple classification tasks. It was difficult for him to follow simple spoken instructions and indicate objects that had been named. The report says: 'Using manual signs has widened Eric's opportunities for interaction and communication, but it took a long time before Eric agreed to sign.' At that time, Eric signed spontaneously DOG, CAR, BIRD, DAD, EAT, SLEEP 'and other primary signs', and imitated some others.

One year later, the report of the same speech therapist states: 'Eric did not learn to use signs at this time and was not even interested in them.'

Eric's hearing was assessed at this time because the speech therapist thought Eric did not react well to speech alone, whereas with accompanying manual signs he reacted adequately. However, the focus was still on speech. 'I feel that he watches my mouth movements very carefully and tries to imitate speech with the help of them.' An adenoidectomy was performed when Eric was 4;0 years old and grommets were inserted in both ears. Soon after that, the speech therapist reported that Eric's speech was developing and manual signing was discontinued, but some months later it was reported that speech was not developing and manual signs were used again, and the parents and the nursery teacher also started to sign. By the time Eric was 4;6, it had become evident that manual signs were relatively easy for him to learn, while his speech was practically non-existent. According to the report, Eric was able to perform the signs corresponding to 72 pictures when he was 4;7 years old. They included mainly signs for objects and actions, but also some other lexical categories: adjectives, interrogatives and negatives (Table 6.1). Eric was also said to use combinations of manual signs when naming pictures.

Table 6.1. Eric's 72 manual signs at the age of 4;7 (translations of Finnish glosses)

EAT	MEAL	CUP
PLATE	BANANA	APPLE
MILK	WATER	SOUP
PORRIDGE	SPOON	FORK
KNIFE	CAT	DOG
COW	HORSE	PIG
HEN	COCK	SHEEP
RABBIT	BEAR	SHOE
MITTEN	SHIRT	TROUSERS
MOTHER	FATHER	BOY
GIRL	HOME	OBJECT
TRAIN	BOOK	BOAT
LAMP	BAG	DOLL
BALL	BICYCLE	TELEPHONE
CUPBOARD	TABLE	BED
BLANKET	CHAIR	HOUSE
SLEEP	SIT	STAND
SPEAK	HEAR	COME
WALK	READ	END
SCOLD	PEE	TOILET
NICE	GOOD	ILL
SMALL	NO	NOTHING
DO-NOT	WHICH	WHAT
WHERE	MORE	SNOW

The change in communication environment

Eric's interaction skills were very good throughout his development. Although he often was shy with unfamiliar people, he was active and confident in communicating with people whom he knew well. His attempts to communicate about matters outside the immediate environment were constantly increasing, but often failed because he did not have the necessary linguistic means. Both parents and professionals agreed that Eric needed an expressive communication form that would grow with him and make it possible for him to communicate in increasingly complex ways with people in the environment. As a result of these discussions, the planned language environment changed significantly. Eric's language intervention was revised when he was 4;7 years old. Manual signs were defined as his primary expressive form of communication and both the family and the nursery teachers were given an important role in the creation of an alternative communication environment. They started to use manual signs along with speech in most everyday interactions.

Eric's father went to a sign language course soon after the decision was made to use manual signs, and when Eric was 4;10 years old, the whole family participated in a one-week intensive course for five families with children who had learning disabilities. The parents received intensive sign language instruction, while there were groups with children – including siblings – with playful interactions and games with simultaneous communication (speech and manual signs). Anecdotal reports indicate that Eric was mostly an observer in the children's group, but he seemed to follow everything very carefully and after some time usually took part in play and games. He also learned many new signs. Eric's parents said that this course was crucial for changing the communication within the family. The experience of having a shared language with four other families was very important for them at that point. Manual signs as an alternative communication form was not something peculiar to their family, it was a real form of communication which Eric would also be able to use with people outside his home.

In the nursery, Eric was the only child using any form of alternative communication. His nursery teacher went to a sign language course when signing was started, and during the first year, she was the only person in the nursery who used manual signs consistently with him. She usually signed without speaking, which did not seem to affect Eric. The other adults in the nursery started to sign gradually. The other children in Eric's group showed interest in the signs used by the adults, asked to learn signs themselves and used signs with Eric. By the time Eric was 6;3 years, his teacher reported that everybody in the nursery signed a lot.

Individual communication intervention continued with a new therapist when Eric was 4;7 years old. The intervention included some direct teaching and in the beginning Eric had often been hand-guided to make signs. He had soon started to imitate new signs made by adults, and when he was 4;7 years old, this was his main way of acquiring new signs. The goal of the intervention was to influence the whole environment, not only Eric directly. In order to increase their competence in signing, the parents, the nursery teacher, and later the staff in Eric's school, received formal sign language teaching. This enabled Eric to learn more signs in the same way as other children learn spoken words, through social interaction with his parents and other adults and children in everyday communication situations.

One way to influence the language environment was to make the intervention a joint venture. Intervention sessions were therefore held once a month in Eric's home, in addition to weekly sessions in the speech therapist's office. The whole family, or at least one of the parents and the younger sister participated together with Eric in the home sessions. The sessions were very informal, as close as possible to normal family interaction. Eric was the focus of attention, but the presence of his sister made the sessions more genuinely shared. Like other siblings, Eric and his sister were rivals for the adults' attention. She tried to use more manual signs when she observed that Eric's signing was the focus of attention. The main goal of the family sessions was thus to help the family learn new vocabulary and improve their signing skills, and to support Eric's development and active use of signs. At this time, Eric seemed to learn new signs easily and in his sessions the emphasis was on sign combinations. The use of vocalizations was also encouraged, but in a playful way with minimal stress.

With the exception of Eric's nursery teacher, the adults in Eric's environment always signed simultaneously with spoken utterances. In the beginning, they signed mostly single key words related to the spoken sentence. Over time, the number of signed words increased and the sign order followed that of spoken Finnish. Finnish language is exceptionally rich in morphological endings added to the stem word, but such inflections were not taught to Eric in sign. It is possible to do so in signed Finnish, but it would slow down the signing significantly. This means that Eric got vocabulary models in both manual signs and spoken words, but a model for grammar in spoken language only.

Sign development

All through childhood, Eric was dependent on manual signs for communication. He often used sign and gesture alone, without any vocalization. Video recordings from his last pre-school years show that he was totally silent most of the time, producing only occasional vocalizations to express affect. His manual lexicon increased to several hundred signs. Most of the signs were nouns and verbs, but his vocabulary included also adjectives, interrogatives and negations. Pointing, combined with gaze shift and manual signs, formed an essential element in his expressive repertory. He also used other gestures, mime and actions to express himself.

There is no record of Eric's very first sign combinations, but it seems that these started to emerge early. In the description of his first 72 signs at the age 4;7 years, it was mentioned that he combined some of the signs when naming pictures. However, according to the notes from the following two years, he used mainly single-sign utterances and some combinations of pointing and one manual sign in his spontaneous communication.

His use of sign combinations increased quickly, however, and at the age of five years, utterances with two signs were quite frequent. For example, during car play at the age of 5;1 years, he signed CAR BROKEN and TABLE UNDER (correct Finnish word order). In more structured situations, for example when he described pictures in individual sessions, he used utterances with two to four signs or more. There seemed to be a development from utterances that were mostly chains of single signs, for example listing up details of a picture, to complex utterances that included the semantic roles of actor, action, patient, location and attribute. These examples are from written notes made when he was 5;1 years old:

BOY BUTTER CRISP.
MAN PLAY-ICE-HOCKEY.
DOG ANGRY BARK BITE YOU I AFRAID.
CHOCOLATE DELICIOUS BUY SHOP.

In his signed sentences, actor usually preceded action and attribute. When other sign orders were used, the utterances seemed to follow a topic-comment structure. Observations from the notes taken when he was from five to six years old confirm that his picture descriptions became more variable. He often signed the topic first, usually the action in the picture, and then often signed the actor. Occasionally he used ABA constructions (Veneziano, Sinclair and Berthoud, 1990), like TOOTHBRUSH RABBIT TOOTHBRUSH, meaning 'the rabbit is brushing its teeth' (age 5;2).

At this age, he also modified the signs to change the meaning, like changing the sign's place of articulation to indicate location. When he was 5;2 years old, he produced PAINT at the picture instead of his hand (Figure 6.1). He would also indicate plural or quantity by repetition, for example BOOK BOOK BOOK BOOK in the meaning 'lots of books' (age 6;3). In individual sessions, signed songs were used a lot to teach Eric to combine signs and he would sign songs with dozens of signs.

Eric used signs spontaneously in play, conversation and narration. When he was 5;9 years, he hurt his finger and signed later in the evening to the therapist that he had been trapped in a door when they were shopping. His signing was active and confident with people he knew well and who under-stood his manual signing and responded to it. However, the parents said that with new people and in unfamiliar situations, he was often shy and reserved, even fearful. The reports and video recordings from the ages of 5;2 and 6;3 years confirm that his expressive communication was imaginative and that he showed good awareness of the communication partner's skills, constantly monitoring the partner's reactions. He was usually persistent and would repeat and elaborate his messages until they were understood.

He often shared his observations and would use manual signs for making fun and sharing jokes. The following transcript from when Eric was 6;3 years old illustrates both his sense of humour, his creative use of signs and the way he used vocalization for sound effects. The speech therapist (K) was singing and signing an emotional song and Eric (E) pretended that he was not attending:

E: (Yawns).
K: (Singing) *And there is {a golden* GOLD} *{forest* FOREST} *and in {the forest* FOREST} *{a golden* GOLD} *{tree* TREE}.
E: (Straightens up) TREE FALL-DOWN (makes the sound of a power saw).
K: *Did {the tree fall down* TREE FALL-DOWN}?
E: 'Yes' (nods).
K: Oh! (Laughing). (Singing) *and the {blue bird* BLUE BIRD}.
E: TREE FALL-DOWN (makes the sound of a chain saw).
K: *Terrible! With a chain saw?*
E: 'Yes' (nods).
K: (Singing) *{bird* BIRD}, *and the {bird* BIRD} *has a*
E: TREE FALL-DOWN (makes the sound of a chain saw).
K: (Singing) *{golden* GOLD} *{mouth* MOUTH}.
E: TREE FALL-DOWN (makes the sound of a chain saw).
K: (Singing) *And the {blue bird of the dreams* BLUE BIRD DREAM}.
E: (Leans his head back on his hands again.)
K: (Singing) *it {lulls the babies* BABY LULL} to sleep and it *{sings a sleepy song* SING SLEEPY SONG}. *La-la-la-la-la-la-la-la.*
E: (Imitates the tongue movement of the speech therapist without any sound.)

During the intervention sessions at his home, one of Eric's favourite games was making 'riddles' for the rest of the family. He described the actions of cards that the others had to guess.

With regard to articulation, the handshape of Eric's signs was usually correct, but with occasional substitutions. He would, for example, use the fist instead of the index finger when signing TOOTHBRUSH, and extend the index finger instead of the little finger when signing COW (see Figure 6.1). The place or articulation and the movement of the signs were also usually correct, but the hands were sometimes oriented in the wrong direction. As in development of spoken language, Eric often imitated signs correctly and

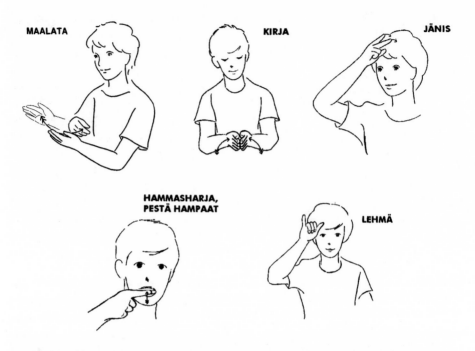

Figure 6.1. Finnish manual signs: PAINT, BOOK, RABBIT, TOOTHBRUSH, COW.

articulated them inaccurately in spontaneous use. When he made errors in his spontaneous signing, he often corrected himself without prompting when somebody else signed the correct form. From an early age, he would notice if people produced signs in a different manner, first mentioned in reports when he was 5;4 years old.

Speech development

Observations indicated that Eric had good comprehension of spoken language in everyday situations. However, no standardized test was used to assess his comprehension of spoken (and signed) language. There seemed to be some minor problems in comprehension and it is possible that these were partly caused by Eric's hearing difficulties. When Eric was 6;7 years old, the speech therapist reported that 'his special language impairment also seems to affect his comprehension of spoken language and he benefits from other people's signing and other forms of visual support used with speech'. The problems were not apparent in everyday communication situations, but they may also have been masked by the tendency of Eric at that time to react in a confirmatory manner or ignore what was said if he was uncertain about what the other person was saying.

There were reports of emerging speech when Eric was four years old, but six months later he showed practically no attempts to speak. In the following two-and-a-half years both the parents and the speech therapist thought that Eric's vocalizations and word attempts were increasing. His vocal output, however, was nearly unintelligible and knowledge about both Eric and the situation was necessary for people should understand it. Articulation was undifferentiated, consisting mostly of vowels or consonant–vowel structures. Unlike his signing, imitation was notably worse than spontaneous production, indicating developmental dyspraxia of speech (McCabe, Rosental and McLeod, 1998; Thoonen et al., 1994). The voice quality was forced and harsh when Eric was attempting to say words. Both articulation and voice quality were more relaxed when he was producing sounds during play. At the age of 6;7, Eric used about five spoken words that people who knew him well could recognize. These included *ei oo* (no, it's not), *mam-ma* (maito, milk) and *Ma*, which is the first syllable of his sister's name.

Eric used vocalizations mainly for affective expressions and in play (for example, car noise). He also liked to play with sounds and mouth movements in front of a mirror. When Eric was 6;3 years old, the speech therapist noted: 'Eric played with his tongue for a long time in front of the mirror. However, when he tried to imitate, he could do nothing, even though he spontaneously made most extraordinary movements.' After Eric had learned a few words, he used them adequately in his communication. After having learned his 'No, it's not', he enjoyed using it for making good-humoured disputes.

The primary school years

The school puts new demands on children's language and communication skills. When Eric began school at the age of seven years, his communication environment outside the home changed in many respects. He was in a special class for children with learning disabilities and manual signs were used with several other children in his class. The teachers used manual signs generally in the class, not only with Eric, as had been the case in his nursery. This meant that Eric shared his communication mode with a larger community. However, he was the most fluent signer in the class, so he did not have any advanced peers he could learn signing from.

The signing competence of Eric's family was important for his language development. When Eric started school, speech therapy became part of the school schedule. This brought an end to the close contact between the parents and the speech therapist, and to her monthly home visits. Teaching signs to the parents had been part of the monthly sessions and new arrangements had to be made. With Eric's growing signing skills, the parents also needed to build up more advanced signing competence. They received individual teaching from a professional sign language teacher at home once a week for about a year. This form of individually designed course was repeated every two years until Eric in his late teens started to express himself mainly in spoken language.

Reports of Eric's communication and language development during the first school years are sparse. He still seemed to have some problems in comprehending spoken language: 'Eric listens, but does not always get the spoken message. Gestures and manual signs help his comprehension.' His expressive repertoire did not develop very fast, but his communication skills seemed to be constantly growing. At the end of Eric's first school year, when he was 7;10, it was reported that both his vocalizations and his use of manual signs had increased. In the second grade, a new boy who used manual signs joined Eric's class and Eric's use of manual signs in the classroom increased notably. There are no reports of possible attempts at spoken words from this period. Because vocalizations and word attempts did not increase, Eric's weekly speech therapy was terminated after the second school year. The last report from his primary school years, at the end of his third grade (age 9;10), says that he had language intervention in a group once a week during that school year.

Manual signs and emergent speech

At the time when Eric was about to finish primary school, at the age of 12;9, his teacher noted that he had started to speak more during that spring. The parents confirmed that Eric had started to speak more at home, and that this had started in the autumn and increased gradually since then. According to them, Eric could produce single words, but 'no real sentences'. He would also put some words together, like when he was chatting with his sister, who was nine years old at the time, and told her: *Mary do this, Mary do that.* The parents said they were unable to judge how intelligible Eric's speech would be to other people, but that the family could understand it. They also mentioned that Eric liked to finger spell everything he saw written. He could also write his own name and a few other words.

At this age, however, Eric was still highly dependent on signing. He was reported to use spoken words in combination with signs both at home and at school, but his communication mode depended on the people and the setting. He was still shy with unfamiliar people and during his visit to the first author he remained silent and used manual signs only in the first part of the assessment. He did not vocalize at all during conversation and picture naming, but produced many mouth movements. However, he later vocalized with great enjoyment using a voice-controlled computer program. When describing pictures, 60 of the 62 picture names (97%) and 75 of the total 82 utterances (91%) were signed. Simultaneously with his signing, he pointed and used mime a lot, and finger-spelled written words. He also used the hand alphabet to indicate the first letter of names.

Sign development

Eric's vocabulary and language structure expanded during the school years. When he was 12 years old, he used several hundred signs. Most of them were articulated correctly, but Eric seemed to have developed some idiosyncratic sign forms. When signing I or ME, he consistently used the thumb instead of index finger. His fine motor skills were good, which was particularly apparent in his finger spelling, but he also signed fluently.

When describing pictures in the assessment, he still used some utterances with single signs and combinations of pointing and one sign, but of his 48 picture descriptions, 31 included utterances with two or more signs (65%). He often produced utterances with 4–6 signs, like WANT I SWEET WANT BAR CHOCOLATE and PLAY-GUITAR I WANT GUITAR ELECTRICITY. The word order was inconsistent. In 7% of his signed utterances he used a topic-comment structure, for example BAG SHOULDER-STRAP, CANDLE UPRIGHT and CAN COFFEE.

He also frequently modified signs to indicate a different meaning, for example: TABLE BIG-TABLE, ROCKING-CHAIR "no" (head shake) WRONG NOT-ROCKING-CHAIR, and HAMMER HAMMER (with an almost voiceless bang) (see Figure 6.2). As many as 22% of the signs showed some elaboration of meaning and, of these, 13% indicated size or shape, whereas 6% of the modifications indicated movement.

His manual signs also included some non-manual features. He used facial expression to convey affect, as when signing WANT CHOCOLATE with raised eyebrows and a smile, and STUPID ME with rounded eyes. He also used facial postures to describe details of pictures, signing for example HAT-WITH-BRIM with furrowed brows and pursed lips (Figure 6.3). Eric's use of non-manual features was especially apparent in his spontaneous jokes. When shown a picture of scissors, he signed SCISSORS and pointed smilingly at the lead of the camera, indicating that he was going to cut it. When asked how he was doing at school, he signed BAD with an amused face.

When looking at pictures at the assessment, he often called the attention of his father (F) to similarities between what he saw in the pictures and what he had at home, as in the two dialogues below:

E: COMB (points at the picture). I SIMILAR (points at the picture).
F: *Is it in your pocket?*
E: HOME.
F: *At home.*
E: HANGER SHELF.
F: *On a shelf.*

E: (Points at the picture) SIMILAR COTTAGE (looks at his father).
F: *At the cottage?*

E: (Points at the picture) CLOCK WRIST-WATCH.
F: *You are right, there certainly is.*

He also described his own experiences but, as before, the structure of his descriptions was simple, more a listing of details than a sequential narrative of related events. However, with the help of his father's questions he reported some of the main events of a school play in which he had recently been acting.

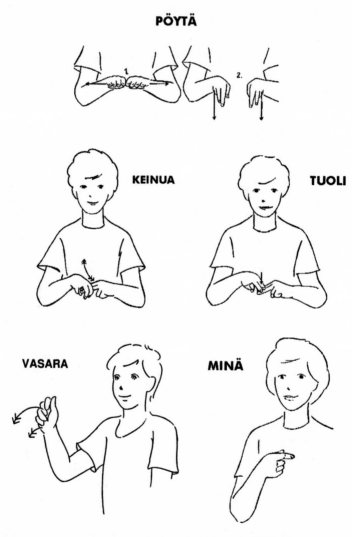

Figure 6.2. Finnish manual signs: TABLE, ROCKING-CHAIR, HAMMER, I/ME.

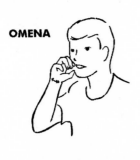

OMENA

BIG-APPLE

Eric first signs APPLE in a normal way, then modifies his handshape to indicate that he has a big apple in his hand. He also makes a mouth movement, pretending that he is biting at a very big apple.

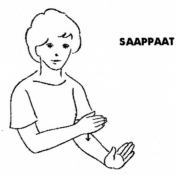

SAAPPAAT

LONG-LEG-OF-THE-BOOT

Eric starts to sign BOOT in a normal way, where the length of the leg is indicated by tapping the arm, then extends the length to the upper arm.

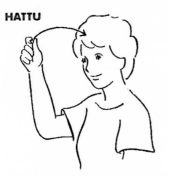

HATTU

HAT-WITH-A-BRIM

Eric starts to sign HAT, but he stops the movement and changes it to one which shows the shape of a brim.

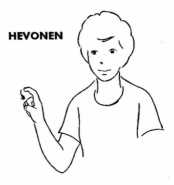

HEVONEN

HORSE-JUMP-OVER

This is about a horse jumping over a fence. HORSE is produced with a high and long curve.

Figure 6.3. Drawings of Finnish manual signs: APPLE, BOOT, HAT, HORSE.

Speech development

At the 12-year assessment, Eric's voice had broken and he had a deep male register. However, he did not use the voice in conversation and picture naming but he mouthed or whispered some words (for example, *comb, sleep* and *teeth*), which he usually signed simultaneously. According to the parents and the teacher, he frequently tried to speak in everyday situations, but for people who did not know him and the situation well, his speech was unintelligible without the support of manual signs. In the second part of the assessment, when Eric was using a computer program, which had to be controlled by vocalizations, he produced vocalizations and exclamations like *Oh no! I did it!* and *Yes!*

As in earlier assessments, at 12 years Eric gave an impression of having good comprehension of spoken language and he seemed to rely mainly on the spoken utterances of others. Observations show that when the communication partner was signing and speaking simultaneously, most of the time Eric was not attentive to the hands of the partner. He would occasionally watch the signing hands, indicating that he sometimes sought to support his comprehension of spoken language with signs. In the 12-year assessment situation, his father consistently signed simultaneously with his speech and if Eric did not understand him he tried to clarify his message by repeating the spoken utterance and emphasizing the most important sign. Eric still had a tendency to react in a confirmatory manner or ignore what was said if he was not sure what the partner was saying.

Secondary school years

Eric started his secondary education in a special school for students with learning disabilities, at the age of 13;0 years. When this school arrangement had been discussed in spring, it had been decided that he should go to a class where manual signs would be used with most of the students and whose teacher was fluent in signing. However, when the school started in August, there was a new teacher whose signing skills were poor. With several manual sign users in the same class, Eric nevertheless had a shared communication system with other members of his community.

Speech therapy was started again when Eric was 13;1 years old and continued for three more years. When he was 15;9 years old, signing was still considered his main communication form. Although Eric was speaking more consistently, his speech was judged to be at about the same level as the autumn before, which indicated that his speech development was slowing down.

It seems, however, that there was a renewed spurt in Eric's speech development during the summer he turned 16. In September, when he was 16;1 years old, reports say that he communicated mainly with speech but used manual signs to augment his spoken utterances. However, in spite of Eric's increasing speech skills, the school reported that their only problems with him were in communication. There were situations in the classroom, when Eric got frustrated because he was not understood. With regard to comprehension of spoken language, he followed instructions if they were clear and short. The report still suggests that he may have had comprehension problems, that at this age he should have understood more complex spoken language than he did.

Because of the positive development in spoken language, it was decided that Eric for a period should receive speech therapy twice a week. This was the last comment on speech therapy in his records.

Total communication in full use

When Eric was 17;3 years old, the parents said that he had stopped using manual signs and was communicating in speech only, using long sentences. They and other people who knew Eric well could understand most of what he was saying but they did not know how intelligible his speech would be to somebody who was not used to it. Observations at home when he was 17;4 years old showed that although speech was his main form of expressive communication, he was in fact using manual signs and gestures with his speech. He gave a vivid presentation about an incident at his school earlier the same day: somebody had accidentally cut his wrist, and they had called an ambulance and showed it where to go. He used manual signs, gestures, and mime along with speech which appeared highly unintelligible to the observer.

Not only Eric, but also others in the family – his father in particular – still often used signs to clarify or emphasize their utterances. It seems that signs and gestures had become such an integrated part of their communication that they were not always aware that they were using them. They were surprised when they were told about it. However, the parents had also thought that they should have used manual signs more consistently to keep this communication mode active in Eric, who would probably benefit from using it when people did not understand his speech, possibly for his whole lifetime.

Eric had changed his communication form but was still very talkative. 'Now Eric talks a lot, for example in the car when I come to take him home from school. He tells me everything that has happened during the day – sometimes I even wish that he wouldn't speak so much', his father said and laughed. At home, Eric did not hesitate to pick up the phone, and if it was somebody whom he knew well, he could have long discussions on phone. Also in the assessment situation he was talkative even when his father was not with him in the room. However, according to the parents, even at this age he was still reserved with new people and in unfamiliar or crowded settings, and would not use his total communicative repertoire: 'In those situations he may come to a total deadlock and not be able to express himself.'

The video recordings confirm that Eric was using speech consistently in conversation and that speech was his main expressive mode: 80 of 129 utterances (62%) were spoken only. There were 49 utterances where signs were used and in 16 utterances the signs paralleled the spoken utterance, whereas the signs in 18 utterances functioned as holistic elaborations of action sequences. Signs were more prominent in the picture descriptions, where signs were used in 24 of the 62 descriptions (39%).

Speech development at 17 years

At this age, Eric could now produce voice without noticeable effort and he showed great enjoyment in hearing and using his own voice. His articulation was unclear and too unintelligible to make an accurate transcription of it and to give his phonological profile. In contrast to his ability to change the production of manual signs, he could not correct his spoken words according to the model given by the partner. He also used natural sounds like a dog barking. He could also spell.

Eric used most of the usual word classes: nouns, verbs, pronouns, adjectives, adverbs and some function words, such as copula and post-positions. The grammar of Eric's spoken language is not easy to analyse because of its limited intelligibility and his simultaneous use of signing. The basic principle of word formation in Finnish is the addition of endings (bound morphemes, suffixes) to stems, and the form of the stem often alters when endings are added (Karlsson, 1987). These features were particularly difficult to determine in Eric's speech. He had at least some use of past tense and of the most common ones of the 15 cases of Finnish (partitive, genitive and the six local cases).

In conversation, more than 70% of his utterances were short sentences or phrases. Many of them were telegraphic and half of them were incomplete. The grammatical subject of sentences was relatively often omitted, as in the example of dialogue below. Word order, when it could be determined, tended to follow spoken Finnish. Word order errors seemed to occur predominantly when he was trying to convey complex narratives, and in these instances, he often used manual signs and gestures, like *leg broken – doesn't get* in the following example:

> E: {*Man* (lifts his finger up)}. *Falls* {*on* ON}. {*That man* (makes a very small pointing movement, probably referring to the 'man' he marked in the beginning)} {*leg broken* (hand is in a waiting position on his right side, palm up)} {*doesn't get* HIT} *gets up* {*to jump* JUMP}. (Looks intensively at the partner all the time, and after having signed JUMP, leaves his hand in that position and waits for the partner's reply.)

Eric used speech with a variety of communicative functions. However, he was not always able to give the information that was critical for the listener to understand what he was talking about (see von Tetzchner and Martinsen,

2000) and did not maintain the sequential structure of narratives. He needed significant support from a co-narrator to retell the story of 'Mr Bean' in event order, even though he knew that particular video well. On the other hand, he could recall numerous episodes and details from the story and describe them very animatedly. When facing situations where he did not become understood, he was very persistent and used different strategies to get his message through. He also showed good awareness of listeners' needs and was constantly monitoring the partner's reactions and checking whether he or she had understood. His mother commented: 'He is so good at it that it sometimes demands real acting talent from the partner to make him believe that you have understood something you haven't. Otherwise he will go on trying forever.'

Eric had also become more aware of his own difficulties in conversations. He had abandoned his strategy of just expressing agreement or ignoring what the other said if he did not understand it properly. He always asked the partner to repeat if he had not understood or heard what was said. In some cases it was difficult to determine whether the problem was in hearing or in comprehension, but he generally gave the impression of having both good comprehension when somebody talked about everyday topics and good hearing in normal noise conditions. When Eric at the age of 17;10 continued his studies in a centre of further education for students with intellectual impairments, the parents bought him a mobile telephone in order to enhance his independence and self-help skills. However, even they still found it difficult to understand Eric when they did not see him. Considering his rich communication in face-to-face interaction, this demonstrates the continued importance of total communication for Eric's social relations and quality of life.

Word-finding problems

When Eric was 17 years old, for the first time it became apparent that he had considerable word-finding difficulties in spoken language. These were most prominent when he was asked to describe object pictures and increased as the session lengthened. Eric had difficulty when describing the first picture (of a milk bottle) to the first author:

    E: *I don't remember* (makes a thinking face). *Glass.*
    K: *Mmm.*
    E: *Milk.*

After that he said the name of objects on the following 15 pictures without any apparent difficulties. Of the next 31 pictures, however, he had problems with 18. For some pictures he said another word of the same category. For example, pictures containing a plate, a cup and a mug were all named *glass*. However, when asked to look more carefully, he said the name of each of them correctly. In six cases, he seemed just to need some time to recall the spoken word, but in two of them he also signed the name simultaneously. In four other instances, he said the word after having produced the correct sign first. Four pictures were named in sign only. It may be noted that the researcher started to prompt him to sign when he did not name the seventeenth picture (an umbrella) and prompted him every time he could not say the name of the picture. However, with some of the pictures, he signed spontaneously. In the next example, the researcher (K) had shown him a picture of a chair.

E: ??? (unintelligible speech).
K: *What?*
E: (Puts his hand on his mouth, looks at his side, smiles.)
K: *What is it?*
E: 'Chair' (indicates the chair he is sitting on).
K: *Mm.*
E: (Puts the picture aside.)
K: {*A chair* CHAIR}. *Isn't it?*
E: 'Yes' (nods).
     (Points at next picture) *I don't remember the name of that one.*
K: *You don't remember the name of that one either?*
E: 'No' (shakes head).
K: *Well, sign it.*
E: CANDLE.
K: *Yes, it is a . . .* CANDLE
E: *Candle.*

By contrast, when asked to describe action pictures, Eric never said that he did not remember, which was his typical answer when he appeared to have problems finding the name of an object in the pictures. He often described details of the picture or referred to similarities in his own life. Signs were often used in these descriptions:

E: *Same that boy.*
K: *Yes, that is a boy, as well. But is he eating?*
E: *No.* SKATE. *Goes. Five* (points at the picture).
K: *Yes, he has a number there in his front. Can you ice skate?*
E: *Yes, I can.*
K: *Do you wear a helmet when you skate?*
E: *Yes.*
K: *I mean, he doesn't have a helmet.*
E: *He hasn't.* FUR-HAT.

In conversation, Eric's possible word-finding problems were less obvious. However, when the videotaped conversations were analysed more carefully, there were many occasions where word-finding problems might be suspected. They consisted of long, clarifying discussions, where Eric was very persistent in getting his message through:

E: *This is the same* (points at picture).
T: *What is the same?*
E: *This ??? here is* (keeps on pointing). *This is* (points).
T: *You mean that computer?*
E: 'No' (shakes head and changes from pointing with his right hand to pointing with the left hand). *That a v.*
T: *This?* (the letters AV are on the monitor Eric is pointing at).
E: *Yes.*
T: *It is . . . Similar to what?*
E: *This is same is home.*
T: *Do you have similar at home?*
E: *Yes.*
T: *Maybe it is a bit bigger television.*
E: 'Yes' (nods).

In the next example, with the help of his father (F), Eric was telling the researcher about Mr Bean's visit to the dentist. *Dentist* had been mentioned several times in the discussion before this:

F: *What happened after he had got himself up from there? Who came then?*
E: *A man.*
F: *Who was that man?*
E: (Makes a thinking face) *I don't remember.*
F: *Well, could it have been that dentist?*
E: 'Yes' (nods).

The parents said they had never thought of word-finding problems in Eric's everyday communication. However, they remembered many occasions where he did not say the right word. Difficulties might have been masked by Eric's use of other communication forms and by the fact that they often knew what the topic was and therefore it was not so necessary to find the exact words.

Sign development at 17 years

Signs had an augmentative role in Eric's language and it is difficult to estimate the size of his sign vocabulary. It is highly improbable that he had started to forget his signs as he was still using them actively, but growth had probably slowed because, according to the parents, Eric rarely saw other people making signs. In conversation he appeared to use a narrower range of signs than when he was 12 years old, usually a mixture of nouns, verbs and attributes. In picture description at the age of 17 he used signs predominantly to fill lexical gaps. When prompted to sign, he could nearly always recall the corresponding sign or one with a close semantic relation to the referent.

Eric rarely had longer utterances with signs only. They were mainly mixtures of speech, gestures and a few single signs. In narratives, he occasionally used several signs in one utterance, almost always simultaneously with the corresponding spoken words:

> E: *Glass. (Glass does not get* GLASS} *(doesn't get broken* NO BROKEN}. *(Is hard* HARD}.
> K: *Good. He has certainly a fine . . .*
> E: *Same that (weapon* GUN} *gets (glass* GLASS} *(broken* BROKEN} *(dhu-dhu* SHOOT}.

Occasionally he combined signs in a sentence-like structure, but simultaneously with similar spoken utterances. For example, he described Mr Bean's morning: *(Teddy bear is sleeping* BEAR SLEEP}. He communicated the size and shape of objects in pictures, but this was now done by tracing the objects' outlines on the pictures, as in the extracts below, instead of inflecting the sign by changing the amplitude of its movements like he had done before:

> E: *Banana. Eh.*
> K: *Mm. Does it look good?*
> E: *Yeah* (takes the picture in his left hand and shows it to the camera, indicating the curving shape of the banana with the other hand, making a funny face).
> K: (Laughing) *You showed it to the camera?*
> E: *Mm. (Moon* MOON} *resembles that (banana* (points at the picture)} *(moon* MOON}.
> K: *The same shape as a moon, or what?*
> E: *Yeah.*

> E: *Boot* (turns the picture to the camera). *Boots go* (shows with his whole hand the boot's legline upwards and then with his forefinger the shoeline to the toe).

Pointing still formed an important part in his utterances, as well as pantomime and looking. He used pantomime to describe complex sequences of movement in 18 of his 129 utterances in the picture description. In his narratives, he used spatial locations, directional movement and handshapes effectively to indicate the manner in which actions were carried out and where they happened, for example when describing actions in his favourite television series, *Martial Law*:

E: (Makes a rolling movement with his right hand) *that man. That jumps, this* STAND (makes the sign on top of the table, and points with his left hand at the signing hand). *This way* JUMP (a bow to the right) *fiiuu* (and ends in a sudden stop, probably on an imagined wall) *doks!*

James Bond was one of his favourite film heroes:

E: Goes. *????* *Door open* (mimicking the movement with his right hand, palm open, towards himself). *Bond hurries to escape* (moves his right hand from his right to his left). *Door closed* (moves his right hand back from the left to the right side). {*Turns* (control device movement)} {*is picture* (shows the shape of screen on his control-device-hand)}. {*Driving road* (repeats the previous sign)} {*turn the same* (control device movement)}. *Goes* {*bumps* BUMP} *in stones* {*downhill, glass broken* DOWN}.

Thus, although he was still producing distinct signs that can be analysed according to handshape, location, movement and orientation, he was also using a lot of gestures and pantomime-like forms, where it is less easy to identify the parameters. In picture naming, his signs were accurate and he still noticed immediately if the partner made the sign in a way different from his. He engaged in discussions about different ways of making signs. For example, after having signed RADIO with two hands (Figure 6.4), he put his right hand down, showing that it can be made with one hand only.

Sign use increased during the assessment session, possibly because the researcher prompted signing when he was unable to relay the meaning through speech only, or because he was becoming tired and reverted to a, for him, more accessible mode of communication than speech.

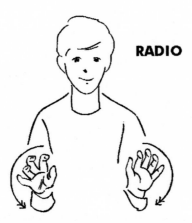

Figure 6.4. Finnish manual sign: RADIO.

Discussion

Some features in Eric's communication, both in sign and in speech, may be explained by his cognitive impairment, for example his inability to maintain sequential structure in his narratives and give necessary information to a communication partner who is not acquainted with his topic, or to reformulate his message if the partner did not understand it. However, there are several features of Eric's exceptional communication and language development that may contribute to the understanding of development in speech and in sign. Firstly, he showed early good interaction skills and was an active communicator despite the severe and manifold difficulties in his speech and language development. He became a proficient signer and developed strategies for overcoming the communication problems caused by his limited expressive repertory. One important question is why he developed such advanced signing skills, exceptional for children with Down syndrome. Secondly, his late acquisition of speech and the subsequent changes in his use of manual sign and gesture appears to be very unusual. Thirdly, his word-finding difficulties which appear to be specific to spoken language suggest that the profile of linguistic strengths and problems may vary according to the mode of expression.

Interaction and language development

A consistent feature of Eric's development has been the interplay between his own personality and behaviour and the reactions and attitudes of significant people in his environment. Throughout his 17 years, Eric has shown how determination to communicate, interest in others and enjoyment of sharing information can enable the individual to circumvent even severe communication problems. His behaviour is the opposite of learned passivity, common among people using alternative communication (von Tetzchner and Martinsen, 2000). The age of 3;6 years, when signing was introduced to Eric's family, would represent a late onset today. In most parts of Finland and in many other countries, families with an infant with Down syndrome are provided with communication intervention including signing already in the children's first year of life. Eric's development shows, however, that beneficial effects can be obtained even if intervention is started a little later, although studies suggest that late onset may lead to non-optimal development (Launonen, 1996, 1998). It may be that Eric established a good foundation for later language development through his successful early non-verbal interactions. This emphasizes the need for communication-oriented early intervention in families with a new child who is known to be vulnerable in the domain of language and communication.

Most early intervention programmes emphasize the provision of information to parents, but the change in children's language environment implied in language intervention requires more than giving information to parents. The whole life of a family is influenced when a new communication form is introduced in the family's everyday interaction. One of the major challenges in alternative communication intervention is to make the transfer from the intervention settings to everyday life. In Eric's case, his parents said that the family course they attended had been important in giving them an experience of a genuinely shared communication system. Other parents who have participated in group sessions with families using the same system have reported similar reactions (Launonen, this volume).

The efforts of Eric's family have been crucial for his communication development. His good interaction skills were mentioned in the reports from the family's first visit to the clinic, and repeatedly thereafter. This suggests that the parents were able to create activities with Eric in a way that supported and encouraged his active communicative role from very early on. Eric was their second child, and because his brother was only one-and-a-half years older, non-verbal interaction was probably a natural part of the family's communication in Eric's first years. Later, manual signs were integrated naturally into their everyday interactions so that Eric's mode of communication was always valid in his environment. This is in contrast to reports that show that many families find it difficult to sustain signing at home and that nurseries and schools provide limited sign input (Grove and Dockrell, 2000; Grove and McDougall, 1991; Launonen, this volume). Signs were abandoned by Eric's family only in response to his own switch in communication form, and even after that they would readily use signs if Eric had problems understanding or if he started to use signs and gestures himself. Eric's exceptional development thus demonstrates that even severe disabilities in communication and language development can be overcome if the child has a communication form that is genuinely shared with other people. Unfortunately this is not often the case. Children who use manual signs often have to construct and adapt their own communication form from the fragmented use of the same form by other people.

One reason for this may be that children's knowledge of spoken language is overestimated when they start to speak. In Eric's case, any possibility of emergent speech led to less focus on signing in the intervention, particularly in the beginning of his intervention, even if signing functioned as a catalyst for the emergent speech. But also in primary school, reports suggested that his manual communication was not considered as important as speech. The reports do not give the reasons for terminating Eric's individual speech therapy when he was nine years old, but it seems as if the professionals thought his progress had levelled off and that the speech therapy would not have any effect any more. However, there is reason to believe that a child with such an exceptional communication development as Eric would continue to benefit from individual language intervention at the age of nine years, and even later, in response to the growing communication demands of school and social life in general. On the other hand, it may also indicate that Eric's natural language environment was considered to be so good that it would be enough to sustain further language development.

It is, however, not only people in the environment who make communication development possible even for children with disabilities. Children contribute to their own development through their influence on the environment as part of a transactional process. Eric's early interaction skills implied resilience because they made it easy for the adults to see when his early non-verbal means of communication failed to lead him to communicative success. This may also explain the parents' exceptionally fast adoption of signing: they had already started to feel that they needed adapted language means to be able to share more complex information and communicate in more sophisticated ways with Eric. Because of the competence of the people in the environment, Eric could use manual signs for a variety of purposes: to ask for objects, people, actions and information, to comment, to relate his experiences and make jokes, which he enjoyed a lot as he got older. His ability to express himself then made it easier for others to adapt their communication to his competence. In this way, they treated Eric as a competent individual and an interesting communication partner. This process is likely to have had cumulative effects on Eric's language and communication development, as well as on his knowledge of the world in general. The responses of his family and professionals to his communication attempts were an essential contributory factor for this development. Hence, Eric's communication development also raises issues for clinical practice, showing the significance of ecologically valid procedures in intervention.

Language development in sign

Eric started to use sign sentences after he had used signs for some time. Neither the time of emergence or the structure of his first sign combinations are recorded in the professionals' reports, like in most other cases. This indicates that professionals tend not to attribute significance to this information, unlike the first spoken sentences of children with delayed speech, which are usually mentioned in reports.

It is a general finding that language-impaired children who use manual signs do not tend to develop a grammar (Grove, Dockrell and Woll, 1996). This does not necessarily mean that they are incapable of doing so. It may also be a result of a lack of language models: adults tend to use only single signs (key-word signing) with their spoken sentences (Grove et al., 1996).

There is no record of the early signing of Eric's parents, but the use of sentences was mentioned as one of the main goals in his individual sessions from early on. The game the family played in the home sessions, where Eric had to sign the content of pictures the others should guess, may have made him aware of their need for more information about the details of the picture, and thus contributed to making him use utterances with more than one sign.

Another contributing factor may have been the fact that his nursery teacher was reported to sign without speaking. If this was a consistent feature in her communication with Eric, it is probable that she used more sentences than the other adults who were using signs. It seems, thus, that Eric was exposed to more sign sentences than is usual for intellectually impaired children acquiring manual signs. These findings support the view, presented by Grove et al. (1996), that the competence of this group of children may be reflected in sign-specific constructions rather than in signed constructions based on the grammar of the spoken language.

Video recordings show that when Eric was 12 years old he signed fluently. He had a wide and varied vocabulary, and he was consistently inflecting signs to indicate changes in meaning in ways that were similar to the instances of 'gestural morphology' described by Grove (Grove and Dockrell, 2000; Grove et al., 1996). In the picture naming task, these were related to descriptions of objects and functioned rather like size and shape specifiers in a sign language (compare Kyle and Woll, 1985). There was no real evidence of any syntax although in many of his utterances, topic appeared to precede comment.

It is not clear how Eric developed sign inflections and structure. Eric's parents used signs simultaneously with spoken Finnish, and although there is no record of their signing, they had no knowledge of the structure of Finnish sign language. However, if Eric inflected his signs to relay specific meaning, it is reasonable to assume that also the other signers in the family or at school, for example, increased the amplitude of the sign to indicate size. It is also possible that this is another example of children 'going beyond the input given', as has been found for deaf children in predominantly non-signing environments (Goldin-Meadow and Feldman, 1975; Singleton, Morford and Goldin-Meadow, 1993) and children with intellectual impairments (Grove and Dockrell, 2000).

Speech acquisition

There is a considerable body of literature relating to the effect of the introduction of manual sign on speech development in individuals with communication difficulties. Although parents and teachers are still often concerned that speech may be negatively affected, all the existing evidence suggests that on the contrary, signing may facilitate the use and development of spoken language (see, for example, Abrahamsen, Cavallo and McCluer, 1985; Kouri,

1989; Launonen, 1996, 1998, this volume; Romski, Sevcik and Pate, 1988; von Tetzchner, 1984c).

Explanations have ranged from the suggestion that sign use relieves pressure on speech, thus making involuntary and spontaneous vocalization more likely, to the suggestion that the motor performance of sign use facilitates spoken articulation (Creedon, 1973; Powell and Clibbens, 1994). There are no other documented accounts of speech development as late as 12 years, although Grove (1995) found some anecdotal reports of late onset of speech in signing children in a survey of special schools in the south east of England.

In order to understand why a problem begins to resolve, one needs some insight into its original cause. The nature of Eric's language impairment is unclear, as is the stimulation for the emergence of speech. The etiology of his difficulties with speaking appears complex, probably involving interactions between different factors. As with many other children with Down syndrome, Eric's speech has remained very unintelligible. It has deviant and imperfect morpho-syntax (see Bol and Kuiken, 1990; Kernan and Sabsay, 1996; Miller, 1988) and many phonological and phonemic errors (see Bray and Woolnough, 1988; Dodd, McCormack and Woodyatt, 1994). Eric's hearing loss, caused by his recurrent secretory otitis media, may be a contributory factor in his difficulties with speech and articulation (Kile, 1996). Processing difficulties may also have been contributory to Eric's problems in speech development. People with Down syndrome have been found to be particularly poor in tasks that demand auditory, sequential processing (Kernan and Sabsay, 1996; Lincoln et al., 1985; Pueschel et al., 1987). The qualitative deviations in Eric's speech meant that it was very difficult to make even a rough transcription of it for analysis, a common problem in studies of people with Down syndrome (Dodd et al., 1994). However, although many children with Down syndrome have severe speech and language problems, the problem cannot be attributed to this condition only because not all children with this syndrome have unintelligible speech.

There are strong indications that Eric had severe oral dyspraxia, which is common in children with Down syndrome (Brown-Sweeney and Smith, 1997; Devenny and Silverman, 1990; Devenny et al., 1990). From the age of four, in periods, he displayed a keen interest in the production of sounds and movements of the lips and tongue. He would watch the speech therapist's face intently and look at himself in the mirror, but any imitations were effortful and inaccurate in comparison with his involuntary vocalizations. He sometimes mouthed words without sounds, not only in intervention sessions but also at home with the family and at school. This was not selective mutism, because he never spoke in any situation and was a confident and engaged communicator in manual sign. At the age of 12, when he began to speak, it was in a bass register and his voice had clearly broken. From this point on, he appeared to find it easier to imitate and sustain vocalization, and when he was 17 years old, he produced voice with ease. It is possible that physiological changes in the vocal folds and larynx may have contributed to the development of speaking.

Word-finding difficulties are defined as problems in the speed and accuracy of naming, possibly due to poorly specified semantic representations (Dockrell et al., 1998; German, 1996). Although children with Down syndrome are known to be delayed in lexical acquisition relative to typically developing children matched for chronological age, evidence suggests that the diversity and size of their vocabularies are comparable to, or even exceed, those of children matched on non-verbal intelligence (Rondal and Edwards, 1997). Word-finding difficulties do not seem to be a characteristic of Down syndrome (Marcell et al., 1998). However, people with Down syndrome may also be affected by other difficulties, such as a specific language impairment (see Chapman et al., 1998). Word-finding difficulties are one of the most commonly reported problems of children with language impairments (Dockrell et al., 1998). Eric's difficulties in spoken language were most marked when he had to name objects on pictures and less obvious in descriptions of actions, narratives and conversations. It might be expected that he would have problems with word retrieval in the more complex narrative tasks, but in these situations and in his action descriptions, he may have compensated for expressive difficulties in both vocabulary and grammar by using mime, pantomime, gesture and manual signs. This enabled him to communicate information he could not relay in speech, particularly about actions and visuo-spatial relations. Word-finding difficulties may thus have been masked in conversation by the compensatory strategies, with help of which he managed to keep up the impression of a smoothly proceeding conversation.

The difficulties seemed to be specific to spoken language. Eric never seemed to have a problem in naming pictures with signs. One possible explanation for this disparity may be that he had unclear phonological representations for the spoken vocabulary. It has been hypothesized that poorly elaborated semantic representations are caused by underspecification of phonological and morphological features (Chiat and Hunt, 1993), which is consistent with Eric's word-finding difficulties being most evident in spoken language.

Another possibility, related to Eric's poor articulation skills, is a specific difficulty with the retrieval and processing of auditory information. People with Down syndrome seem to perform poorly on auditory retrieval tasks (McDade and Adler, 1980), and their retrieval of lexical information from long-term memory is often slow (Varnhagen, Das and Varnhagen, 1987). The fact that Eric was sometimes able to name an object after a period of time is consistent with the hypothesis of slow auditory processing. Observations in the picture naming task also suggest that manual signs sometimes functioned as cues for word retrieval and the fact that he sometimes could say the word after having signed the name indicates that signs had a priming effect on his spoken word retrieval (see German, 1992). Similar findings have been found with other language-impaired children. Creedon (1973) found that some children who started to speak after having been taught manual signs could say, for example, *baby* when simultaneously signing BABY, but were only able to produce *buh* when asked to sit on their hands. Thus, it is quite likely that manual signs not only gave Eric an expressive foundation for learning to speak, but that the motor production of signing also helped him activate and produce spoken words.

Finally, Eric learned the one-hand alphabet and enjoyed spelling written words that he saw. In a study of children with articulatory apraxia, Morley (1972) found that half of them learned to read and began to speak more intelligibly when they were taught spelling, while the other half developed reading disorder. It is probable that the first group made their production of speech more distinct by allocating sounds to letter categories, while the other half of the children may have tried to allocate letters to their unclear articulation categories. Similarly, Eric's finger spelling may have helped develop his phonological awareness and speech production.

It is unlikely that the relationship between signing and speech development is simple. The discussion above suggests that several factors may have interacted in contributing to the emergence of speech, in a way that best may be described as a dynamic systems model (Thelen and Smith, 1994). Within this framework, simple processes combine in a process that is more complex than the sum of a simple addition of the individual processes. Whatever the processes underlying Eric's deviant and exceptional speech development were, the fact that he developed speech in adolescence and came to use it as his primary means of communication provides additional support to studies that show that the use of manual sign will not prevent the production of speech, and rather support the emergence of an ability to speak if the individual has the opportunity to do so.

Changes in communication form

Grove and McDougall (1991) introduced the concept of modality dependence as a way of describing patterns of sign and speech use in children with intellectual impairments. Modality dependence can be calculated as a ratio of the number of signs to the number of words produced by a child. This makes it possible to track changes in communication form across different situations and over time.

Eric was clearly sign dependent in all situations until he was 12 years old. He did occasionally vocalize and when he did so it was to express affect or use imitations of natural sounds as part of the utterance. His vocalizations were vocal gestures rather than word approximations (see Grove, 1997). At the age of 17, Eric seemed to have made a total switch in modality dependence. He was mainly speaking, and signing had assumed a complementary role. Thus, manual signs and gestures changed character and function over time.

It is not the case that Eric was using a true sign language, which can only develop through exposure to linguistic and rule-governed input. However, McNeill (1992) has shown that when individuals become dependent on the manual mode for communicating complex meaning, their gestures start to evince some of the features of a sign language – the individual starts to exploit correspondences in form and meaning, which result in a principled and contrastive use of handshapes, movements and spatial locations and orientations. McNeill suggests that one of the criteria that can be employed to distinguish sign from gesture is that the components of sign can be clearly identified, whereas gestures are holistic, and less easy to analyse into their separate parts.

Eric's development seems to reflect this process of mode dominance but in reverse: he started by using manual signs as his primary communication mode but as speech became more dominant the signs began to take the form of gestures. It was noticeable that when he was 17 years old, he produced more manual behaviour that was difficult to identify as the separate parameters of hand-shape, movement, location and orientation. This is exactly what McNeill's model would predict. A particular feature was the change in how he described the size and shape of objects. At 12 years, when signing was the dominant mode, he made internal changes to the form of sign. At the age of 17, he still communicated information about the pictures, but did so by tracing the outline on the photograph – in a way that is far more suggestive of gesture than of sign. Like the children described by McNeill, Eric used gesture to communicate visual and dynamic information he did not encode in spoken language, and the analogue inflections of signing had no parallel in speaking. He may also have lacked sufficient grammatical skills in Finnish to convey the kind of information that he wanted. He did, however, show some evidence of grammar in Finnish. We suggest, therefore, that Eric's profile is consistent with the hypothesis that there is a complementary relationship between the vocal and manual modalities (Singleton, Goldin-Meadow and McNeill, 1995). When signing is the dominant mode, vocalizations may assume a complementary gestural role. Eric used vocal expressions mainly for affective and onomatopoeic meaning. When the vocal mode became dominant, the situation was reversed, and the manual mode assumed the complementary role.

Conclusion

Eric's development suggests that the use of alternative means of communication is a dynamic phenomenon, which changes and grows throughout the lifespan of an individual. His unique pattern of development was the result of the interaction between individual characteristics and influences of the environment. Intrinsic factors may have been critical in determining his uptake and output in different communication modes. These include cognitive impairments related to the chromosome deviance, possible associated disorders and dyspraxia; maturational factors leading to a change in vocal physiology and factors related to temperament and emotion regulation, including his sociable personality. As Eric grew up in a supportive environment, where all forms of communication were always accepted, he was able to shift his pattern of communication mode use in ways that were appropriate to him. This may seem obvious, but is not the case for many individuals, where communication form is decided by others. For example, Grove and McDougall (1989) found that teachers often determined that sign was no longer the appropriate option for a child because the child had started to speak, and that day centres sometimes refused to support signing because they believed it made the service users conspicuous. At the conference of the International Society for Augmentative and Alternative Communication in 1998, a speech therapist was heard to tell colleagues that she advised against the use of manual signs because it was too difficult to get staff to sign themselves. We feel that this is a violation of the rights of individuals to use the modes of communication with which they are comfortable and which allow them the best way of expressing themselves.

Acknowledgement

The authors acknowledge with gratitude the participation of Eric and his parents in the research which led to the writing of this chapter.

CHAPTER 7

Environmental influences on aided language development: the role of partner adaptation

MARTINE M. SMITH

To paraphrase the words of Katherine Nelson (1997, p. 101), the process of development is largely an elusive, underground process, hidden from view. Development is discussed generally in terms of its outcomes with associated inferences about the changes underlying such outcomes. Developmental theories are still somewhat lacking at the level of descriptive adequacy, and fall far short of explanatory adequacy (Bennett-Kastor, 1988). Despite this limitation, interventionists working with children with developmental difficulties bring to their work an implicit assumption that the developmental process can be influenced, and that such influence can be exerted through the manipulation of factors external to the individual.

Such a position has little resonance with strong nativist views of development (such as Chomsky, 1972), where the path of change is largely predetermined, either by innate knowledge structures (Fodor, 1983) or by pre-specified constraints that limit the possible paths of development, and hence the knowledge structures which can evolve (see, for example, Markman, 1990). By contrast, a constructivist position, as exemplified by the work of Jean Piaget (1977), views the environment as an essential stimulus to children's construction of knowledge. Within a constructivist approach, attempts at intervention may influence development, provided a cognitive state in equilibrium is challenged by an appropriate 'disturbance' – that is, a previously unpredicted effect. In his 'new theory' Piaget attributes even more importance to empirical experience in development, influencing the relationships which are abstracted and re-represented by children (Barrouillet and Poirier, 1997). The environment can provide the raw materials to stimulate the construction of children's knowledge. However, the child remains largely master of the construction process. Intervention may stimulate the desired question or disturbance, but the resolution of the disturbance is a problem for the child to solve internally.

Within a social constructivist framework however, as exemplified by the work of Vygotsky, development proceeds 'from the outside in':

> The entire history of the child's psychological development shows us that, from the very first days of development, its adaptation to the environment is achieved through social means, through the people surrounding it. (Vygotsky, 1993, p. 116)

Development is not merely a process internal to the child, but is situated in, and mediated by, the social context within which the child is developing. The social context is not simply a stimulus, but a powerful force in shaping development.

Over the past 20 years, intervention programmes to support communication development have increasingly focused on the social context, and the role of communication partners as potential agents of change (for example, Fey, 1986; Nelson, 1991). Although the seeds of social constructivism are implicit in many such intervention programmes, the theoretical principles may not be made explicit. Within such approaches, there is a fine balance to be drawn between developing effective communication strategies to support interaction of both partners in a dyad, and implying, however unintentionally, that one of the communication partners is responsible for the other partner's communication difficulty.

As yet, science is at the early stages in determining how much skilled communication partners can influence the development of less skilled communication partners. Common sense would suggest that a developing language system should tolerate a wide range of interaction styles. There is initial evidence that parent interaction styles may have an effect on their children's communicative development (Nelson, 1997); it is a giant leap to suggest that parental behaviours in some way cause the development or lack of development of particular communication behaviours. Furthermore, we do not as yet know whether features of development observed with typically developing children (i.e., the influence of parental communication behaviours on language development) necessarily apply in the same way to those children whose development is atypical, such as children acquiring language using manual or graphic signs. We have considerable data to profile typical linguistic development, but similar developmental indices are not yet available to track atypical development. Indices from spoken language development may be applied, without clear evidence as to how these indices are relevant or appropriate.

Parents of children who are developing atypically are in a particularly vulnerable position. They may blame themselves, or perhaps even be considered by others as contributing, however unintentionally, to their children's presenting difficulties. They may feel a responsibility to 'improve' their child's development, while lacking any real sense of how development can be influenced. In such a situation they may simply intuitively work with strategies they have observed, or remember from other situations. While therapists may seek to support them by providing guidelines for 'good interaction behaviours', a shared frame of reference to interpret such guidelines may be lacking. Without a shared understanding of the process of development, the promotion of parents as 'primary agents of change' in the developmental process may leave them vulnerable to the inference that they are also a primary cause of any presenting problem.

A focus on modifying parental interaction patterns in order to support a child's communicative development only makes sense if linguistic input is viewed as a powerful influencing factor. There is still considerable disagreement, however, about the role of linguistic input in development.

Linguistic input in typical development

In typical language development a triad of influences converge: the input provided to the child, the uptake by the child from the input provided (Harris, 1992) and the communication efforts by the child, which in turn influence the input subsequently provided (Locke, 1995). Whilst the relative importance of each of the sources of information is controversial, nonetheless there is little argument that all three set the context and influence the process by which the child becomes a linguistic communicator. Across many different cultural settings primary caregivers adopt particular communicative styles in interacting with infants and young language-learning children (for example, Locke, 1995; Pine, 1994; Snow, 1995). Caregivers exaggerate prosodic information, use generally higher pitch, emphasize eye-gaze behaviours, facial expression and gestural input, and reduce utterance length. They maintain contingency with a child's previous communication, even if this means doing more of the conversational work and assuming responsibility for conversational repair. Comparable behaviours have been reported also in interactions with infants acquiring language through the manual modality (Masataka, 2000). Such behaviours are often referred to as 'fine tuning' and are most commonly described in interactions between mothers and their children (Snow, 1995). Fine tuning is a dynamic process, with mothers modifying their input in accordance with the response from the child. In this sense, Locke (1995) argues that it is the child who drives the process and determines the nature of the input that is provided for further learning.

An alternative view is that from the start, the two forces shape and influence the child's development – 'the child's cognitive construction and the provisions of the social-cultural world of people and things' (Nelson, 1997, p. 100). In Nelson's view, the child contributes 'knowledge based on direct experience . . . (with) the adult "other" contributing support, scaffolding, modelling, directives and eventually new semantic symbolic representations to the child's cognitive models' (1997, p. 100). Irrespective of the relative import imputed to the child or social partner, such scaffolding is interpreted by many as facilitating language acquisition, influencing not only the speed and range of lexical development, but also the communicative intents expressed by the developing child (Ninio, 1992), mastery of syntactic structure, and the development of narrative skills (Snow, 1995).

However, despite the prevalence of tendencies such as phonological simplification, prosodic exaggeration, lexical and grammatical reduction and communicative clarity in interactions with young children, by no means all communication partners engage in such closely fine-tuned styles of interaction. Snow (1995) suggests that fathers (or secondary caregivers) and older siblings produce child-directed speech that is less finely tuned to the child's developmental level. The less discriminative tuning may result in lower levels of contingency responsiveness to immature child utterances; communication breakdown may occur more frequently and be less effectively repaired; child topics are less likely to be expanded and continued, and fathers are also more likely to use unusual vocabulary than are mothers (for example, Rondal, 1980; Tomasello, Conti-Ramsden and Ewert, 1990). Barton and Tomasello (1994) suggest that fathers engage in fewer and shorter conversational dialogues with their children. They respond less than mothers to child utterances, and tend not to initiate a conversation, but wait for the child to make the first overtures. Fathers' child-directed speech is reported as containing more imperatives and directives, and fewer conversation-eliciting questions. Furthermore, it is more lexically demanding, evidencing a higher level of linguistic diversity, with more low-frequency words, fewer 'yes/no-' and more 'wh-' questions, and an increased proportion of requests for clarification.

It is not clear at this stage whether the differences noted between mothers' and fathers' child-directed speech reflect gender differences in interaction style (see, for example, Tannen, 1996), or are related more to familiarity with the child. In instances of bilingualism – for example, where the father is the only interaction partner using a particular language – fathers and mothers differ little in their interaction style, at least until the child has progressed beyond the early stages of language acquisition (Goodz, 1989, cited by Barton and Tomasello, 1994).

Whilst secondary caregivers' child-directed speech may be characterized as less supportive or facilitative of early attempts at communication through language, Snow (1995) argues that the less precise tuning may carry with it some developmental advantages. The more demanding style may provide a contrasting interaction experience, and expose the child to conversation situations more typical of those in the 'outside world', as suggested by the *linguistic bridge hypothesis* put forward by Berko-Gleason (1975, cited by Barton and Tomasello, 1994; Mannle and Tomasello, 1987). Although children may experience more disruptions in interacting with secondary caregivers, they are consequently afforded potentially important opportunities to learn skills needed for communication with 'more distant or unknown audiences, without the contextual and conversational support very young children enjoy in interaction with mothers' (Snow, 1995, p. 183).

The relative long-term importance of differing interaction styles for children's language development remains speculative. However, immediate effects are nonetheless to be found in children's linguistic efforts. Rondal (1980), for example, reports that in the dyads he studied, the children produced longer utterances with their fathers than with their mothers. He interprets this finding as consistent with the bridge hypothesis, because the fathers' higher proportion of clarification requests led the children to adapt their language. In a study of 12- to 18-month-old children, Tomasello, Conti-Ramsden and Ewert (1990) found a higher proportion of clarification requests in interactions with fathers than with mothers, placing an onus on the child to repair linguistically the communication breakdown. Furthermore, they note qualitative differences between the types of clarification requests issued by both parents. Fathers were more likely to use a non-specific query (for example, what?), while mothers tended to use specific queries (for example, put it where?). The non-specific query may force children to re-evaluate their utterances and modify them, whereas a specific query highlights a particular gap in information that may be resolved either through simple repetition or through provision of new information. Tomasello and his associates (1990) report that children respond differentially to the various types of requests, tending to use repetition as a repair strategy when interacting with mothers, while revising or recasting utterances in response to lack of comprehension on the part of their fathers. Barton and Tomasello (1994) conclude that secondary caregivers 'encourage the development of more linguistic means of communication (using language to serve a conventional referential function) via their lexically demanding style' (p. 133).

Linguistic input in atypical development

If reciprocity in conversational dyads is important not only to the immediate unfolding of a specific interaction, but also as a link in a developmental process, what are the implications for children with significant communication difficulties? If children are unable to participate as expected in spoken interactions, do caregiver interaction patterns differ from those reported above? If so, what is the significance of such differences?

Some children experience serious difficulty in acquiring the language of their community, despite intact sensory and motor systems, access to language input, and generally appropriate abilities in other aspects of cognitive and social functioning (Conti-Ramsden, 1994). Research suggests that language input to children with specific language impairments may differ from that provided to either language-matched or age-matched peers. Two key differences are commonly reported. The first is increased maternal directiveness, reflected in increased use of demands, imperatives and a tendency to initiate conversations. A highly directive parent may tend to use language primarily to control a child's attention and behaviour, rather than as a medium for reciprocal communicative and informational exchange (Conti-Ramsden, 1994). A second difference commonly reported is of reduced semantic contingency between maternal and child utterances (Conti-Ramsden, Hutcheson and Grove, 1996), possibly due to difficulties in intelligibility. High levels of directiveness and low semantic contingency are patterns associated with slower progress in language development in typically developing children (Conti-Ramsden, 1994).

The nature of the relationship between altered maternal input and language problems in children with specific language impairment remains somewhat unresolved. Conti-Ramsden argues that the altered input provided to children with specific language impairment may reflect many factors. Such children may be more passive conversational partners, thereby shifting responsibility for initiation to their partner. They may have attention difficulties requiring more explicit management of their attentional focus. Conti-Ramsden (1994) suggests that parents may not be able to gauge their child's language level, and identify its needs, as the typical pattern of development has been disrupted. 'By definition, atypical language learners present a mismatch of characteristics to their parents in terms of their physical and cognitive maturity, age and language ability which may have stronger effects than we have so far contemplated' (p. 196). In general, therefore, interest in linguistic input to children with language difficulties has shifted from a focus on the potential causative effects of the distorted input (Snow, 1995) to a recognition that, where changes are noted, the altered input may constitute an adaptation by parents to the language learning difficulties of their children. Such findings have led to a variety of intervention programmes focused on changing communication partner behaviours, and developing facilitative acquisition strategies to replace a directive style (for example, Nelson, 1991; McCathren, Yoder and Warren, 1996). Such approaches are premised on the view that some element of collaborative constructionism, in Nelson's (1997) terms, is implicit in language development.

To summarize, in many cultural settings parents accommodate to their children's levels of linguistic sophistication. Primary caregivers frequently interact in a highly responsive, semantically contingent way, apparently providing maximal support for children's emerging abilities. Secondary caregivers use less finely tuned and more challenging interaction styles, demanding greater linguistic efforts, more initiation and greater lexical diversity. In at least some cases, the effects of the contrasting interaction patterns is that children use longer utterances when interacting with secondary caregivers, and a more referential style of communication, to accommodate the lesser degree of familiarity of the communication partner.

Children with language impairments present with an apparent asynchrony across domains of development, creating a challenge for parents trying to gauge an appropriate level of linguistic input. Under such conditions, parents may use more directive and less semantically contingent responses, in an effort to maintain a conversational focus and topic. These altered input patterns suggest that atypical contexts elicit adaptations in the interaction style of communication partners, even if the adaptations cannot be presumed to be any more facilitative of linguistic development. Children with language impairments are typically able to use spoken language, even if this is difficult for them.

Children who have unintelligible speech and use communication aids to express themselves may present an even greater challenge to attempts by partners to 'fine-tune' their communication. Their form of communication is unusual and may be difficult to interpret. Message construction and interpretation may take an inordinate amount of time, relative to the content of any given message. Speaker–listener role boundaries may become blurred with an aided communicator – natural speaker interaction. Two important questions are how children acuiring language in this situation influence the input they receive and how they can collaborate effectively with communication partners in order to develop language and communication skills. These issues are addressed in the investigation of Yvonne.

Yvonne

The focus in this chapter is on Yvonne, a young communication board user, and interactions between herself and her parents over a two-year period. Yvonne presents with severe cerebral palsy and very limited speech production abilities. Her comprehension of spoken language is relatively sophisticated, at least as far as can be determined through formal assessment. At the time of the study she was aged between five and seven years. On the Test of Reception of Grammar (Bishop, 1982), she achieved an age-appropriate score, although her receptive vocabulary as measured by the British Picture Vocabulary Scales (Dunn et al., 1982) may be relatively more limited. Her primary formal means of communication during the time of the study was a communication board, with approximately 250 Picture Communication Symbols (PCS) (Mayer-Johnson, 1981, 1985). She accessed the board directly through finger pointing. At that time, she had been assessed educationally as functioning within the average range and was attending her local mainstream school. She was seen on request by a local speech therapist and for consultation by a specialist centre. According to parental report, the focus of intervention at the time of the study was on increasing Yvonne's use of her communication board and on extending the length of her board-based utterances.

Yvonne presents a clear asymmetry in development in that her receptive language development far exceeds her observable performance in expressive communication. As discussed below, her parents appear to adopt both similar and contrasting strategies in interacting with Yvonne. Parallels to their interaction styles may be found in input styles with typically developing children and children with specific language impairment. The discussion explores the interaction patterns and the reciprocal influence of each partner in the dyad, and considers possible explanations for, and implications of, the patterns observed.

Yvonne was visited in her home every four months over a two-year period and was recorded in interactions with one of her parents. No attempt was made to determine in advance which parent was available as the interaction partner. During each visit, a range of structured and unstructured tasks were presented. Attempts were made to include tasks requiring communication of both simple and complex messages with shared and unshared information, following Nelson (1991). Several dialogue excerpts are discussed below. These excerpts have been selected to highlight particular interaction strategies rather than for their relative representativeness of the total data set.

Interactions with the mother

For visits 1, 2 and 5, Yvonne's mother was present, while for visits 3, 4 and 6 Yvonne interacted with her father. The first dialogue excerpt is taken from the first visit to Yvonne, where the researcher had been playing with bubbles while Yvonne's mother was out of the room. The bubbles were then hidden behind the television, and Yvonne's task was to tell her mother where to find the bubbles (complex, unshared information).

M: *Excuse me* (points on chart) *can I, can I have a verb? Can I have verbs first so?*
Y: 'Yes' (nods head, looking at chart).
M: *Tell me what I'm supposed to do with the television.*
Y: *TELEVISION.*
M: *What? Something about the television. What about it?*

Y: (Looks at mother, lifts hands, smiles).

M: *I don't know. Come on and tell me about the television so* . . .

Y: 'Yes' (nods head) *Eh.*

M: *What I'm supposed to do? Is it me?* (points to self, holds verb section of chart).

Y: 'Yes' (nods head) *Eh.*

M: *And something to do about the television.*

Y: 'Yes' (nods head).

M: *Alright. I, so, is mammy* (points to self) *MAMMY. Yes, give me a verb please. What? Something up here* (points to upper section of chart). *You want me to do something about the television do you?*

Y: 'Yes' (nods head) *Eh.*

M: *Yeah well, there is a verb but* . . . *I want it from you please* (puts down verb section of chart). *Come on. OK. It's up here, it's up here* (points to upper verb section on chart).

Y: (Looks at chart) *GO.*

M: *Oh. You have your finger on it. Go. You want {I ME} {to GO go} to the {TELEVISION television}.*

Y: 'Yes' (nods head, smiling).

M: *OK, I'll go to the television so, yes. I'm at the television. there's nothing there. oh, down this side. Oh, look. There's a bag. Will I bring it over?*

Y: 'Yes' (nods head) *Eh.*

In this dialogue, several features of the interaction style are noticeable. In common with findings from much of the research on interaction with children with language impairment, the mother's style is directive, with all exchanges initiated by her, and containing utterances such as; *Tell me what I'm supposed to do with the television*; *Come on and tell me about the television so*. The mother's requests for clarification in the dialogue are specific, as is commonly reported for child-directed speech:

- *Something about the television, what about it?*
- *What I'm supposed to do? Is it me?*
- *And something to do about the television.*
- *You want me to do something about the television, do you?*

Some of the features of the interaction are unique to aided communication. For example, the mother attempts to model use of the communication board. In the final exchange sequence, she models and expands on Yvonne's output, effectively combining the three elements into a single clausal structure: *You want {I me} to {GO go} to the {TELEVISION television}.* However, one of the most striking features of the interaction in the dialogue above is the explicit specification of a grammatical structure at certain points: *Can I have a verb? Can I have verbs first so? Give me a verb please... There is a verb but I want it from you please.* In effect, it would seem that Yvonne's mother is acknowledging the relative linguistic sophistication available to Yvonne, expecting that the metalinguistic message will be comprehensible to her, even though her output is limited primarily to single signs.

In the following dialogue excerpt, taken from the second visit, Yvonne and the researcher had played with a boat that squirted water. Yvonne's task was to tell her mother, who had not been in the room, about the activity.

M: *Don't mind them. They're not here. Who else is here? Who else is here? It wasn't me. So who else is here? Who else is here? Is it a {BOY boy}?*
Y: 'No' (shakes head).
M: *Is it a {GIRL girl}?*
Y: 'Yes' (nods head).
M: *Or a {WOMAN woman}?*
Y: 'Yes' (nods head).
M: *Which one? {GIRL girl} or {WOMAN woman}? Show me with your finger.*
Y: *GIRL.*
M: *A girl is it?*
Y: (Smiling, looks at Mother) 'Yes' (nods head, laughing).
M: *Right. Did ye do? What did ye do?*
Y: (Looks to right of chart.)
M: *Uhuh. Excuse me. Verb first* (points to green section of chart).
Y: (Looks to left of chart) *Eh. ALLGONE.*
M: *Allgone. That's the wrong one. You something allgone. Somewhere up here so.*
Y: *OPEN.*
M: *OK, you opened it.*
Y: *PUT.*
M: *Oh, you put. Put what so? Sorry. It's open. I thought it was open you were going to go for. What did you put?*
Y: *WET.*
M: *Wet? Your board is wet alright. But what did you put?*
Y: (Hands out either side, vocalizing.)
M: *You have water on the board. Where's your water picture? Your finger??? (unintelligible). Where's the water picture?*
Y: *ABC.*
M: *This one? ABC? That's not the water picture. Where's the water picture? You should know it by now. Definitely you know your water picture.*
Y: *WATER.*
M: *That's it. Water. Where did you put the water? Where's the water? Where is the water? Is it on? Upside down?*
Y: *BOAT.*
M: *Excuse me. Wait a minute. You forgot your prepositions again. I told you. You have to use them I'm afraid.*
Y: *UP.*
M: *Now. Look at your book.*

Again, the mother's focus seems to be explicitly on eliciting a particular syntactic structure, with little apparent attention to the content of the message. She models use of the board, and specifies the need to include a verb. At the end of the sequence, she draws attention to the need to include a preposition in the structure, reinforcing the notion that Yvonne should be able to understand syntactic categories and their relevance. The thrust of the interaction seems to imply that the goal is to practise use of a particular structure, rather than to engage in a reciprocal communicative exchange of information. This is particularly evident where she indicates that Yvonne has selected an 'incorrect' sign, although the mother did not know what the intended message was supposed to be, and therefore could not have known whether or not the selection was appropriate. At one point, there is a real sense of a 'teaching' sequence, where the mother tries to elicit a sign for water, although the message has clearly already been received: *You have water on the board. Where's your water picture? Your finger ???* (unintelligible). *Where's the water picture?* When Yvonne indicates *ABC*, the mother continues: *This one? ABC? That's not the water picture. Where's the water picture? You should know it by now. Definitely you know your water picture.* The mother spends a full 60 seconds trying to elicit the specific PCS desired, and the implicit message seems to be that form takes precedence over the content of this particular communication exchange.

In the final dialogue excerpt with the mother, taken from visit five, Yvonne and the researcher (R) had read a story about going to bed, and Yvonne was asked to tell her mother about the story.

Y: *BED.*
R: *Bed, OK, to go to bed, is that right?*
M: *How do you say to go to bed? Where's the word go? Where's the word go? Where's the word go? Could you find the word go for me. Ah, come on Yvonne find the word go for me. Take one finger only Yvonne. Now where's go? Where's the word go?*
Y: *GO.*
M: *Thank you.*

Again, the interaction above suggests an explicit attempt from the mother to elicit a particular structure although the content of the message has already been received. In fact, at the end of the sequence her mother thanks Yvonne for co-operating and selecting the appropriate sign, reinforcing the idea that the important element of the task relates to the structure, rather than the content of the communication.

Overall then, certain features are noticeable in the above interactions between Yvonne and her mother. There is an implied emphasis on form over content. The style adopted by Yvonne's mother is directive, and at times didactic. Her attempts to elicit more 'appropriate' syntactic structures at times drive her to draw on quite sophisticated metalinguistic messages, such as specification of word categories. It is hard to imagine an interaction between a mother and a speaking child including corrective responses such as: *You forgot your prepositions again.*

Interactions with the father

On three visits, Yvonne's father was the main interaction partner. In the following dialogue excerpt, Yvonne is telling her father about a story that had been read to her by the researcher while the father was out of the room.

> F: *What did the witch do?*
> Y: *PUT.*
> F: *Put? OK, put what?*
> Y: *CAT.*
> F: *The cat? Where did the witch put the cat?*
> Y: (Points to garden.)
> F: (Opens chart) *Where did the witch put the cat?*
> Y: *OUT.*
> F: *Put the cat out?*
> Y: 'Yes' (nods head, smiles).

Father–child interactions are reported to be more linguistically challenging than interactions with mothers, placing a greater onus on the child to expand and reformulate linguistic expressions, through non-specific requests for clarification. The pattern presented by Yvonne's father fits these reported features in some respects. Overall he labels the PCS selected by Yvonne, confirms the selection, and then seeks further information, as in the dialogue above, where *PUT* is answered with *Put what?* and *CAT* with *Cat where.* Von Tetzchner and Martinsen (1996) refer to such exchanges as topic setting by the communication aid user with subsequent co-construction of the comment related to the topic. Yvonne's father typically then repeats the communication output, and expands the utterance: *Put the cat out.* His queries in the excerpt are specific, and in fact are initiated without waiting for Yvonne to indicate whether or not she has finished her message. For instance, in the example above, Yvonne has already started to search her board for another selection when her father asks *Put what?* in a sense creating an overlap in their conversational exchange. Furthermore, although Yvonne had responded to his query, *Where did the witch put the cat?* by pointing to the garden (in fact corresponding exactly to the story line), her father either did not notice this unaided communicative attempt, or ignored it, focusing instead on opening her communication board for her to respond.

In the following dialogue excerpt, also from the fourth visit, Yvonne has been offered a choice of activities while her father was out of the room and her task is to tell him about her chosen activity.

Y: (Looks down at chart.)
F: *In here is it?* (turns over action section). *Do you want me to hold it up?*
Y: (Looks to the father and smiles) 'Yes' (nods head) *READ.*
F: *Read. You want me to read something?*
Y: 'Yes.'
F: *You want me to read for you?*
Y: 'Yes' (nods head, eyes down) *READ.*
F: *What've I to read?*
Y: *READ.*
F: *Yeah, I've to read. Read what? Read what?*
Y: (Looks to L, pointing to action section.)
F: *Something here? I don't think so.*
R: *Maybe it's on the other page is it?*
Y: (Closes action section.)
F: *On the back page, OK, read what? Read what? What've I to read?*
Y: *BOOK.*
F: *A book.*

In this instance, Yvonne initiates the interaction, by looking at her chart and selecting *READ*. Her father responds by labelling and confirming the selection and offering possible expansions in the form of yes/no questions, before a specific query *What've I to read? . . . read what?* (There were several types of reading materials present, and selection of *BOOK* was referential, and not redundant in this setting.)

In the final excerpt, Yvonne has been shown a video of herself, on the camcorder, while her father was out of the room. Her father has now come in, and she indicates that she has something to tell him, initiating the sequence below.

F: *Something in here.*
Y: *I.*
F: *You.*
Y: *Eh.*
F: *Yeah?*
Y: (Looks at chart, points.)
F: *This one?*
Y: 'No' (shakes head).
F: *Which one?*
Y: *GO.*
F: *You go?*
Y: 'No' (shakes head).
F: *What, where is it? Down here? This one? You talk?*
Y: 'No' (shakes head). *LOOK.*
F: *Look.*
Y: 'Yes' (nods head).
F: *You look. Don't be tearing.*

Y: *I.*
F: *You look at yourself?*
Y: 'Yes' (nods head).
F: *You're looking for me?*
Y: *VIDEO.*
F: *Video?*
Y: 'Yes' (nods head).
F: *Is that it?*
Y: 'Yes' (nods head).
F: *What?*
Y: (Points to camera.)
F: *You look at the video? At yourself?*
Y: 'Yes' (nods head).

In this last sequence, Yvonne and her father share the construction of the utterance over several turns. Each PCS selection is confirmed, and the cumulative output is recast for Yvonne after each new selection, before the completed utterance is produced. The father's responses are highly semantically contingent, with a non-specific request for clarification, what, near the end of the sequence, putting the onus on Yvonne to add further information. This particular interaction sequence is somewhat exceptional in the overall range of interactions recorded. The rate of communication is relatively rapid, with a high 'density' of PCS productions for the time unit. The interaction sequence lasted 91 seconds, including almost half a minute taken with attempts to indicate *LOOK,* due to Yvonne's motor limitations. Transition between PCS selections was tight, in terms of a spontaneous initiation of a search for a new graphic sign following confirmation of a previous selection. The pause time of such transitions did not exceed two seconds for any selection. There is a sense of Yvonne leading the interaction, and of dynamic communication within the interaction.

Contrasting styles?

Both similar and contrasting features are present across both interaction contexts. Yvonne's mother adopts primarily directive interaction strategies similar to those reported for parents of children whose development is atypical. She draws explicit attention to the communication board, prompts Yvonne to specific sections and models use of the board. She requests specific syntactic structures and focuses on metalinguistic aspects of development – acknowledging Yvonne's receptive language skills. At times she emphasizes form over content.

By contrast, Yvonne's father does not use the board himself at all. He recasts board output into a spoken form; he uses direct, highly contingent questions. His attention overall appears to be on the communication message, with fewer direct language support strategies being employed. How do these contrasting patterns affect Yvonne's communication output?

Proportion of multi-term utterances

Determining utterance boundaries, or even defining the unit of analysis itself is an area fraught with difficulties in aided and multi-modal communication (see Smith and Grove, 2001 for further discussion). Several possible analytical approaches have been suggested. In relation to aided communication, one useful framework is to contrast vertical structures, where an utterance is co-constructed over several turns through collaboration between both partners, and horizontal structures, where the temporal contiguity is tighter, and the partner dependence reduced (von Tetzchner and Martinsen, 1996, based on Scollon, 1976). However, even this proposal is difficult to tie down definitively, given the time often required to select a PCS, and the possible 'intrusion' of partner behaviours such as labelling selections. Frequently, the distinction between utterance and turn is difficult to disentangle.

The term 'turn' is used in this chapter to refer to the confirmed selection of single or multiple PCS bounded by 'strong' turn completion behaviours. For Yvonne, such completion behaviours consisted in the main of eye gaze towards the speaking partner, a smile, head nod and/or vocalization, but occasionally she pulled both arms back and folded them, placing her head on the communication board or pushed the board away. Most of Yvonne's turns consisted of single-PCS selections. Occasionally she selected sequences of PCS. Such sequences were regarded as occurring within a single turn if, at the message level, they shared a contextual framework and if, at a pragmatic level, Yvonne searched for another PCS after confirmation of a previous selection. Searching behaviour consisted primarily of a return of eye gaze to the communication board, occasionally with gestural or manual cues. In some instances, such search behaviour was unprompted, akin to the horizontal structures described by Scollon (1976). On other occasions, the partner supported or prompted a search for a further selection, analogous to Scollon's vertical structures.

Yvonne produced a total of 208 utterances using PCS over the six visits. Of these, 63 were produced with her mother as a speaking partner and 51 with her father. The remainder were produced with either the researcher or another visitor. It might be expected that different conversation styles would affect overall complexity of Yvonne's expressive output – that, for instance, specific requests for a verb phrase element might encourage a wider range of syntactic structures and more multi-PCS utterances. In fact, Yvonne's mother was least successful in eliciting multi-PCS utterances. Of the 63 PCS utterances produced by Yvonne in conversation with her, only one included more than one PCS. By contrast, 11 of the 51 PCS utterances (21.5%) produced with her father contained more than one PCS, with one four-PCS utterance recorded (see Table 7.1).

Yvonne was least likely to produce multi-PCS utterances with her mother, where much of the interaction centred on attempts by her mother to elicit specific information, often through long sequences of questions. Of a total of 515 mother utterances during the first visit, 211 (41%) consisted of questions.

Discussion

In typical development, increase in utterance length yields considerable communication advantages. Children encode new meanings and are able to express new relationships through their early word combinations. In the interactions above between Yvonne and her mother however, relatively less attention is paid to the information yielded by PCS selections than to the structural 'accuracy' of such selections. There is a strong sense of 'teaching' rather than of communication. Yvonne's mother adopts both modelling techniques, and verbal directives to guide 'appropriate communication'. These features are present across all three excerpts, taken over a period spanning 18 months. There is little change to see in interaction style over this period, the teaching emphasis being evident in each case.

This teaching mode may arise from the mother's understanding of how language is learnt by all children – that is, that rules must be explicitly taught and that they are taught by drawing on metalinguistic resources. Alternatively, it may be that she considers 'teaching' most appropriate, given that Yvonne is not developing typically. The teacher role may be relatively unconscious, or it may be her understanding from her contact with professionals that this is the role she should assume. In other words, it may represent her understanding of how she is expected by others to support Yvonne in developing her use of PCS. A teaching strategy may be the best match she can think of to meet the developmental goal of increasing Yvonne's use of her board – the stated therapeutic goal. If the latter is the case, then there is

Table 7.1. Number of utterances with 1, 2, 3 and 4 PCS

PCS utterance length	Mother (63 utterances)	Father (51 utterances)
1	62 (98.4%)	40 (78.5%)
2	1 (1.6%)	8 (15.6%)
3	–	2 (3.9%)
4	–	1 (2.0%)

an implication that use of PCS will mirror spoken language structures and that development can be evaluated using indices drawn from spoken language development. At present, it seems far from clear that either of these propositions is valid (see, for example, Smith and Grove, 1999; Soto, 1999; Sutton, 1999).

What are the possible implications of the adoption of such a 'teaching' emphasis? Yvonne may well perceive her communication board as an educational rather than a communication tool, where 'correct' rather than effective use is important (for example, Smith, 1991; von Tetzchner, 1988; von Tetzchner and Martinsen, 2000). Indeed, this may be a perception shared by her mother. The teaching strategies adopted may interfere with 'good' aided communication strategies (von Tetzchner, 1988), for example, where potential genuine communication attempts are ignored, because they do not match the expectations of the communication partner, as in the second dialogue excerpt. The learning opportunities apparent in the above excerpts restrict both the control Yvonne can exert on the interaction, and possibly the potential roles that a communication board may fulfil. Partly because of the directive and disjointed nature of the interaction, there is little time for Yvonne to generate multi-term utterances, or for a flow of communication to emerge. Thus, there may be significant limitations on aided language and communication learning opportunities available to Yvonne, at least in interactions with her mother.

Yvonne produced more multi-PCS utterances with her father than with her mother. Typically, Yvonne's father seeks further information following a PCS selection, rather than a particular sign. There is a greater sense of real communication, with semantic contingency maintained over several exchanges. Exchanges such as that below conform to the co-construction described by von Tetzchner and Martinsen (1996), the topic set by Yvonne, and the subsequent comment co-constructed with her father:

F: *What did the witch do?*
Y: *PUT.*
F: *Put? OK, put what?*
Y: *CAT.*
F: *The cat? Where did the witch put the cat?*
Y: (Points to garden).
F: (Opens chart) *Where did the witch put the cat?*
Y: *OUT.*
F: *Put the cat out?*
Y: 'Yes' (nods head, smiles).

However, at one point in the above example Yvonne's father did not respond to apparently appropriate unaided communication, instead directing attention to the communication board. This oversight may simply have arisen because of a momentary distraction. Alternatively, it may reflect a reduced sensitivity on his part to Yvonne's multi-modal communication. Finally, he may have chosen to ignore the unaided communication in order to maximize Yvonne's communication board use as an explicit intervention strategy. The last interpretation is somewhat difficult to reconcile with the observation that he did not himself use the board at all. Assigning board use as exlusively Yvonne's responsibility may be far from trivial in its implications for Yvonne's development of aided communication.

Cultural tools play a key role within a social constructivist approach. Children adapt to the world through and with other people, mediated through cultural tools, which are themselves patterns of social interaction, sometimes highly abstract such as symbol systems, and sometimes highly tangible, such as a spoon. Cultural tools entail both social conventions and a logic of social use. Scribner (1997, p. 285) proposes:

> In acting with objects the child is not merely learning the physical properties of things, but mastering the social modes of acting with those things. These socially evolved modes of action are not inscribed in the objects themselves and cannot be discovered independently by the child from their physical properties - they must be learned through a socially-mediated process.

If a communication board is a cultural tool (see Hjelmquist, 1999) then the absence of models using the tool within the immediate social context may suggest to the child that this particular tool operates on the periphery of social interaction (Woll and Barnett, 1998). Yvonne's father acknowledges her use of the board, and physically manipulates the board to ease her access to it, but he responds to her communication with speech and does not attempt to 'share' her convention of use. The socially mediated process referred to by Scribner (1997) above, may suggest that the communication board is a tool for Yvonne to use and to which others respond. The question then arises as to how development in use of the board can be sustained, if 'expert' models are not present in the immediate social context, or if enculturation into use of graphic signs for communication is not a realistic possibility?

Overall, Yvonne was less likely to use aided communication with her mother than with her father, even though her mother modelled use of the communication board and incorporated it into her own communication, while her father did not use the board himself at all. It is tempting to suggest that the mother's tendency to directive and questioning interaction restricted the communication opportunities available to Yvonne. However, with any conversational dyad, both partners influence the structure of the exchange, even if their relative status may tilt the power scales in a particular direction.

Just as input to children with language impairment may reflect caregivers' attempts to accommodate to a perceived problem in conversational management, the 'teaching' style adopted by Yvonne's mother may reflect her difficulty reconciling the apparent gap between Yvonne's receptive and expressive language skills. Pine (1994) points out that child-directed speech typically accommodates to children's receptive, rather than their expressive language abilities. Certainly, some of the cues offered to Yvonne suggest an expectation of relatively sophisticated receptive language. The effect of the didactic style however is that, when compared to interactions with her father, Yvonne's communication attempts are less spontaneous, and are limited almost exclusively to single PCS-utterances, with little evidence of change over the period of observation. When interacting with her father, Yvonne is more likely to initiate, and to produce, longer utterances.

The immediate effects of the contrasting interaction styles are therefore relatively easy to identify. The developmental importance of such effects is much more difficult to disentangle. At a general level, it seems clear that the relationship between the nature of child-directed speech and the process of language acquisition in a typically developing child is complex (Pine, 1994). Parents do not adopt a particular style of interaction in order to teach their child language but rather in order to be better able to communicate with their child. However, where a child apparently requires some assistance in learning language, difficulties arise. Caregiver interaction patterns may change, not only out of an assumption of responsibility for maintaining communication, but also because of specific intervention attempts. The added dimensions of atypical communication means, a cultural tool outside the 'normal' range, make Yvonne's situation even more complex.

It is clear, and hardly surprising, that Yvonne can 'perform' at different levels depending on the interaction context. The observations also suggest that a specific emphasis on teaching form or structure of communication output may limit her attempts at communication. In the longer term, repeated encounters with such aided communication settings could influence not only her learning opportunities, but also her interest and focus within potential learning opportunities, and hence profoundly affect the developmental process. It is possible that her father's strategy of speaking aloud the label of each PCS selection and then expanding the selections into a more elaborated spoken utterance has two benefits: it may support development of cross-modal translation and it may also provide scaffolding for expressive language development. His participation may therefore be particularly critical for Yvonne in varying the learning opportunities available to her. At this stage, such speculations remain tentative. There are several factors that suggest that caution is warranted in interpreting longer-term implications from the above observations.

Firstly, linguistic input is only one component in the language acquisition process. The relationships between certain types of child-directed speech and subsequent language acquisition by the child are far from resolved, even in typical development. Secondly, given that Yvonne's development is atypical, the relevance of findings from typical development is unclear. Even comparisons with other atypical development contexts, such as children with specific language impairment, must be tempered with caution, given the nature and extent of Yvonne's difficulties and means of communication. Finally, it is possible that the interactions recorded between Yvonne and both of her parents may not be typical for them. Yvonne's mother, being aware of the researcher's speech and language therapy background, may have felt compelled to encourage Yvonne to produce 'correct' utterances, to demonstrate her awareness of a therapy goal. Such a structural focus may not have been typical for other interactions. However, even in this scenario, this adaptation in itself would suggest that the mother has understood that the goal of intervention is to elicit 'correct' spoken language-based utterances. Furthermore, it may highlight an interpretation that the goal can be accomplished by 'teaching' specific forms, even if communicative efficiency is sacrificed in the process. In this sense, the therapeutic goal, as understood by Yvonne's mother, may actually inhibit her natural interaction style, and reduce the level of communicative support she offers in interaction. Yvonne's father may have been less susceptible to external pressure as he had less contact both with Yvonne's speech therapists and with her school. He may not have felt a need to demonstrate that Yvonne could 'perform' at a certain level. To this extent, he may have felt more free in his interactions.

Implications for intervention

Parents are assumed to play a key role in supporting their children's communicative development. As such, they are 'privileged' communication partners. For this reason, parental interaction behaviours have been the focus both of analysis and of intervention. Parents come to the language learning situation with a particular understanding of how children learn to become proficient communicators. It is not yet known how particular interaction styles affect the process of language development of children. However, it is clear even from the limited observations above, that interaction styles can affect the language performance of both participants in any dyad.

The observations discussed here show the potential interaction tension or dissonance created when a child presents with a severe speech impairment. They also serve to highlight the reciprocal influence each partner in the interaction dyad exerts on the overall structure and content of communication within the dyad. In this last regard, children using communication boards are no different to children with language impairments or young children acquiring language in a typical manner. Given the potential importance of parent–child dyadic interactions as a source of learning, it is important that any attempt to modify such interactions yield an outcome which is more favourable to the developmental process than pre-existing interaction strategies. The case of Yvonne raises questions about the most effective way of incorporating aided communication into naturalistic parent-child interactions. There is clearly a need for reliable information about the costs and benefits of asking parents to assume particular intervention roles. It may be that, in some cases, a communication board has more value as an educational rather than a communication tool. There may be important benefits at certain points in development in allowing parents to simply be parents, and to interact in the way they find most natural and most nurturing.

CHAPTER 8

Co-construction in graphic language development

KARI MERETE BREKKE AND STEPHEN VON TETZCHNER

Language acquisition is the process by which children come to share not only a means of communication but a form of life (Wittgenstein, 1953). Language cannot be created independently by an individual, it is both created and shared through the communicative activities of the members of a culture, and human children seem to have a species-specific ability to acquire language through social interaction with other people (Lock, 1980; Tomasello, 1999).

Hearing children with motor impairment who lack the ability to speak have to follow developmental paths in their language acquisition that differ significantly from both those of normally speaking children and those of deaf children who grow up in a signing environment. The communication form and the structure differ, as well as the communicative strategies applied. One typical path for this group of children would be from pictographic representations, like Pictogram Ideogram Communication (PIC, Maharaj, 1980) and Picture Communication Symbols (PCS, Johnson, 1981, 1985, 1992), via more complex graphic signs like Blissymbols (Bliss, 1965) to orthographic writing. For children with limited speech, reading and writing are not only skills for accessing material like books, posters and magazines and producing notes, electronic mails and school assignments, but are integral elements of their expressive communicative development. Orthographic writing represents the highest level of expressive competence because it maps onto spoken language and hence in principle gives non-speaking children access to an infinite vocabulary and the grammar of spoken language, as well as to less planned acquisition strategies more similar to typical language development. Writing, however, is also a result of education: writing is a cultural tool that is not usually acquired implicitly through communicative interactions. Although reading and writing are promoted in different ways at home, they are essentially skills resulting from an instructional task assigned to the

176

educational system of the society. A common exception is children who learn to read and write by watching their older siblings doing homework.

Children who acquire spoken language are surrounded by a community of speakers, even if there may be several languages spoken in their environment. For children who have to express themselves with graphic signs, there is no natural language environment of communication aid users. Unlike speaking children, their 'language acquisition support system' (Bruner, 1983) is, to a large extent, planned. They typically learn to express themselves through instructional activities in communicative settings provided by professionals who do not themselves use graphic signs for everyday communication and who are not proficient users of graphic communication. Both non-speaking children and the significant people in their environments have to learn the tool the children will depend upon for expressive development. The asymmetry between children using communication aids and normally speaking adults is both larger and smaller than for other children: larger because of the adults' ability to speak and smaller because the children's communication partners may have only marginally higher – or even lower – graphic language competence than the children. This is likely to lead to very few interactions with competent users of their own communication form. This may hinder the children's development of communicative skills.

A few studies have investigated the nature of the expressive communication of children who use graphic communication (for example, Gerber and Kraat, 1992; Harris, 1982; Kraat, 1985; Light, 1985; Smith, 1996; von Tetzchner and Martinsen, 1996). There are also case studies that describe the intervention history of young communication aid users (Blischak and Lloyd, 1996; Brookner and Murphy, 1975; Bruno, 2001; Gossens', 1989; Hooper, Connell and Flett, 1987; Locke and Mirenda, 1988; Pecyna, 1988; Romski et al., 1984; Spiegel, Benjamin and Spiegel, 1993). However, longitudinal descriptions that focus on the development of graphic language produced by motor-impaired children appear to be totally lacking. Such studies are necessary for obtaining developmental descriptions and gaining insight into the 'natural' course of this form of language development.

The present case study describes the expressive language development of a severely motor-impaired boy, Sander, from the age of five to 13 years of age. The description is based on notes from regular conversations with his parents; assessments and reports from professionals who worked with Sander over the years; notes from meetings in multidisciplinary teams and responsibility groups (in Norway, a responsibility group is a board made up by the parents and representatives of all relevant agencies); individual education plans; class reports; and the observations and notes made by the first author during her years as Sander's teacher. Video-recordings were made regularly in the classroom and used by the teacher for teaching purposes and as a basis for joint reflection with other professionals and the family. Conversations with Sander were time-consuming, and were often interrupted before they were completed, and continued over several lessons and sometimes days, so they were habitually written down. Hence, many of the language constructions made by Sander have been recorded over the years. They include both shorter exchanges and longer narratives. Some of the long conversations evolved into homework assignments for his lessons in Norwegian and graphic communication, and in subjects like geography and social studies. During her work with Sander's individual habilitation plan (see Hesselberg, 1998) the first author interviewed Sander about the instruction he had received. As a supplement to reports and other forms of journal data, several of the professionals who worked with Sander prior to the first author were also interviewed.

Sander

Sander is a boy with severe cerebral palsy. He has poor motor co-ordination and is unable to speak. His movements are unco-ordinated and he needs appropriate positioning for effective motor performance. He has swallowing difficulties and regularly received nutritional supplements, but still has problems obtaining sufficient nutrition. He has short stature, is often ill, has periods when he vomits several times a day and becomes easily exhausted. His poor health and lack of energy has had a significant influence on his education and language development. He has always attended ordinary educational settings (pre-school and school), but it has been necessary to regulate the amount of both education and other activities. There have always been large variations in performance from day to day, related to his health status, and observations revealed that even on good days, he rarely had more than about two-and-a-half hours of classroom time, much less than his classmates. In the early school years, he was very dependent on structure and overview, and often had strong negative reactions to changes in routines and plans. This was probably related to frequent misunderstanding and a lack of means to repair them (see below).

Early development and intervention

When Sander was between six and 18 months old, he and his mother met two hours twice a week with three other disabled children and their mothers. After that, he attended an ordinary pre-school until he started in an ordinary primary school at the age of seven.

In the reports written shortly after his birth, Sander was assumed to be intellectually disabled, but by the age of six months his social attentiveness and eagerness to grasp toys were already being noted. The report at 14 months describes him as a child who likes action but who also needs regular breaks. Just after his second birthday, the multidisciplinary report concluded that he had poor motor control, while his communication and cognitive resources were good. This led to the conclusion that he would need a computer. At an assessment at 3;10 years, Sander's comprehension of spoken language was estimated as age-appropriate.

The intervention in Sander's early years failed in fundamental ways to take his limitations and possibilities into account. His early experiences with expressive communication intervention seemed to be based on means and strategies that created frustration. Despite his obvious inability to produce manual signs and mouth movements, the early communication intervention focused on motor skills. From his second birthday to when he was 3;4 years old, Sander had to take part in speech therapy based on the principle that voluntary sound production could be stimulated by provoking him. He was offered rewards for producing sounds. If he failed, which he did most of the time, the reward was held back. He was also taught to open the mouth to say 'yes' or 'will', and to tighten the lips to say 'no' or 'will not'. However, these expressions gave rise to some problems. When Sander was eager or excited about something, involuntary mouth movements would appear. In such situations, it was difficult to decide whether he said 'yes' or 'no'. When his expression was interpreted as 'yes' for example to a particular activity and he later protested against it, this was perceived by the adults as stubbornness or lack of comprehension. The result was often scolding and he had to do the activity that the adult thought he had chosen. At the same time, attempts were made to teach him manual signing. The first manual signs taught were TOILET and FINISHED, which never achieved functional use due to his problems with co-ordinated movement. Moreover, at this age he was unable to control when he needed to go to the toilet.

Sander also had a switch-operated scanning device with seven photographs that he was supposed to use for playing lotto and for choosing between activities, but demands on his motor skills were too high. Only when he was 3;4 years old, he gained access to graphic communication in the form of pictograms. He got his first communication aid with speech output when he was 4;3 years old and later received a string of small and large communication devices with digitized speech. However, his motor disability made independent use of these devices impossible. They were only used in a few situations and did not come to have any positive influence on his language development. On the contrary, the many wrong keys he hit made him lose motivation for using the devices for communication. Thus, during the early pre-school years, in most situations Sander's communication consisted of answering yes/no questions.

Table 8.1. The first 49 pictograms taught to Sander

EAT	DRINK	TOILET	OUT	PLAY
SING	FOOD	MILK	SLEEP IN	BUILD
MUSIC	BREAD	POP	TIRED	SAND-BOX
BLOCKS	TELEVISION	CAKE	MOTHER	REST
SLIDE	BALLOON	RADIO	PAINT	BUTTER
FATHER	SWING	READ	CHEESE	UN/DRESS
ANGRY	SIT	BICYCLE	BOOK	JAM
SAD	CHAIR	DRIVE	DRAW	APPLE
HAPPY	KITCHEN	TRIP	ORANGE	LIVING-ROOM
BANANA	AFRAID	COLOUR	PENCIL	

The pictogram period

Vocabulary development

The period where pictograms were Sander's main form of expressive communication lasted from when he was three to nine years old. The first 49 pictograms are listed in Table 8.1. They reflect the limited activities in which he was given opportunity to express anything beyond 'yes' and 'no'. Thirteen pictograms referred to food and drinks and were used during meals. He did not like to eat because of his physical problems, so a large part of the early vocabulary involved choices between things he did not like. Twenty-one pictograms related to activities and play, three to emotional states and the rest to locations and care activities. Pictograms were also used on his daily activity schedule that was presented on a board on the wall and that the pre-school teacher went through with Sander every morning.

During the first months of pictogram use, Sander used a seven-item scanning device to choose from various sets of seven pictograms selected by the communication partner. Because this device proved difficult for him to operate, when he was 3;6 years a 'dependent' selection mode was chosen (see von Tetzchner and Martinsen, 2000). The pictograms were organized in a book with four pictograms per page and the communication partner would turn the pages in accordance with Sander's indications. The adult would for example ask *What do you want to play?*, whereupon Sander touched the pictogram that represented what he wanted to do. Due to his poor co-ordination, touching was often imprecise and the adult might have to ask several yes/no questions before Sander's choice was clear.

It was nearly impossible for Sander to take initiative and any communication on his part depended on another person initiating communicative inter-action. He would touch the communication board and sometimes try to initiate contact by staring at a person but these strategies would only be successful if he had the visual attention of the other person. A doorbell was mounted on his wheelchair to give him opportunity to attract attention when he wanted to express something, but this was soon taken away because the staff found the sound annoying and Sander 'too insistent'. This indicates that the adults in the pre-school environment did not accept Sander's ability to talk when he wanted to do so and put physical restrictions on his talking that would have been completely unacceptable for the other children in the pre-school. When he tried to initiate without being understood, he typically reacted either with passivity and a 'folded' posture, or with strong affect. When Sander was 5;6 years old, he was given a 'caller', a device with both light and sound for gaining attention, which he immediately started to use a lot. Again, the pre-school staff regarded his initiatives as too frequent and demanding, and the caller was frequently taken away from him or the sound shut off. However, after some time, people in the environment became accustomed to the caller and Sander became so dependent on it that he had to have a replacement when it was sent away a few days for repair. Similar observations where people in the surroundings react negatively when non-speaking children and adults use new opportunities for taking communicative initiative have been noted (see, for example, Bird et al., 1989; Møller and von Tetzchner, 1996).

When Sander was nearly four years old, his communication board was reorganized into one main board and a book with topics. However, for the next one-and-a-half years, few additions were made to his expressive vocabulary. After that age, the vocabulary was regularly expanded in order to make it possible for him to communicate about more topics and in new situations. His main board at the age of six years consisted of 72 photographs and pictograms (Table 8.2). There were 14 names of children and adults, including *MOTHER* and *FATHER*. Only five pictograms referred to eating and drinking (*DRINK, EAT, CHOCOLATE, HUNGRY* and *FULL*). Twenty-four pictograms were related to toys, activities and play, four to emotional states, seven to locations, two to care activities, and 13 pictograms belonged to other categories, including one that signalled the need for the topic book. This book contained about 50 pictograms, including pictograms related to shape and size and for prepositions. The pictograms in the topic book were related to books he liked to talk about, birthday celebration and doctor play which was popular among the children in the pre-school. When Sander had participated in an activity, the teacher would involve Sander in conversations where the topic sheet was used to talk about the activity. Similarly, adults would initiate use of the communication board when they talked with Sander about his experiences that were known to them – mainly about pre-school activities and recent events that the parents had written about in Sander's message book. The adult would ask questions to which Sander replied with a

Table 8.2. The vocabulary at the main board when Sander was six years old

NAME 1	GIVE	BATH	HOME	LOTTO	CHOCOLATE
NAME 2	HAPPY	BUILD	GUN	TOYS	WALKMAN
NAME 3	ANGRY	UNIT	GUITAR	DRINK	TELEVISION
NAME 4	MOTHER	VIDEO	TOILET	FINISHED	PRESCHOOL
NAME 5	TAKE	BEDROOM	BICYCLE	QUESTION	TELEPHONE
NAME 6	AFRAID	OUT	WALKER	LETTER	WHEELCHAIR
NAME 7	HUG	SHOP	SING	HUNGRY	COMPUTER
NAME 8	FATHER	KITCHEN	WEAVE	FULL	LIVING-ROOM
NAME 9	BROKEN	VISIT	READ	TIRED	TAPE-PLAYER
NAME 10	SAD	VAN	CARDS	WASH	PICTOGRAM
NAME 11	HELP	BOOK	TALK	STAIRS	ILL/HURT
NAME 12	REST	TRIP	GAME	PUZZLE	DIFFICULT

single pictogram, which was then interpreted and a full sentence was formulated by the adult. Although the communication was about events more or less known to the adult, these conversations were often frustrating: they took a long time and ended often in communication breakdown.

As has been the tradition in alternative language intervention, in the early period it was mainly the adults who decided which pictograms Sander had access to at a particular time. In order to promote a wider and more spontaneous use of pictograms, this practice changed when Sander was six years old. The teacher and Sander would regularly go though the book containing the pictograms that were available in Norwegian at the time (about 500), and the teacher would name each pictogram. In this way, Sander became aware of the use of the pictograms that were available and had an opportunity to make his own vocabulary selections. He would also ask for the book with the full set when he lacked pictograms for what he wanted to say.

The understanding that there were more pictograms than those he had on his own communication board also seemed to make Sander aware of the fact that there were meanings he could not say even if he had used all the existing pictograms. Through eye pointing at real objects, he relayed the message that he wanted graphic signs for 'kick-bicycle' and 'standing brace'. By pointing at CHURCH, BOOK and TALK, he made the teacher make the pictograms BIBLE and PRAY. When Sander started to attend school at the age of 7;6 years (normal age in Norway at the time), he used 270 pictograms. During his first school year, 300 new pictograms became available in Norwegian. At the end of this school year, he had 500 of the 800 available pictograms in his main communication board or the topic book. He also had 20 home-made pictograms and eight written words.

Despite the significant increase in vocabulary after Sander was six years old, his vocabulary remained low compared to his peers. He often encountered communicative challenges where he lacked vocabulary and started to use his pictograms in unconventional and untaught ways in order to get his message across. He would look at objects and people in the room when he needed to say something about them. He would also use objects in the environment in a more symbolic sense – for example, looking at the door when he wanted to direct the adult's attention towards something outside. Another strategy was to use details of the pictograms. For example in order to say 'Red cross', he pointed to the cross at the pictogram *HOSPITAL* (Figure 8.1). Another time, he indicated *TOES* to inform the teacher that his father had a bad back. The background for this was that the father, who was a tall man, would lie on the sofa with his feet stretching outside the sofa when his back hurt, and the toes became a very salient feature of this situation. Sander's use of idiosyncratic associations made it difficult for people to understand him, and the pre-school staff often needed help from the parents to interpret this kind of utterance.

One pictogram Sander selected in the pre-school was *GUN*. The pre-school teacher and the other staff members thought he wanted to play or to talk about cowboys and Indians, but he firmly rejected this interpretation. After they had been on a boat trip together, the teacher told Sander how nice she thought the boat trip had been. Sander protested and indicated *GUN*, *AFRAID* and *ILL*. It was an open boat, there had been some waves and the boat had rolled a little. Sander had been unwell, experienced the situation as dangerous and been afraid. Thus, he mostly used *GUN* as meaning 'dangerous', a word he did not have in another form on his communication boards.

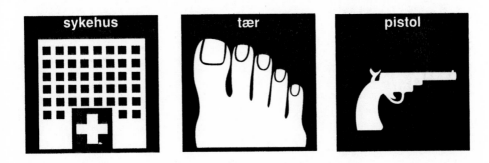

Figure 8.1. Norwegian pictograms: *HOSPITAL, TOES, GUN.*

Sentences and text

Until Sander was 5;6 years old, he only used single-pictogram utterances, which made him dependent on the guesses of the communication partner. In order to scaffold the development of more varied and specific utterances and his ability to relay information about events and tell stories, and promote an active role in conversations, several changes were implemented in his language environment. These included advising communication partners to wait before they provided Sander with interpretations and guesses about what he wanted to say.

In the pre-school, structured conversations between Sander and the teacher were an important part of the planned language environment. These conversations were based on a topic–comment framework, where Sander and the teacher first negotiated a topic, whereupon Sander was encouraged to provide more information and the following turns would function as comments on the topic. In this way, Sander participated in long conversations about events he had taken part in, read about or seen in television; about where he had been, who he had been with and how he had felt. In the first dialogue, Sander is 5;10 years old and initiates a conversation about somebody in the kitchen.

S: 'Bring the communication board' (uses the caller).
T: (Brings the communication board).
S: *TALK.*
T: *What do you want to talk about?*
S: *UNIT.*
T: *Do you want to talk about what happened in the unit?*
S: 'Yes' (mouth movements).
T: Tell me.
S: *LOTTO.*
T: *Did you play lotto?*
S: 'Yes' (mouth movements).
T: *Who did you play with?*
S: *KITCHEN.*
T: *Did you play in the kitchen?*
S: 'No' (mouth movements).
T: *Can you indicate the name?*
S: (Indicates several names without making any choice).
T: *Do you have the name on your board?*
S: 'No' (mouth movements).
T: *Can you see the person you played with?*
S: 'Someone in the kitchen' (Looks at the kitchen door.)
T: *Did you play with Mari who works in the kitchen?*
S: 'Yes' (mouth movements, smiles).

Sander was also exposed to graphic sentences in well-known picture books, which had been supplied with pictogram text. These would contain sentences like *BOY LOOK WARDROBE* ('Ole looks into the toy closet') *NO DOLL* ('the doll is not there').

In the initial period of pictogram use, the communication partners focused on giving Sander choices related to food, toys and activities. Communication about wants and needs was the easiest for communication partners to understand and there was a tendency to interpret all Sander's utterances as expressions of these kinds of requests. When the object or activity was identified, the conversation was mostly over. In some periods, nearly all his communications were interpreted in this way. However, choices comprised only a minor part of what Sander wanted to communicate. In order to direct the communication partners towards conversation, Sander started to use *QUESTION* and *TALK*. This is a conversation from when he was 6;8 years old:

S: *QUESTION.*
T: *Question.*
S: *BOOK.*
T: *Book. Can you say more?*
S: *HOUSE.*
T: *House.*
S: *FINISHED* 'End of topic turn, try to interpret'.
T: *Is there a book you want?*
S: 'Yes' (mouth movements).
T: *Can you say which one it is?*
S: (Looks at project book.)
T: *Do you want your project book?*
S: 'Yes' (mouth movements).
T: *You said house, do you mean your home?*
S: 'No' (mouth movements).
T: *Do you mean the respite home?*
S: 'Yes' (mouth movements).
T: *Do you ask whether you can take the project book to the respite home?*
S: 'Yes' (mouth movements).
T: *Yes, of course, it is your book (gives Sander his copy).*
S: *'No','yes', 'no', 'yes' (mouth movements).*

This conversation broke down because, as it turned out several days later, Sander wanted to bring the original project book the class had worked with because it had colour photographs, while he only was given his own copy with black and white photographs, like the other children in the class.

The first sentence structures were vertical, often prompted by conversation partners (see Scollon, 1976; von Tetzchner and Martinsen, 1996). However, the vertical structure may to some extent have been a result of the communication partner acknowledging each pictogram that was indicated. Horizontal structures appeared first when Sander started to write letters and the partners began to wait before they started to interpret and guess what Sander wanted to say. When he first directed the communication partner to collect certain pictograms and then asked him or her put them in a certain order, one may metaphorically say that the pictograms were within the same intonation contour.

Just before he was seven years old, Sander began to produce sentences with several pictograms that were difficult to interpret, like this:

JACKET CAP BOOK-SHELF WARDROBE.

With the help of the parents, the sentence was interpreted as 'I have visited fatherfather' an interpretation that was acknowledged by Sander. JACKET was here used in the meaning 'going out' or 'visit'. The pictogram CAP looked like the cap Sander's grandfather used to wear and there were a bookshelf and a wardrobe in the grandfather's hall. Sander had *GRANDFA-THER* on his communication board, but in Norway it is usual to distinguish between *bestefar* (grandfather) and *farfar* (fatherfather), and for Sander this was not the same person. This example illustrates Sander's creativity in using pictograms, but also the necessity of the communication partner having sufficient knowledge about Sander's world in order to understand the idiosyncratic associations he often used when producing new meanings. He would use *HAVE* to indicate 'past tense' because there was no pictogram with this meaning.

In order to make his spontaneous sentences more comprehensible, Sander was explicitly taught to construct sentences with a stable structure of subject, verb and object, with patient and attributes sometimes added. In these lessons, he would often be given a scrambled sentence and asked to put it in order. An important aspect of this explicit teaching was to talk about the different ways the same set of pictograms could be interpreted when put in different order.

At the end of the pre-school, Sander started to 'write' small messages and narratives. He would select five to 12 pictograms, of which the teacher made photocopies, and then indicated the order of the pictograms. When all the pictograms were put in the order indicated by Sander, interpretation began. Some of these writings were quite similar to the description of events in the message book that went between the home and the pre-school, which he often asked to be read:

ANGRY REMEMBER SWEATER JOGGING-SUIT HELLO PICTOGRAM UNIT CUT-HAIR HAIR

'I am angry. Remember to bring sweater and jogging suit to nursery tomorrow. Hello, by the way, I have got new pictograms today. I want to cut my hair. Somebody in the unit said I have so long hair.'

HELLO MOTHER CASSETTE COMPUTER KIWI FOOD FACE GLASSES.

'Hello mother, I want a cassette to show in nursery tomorrow. I have worked with the computer alone today. I tasted kiwi and it was good food, mother and father.'

For some reason, he often used *FACE* and *GLASSES* to indicate 'mother' and 'father'. These examples also illustrate the influence the written messages that were read to him had on the utterances he produced himself. The message book between home and pre-school, typically contained a mixture of messages and information about things that had happened or should happen. The strategy of collecting pictograms and then putting them together may also mirror the lessons he had in sentence analysis and synthesis.

The following example is a letter that Sander wrote to his mother after he had watched her quite upset in the kitchen writing a complaint about the number of teacher hours having been reduced in the pre-school. She interpreted the message as an attempt to comfort her.

HELLO WOMAN FACE KITCHEN TYPEWRITER SAD PEN LETTER GUN FLOWER BATHTUB LEG WALLET BODY DOLL.

In addition to messages, Sander also wrote about events, like this narrative about the session he had with his special teacher the day before from when he was 7;6 years old:

WOMAN SHOE FEET SEE CUT-HAIR HAIR JACKET CLOTHES BOX BOOK.

'Eva took her shoes off and walked with bare feet. I saw she had cut her hair. When she took off her jacket, I saw she had got new clothes. We worked with the "strange box" and read a book.'

The conversations around the narratives were often very complex. Many of the narratives Sander produced were never properly understood – that is, they never achieved an interpretation that he acknowledged. However, the difficulties people experienced in understanding him was an important basis for supporting his ability to express himself. They were also the reason for introducing structured pictogram writing with scripts and narratives about at least partly known events.

Breakdown and repair

Quite often Sander changed topic without any indication of topic change. In particular because of his minimal sentences, this usually led to communicative breakdown because the communication partner would interpret Sander's utterances within the context of the preceding conversational topic. In order to avoid such problems, Sander was advised to use *FINISH* when a topic was terminated and he started a new topic or commenting the established topic. The result was a significant reduction in breakdowns caused by topic changes. Sander also used it to signal end of turn, as in the dialogue on page 185.

Another common cause of communication breakdown was the similarity between his ordinary emotional expressions and the mouth movements for 'yes' and 'no'. Moreover, communication partners often used questions with double negatives. In order to have means to lead the adults' questions during negotiations of meaning, *CORRECT, WRONG* and *DO-NOT-KNOW* were added to his vocabulary as repair items.

Reading

It was first suggested that reading and writing instruction should start when Sander was four years old, but this was postponed until the last year before he started school at the normal age of seven. The reading instruction was mainly related to articulation and recognition of named letters presented individually or as part of spoken words, and putting letters together in short words like is (ice), sol (sun), far (father), mor (mother), ri (ride) and lese (read). When he started school, he could point correctly at 10 letters and had a few written words on his communication board, which he mainly recognized by location. In the first grade, he used the same book for reading as the other children in the class. However, progress was slow and he seemed to distinguish words mainly by their vowels. Consonants were difficult for him to distinguish.

At the end of the pictogram period, Sander also produced messages and small narratives with pictograms and thus had experience with producing text, even if non-orthographic.

The Blissymbolics period

Blissymbols were introduced when Sander was 9;0 years old. Pictograms were now regarded as being too limited both in vocabulary size, syntactic possibilities and meaning construction in general. Reading acquisition was going too slowly for him to use orthographic writing as his main form of expressive communication. Blissymbols made it possible for him to create a wider range of vocabulary items without making demands on orthographic spelling, which had proven difficult for him to learn. However, Sander was quite reluctant to change to a new communication system. He thought pictograms functioned quite well as long as the teachers would draw new pictograms for meanings that did not exist within the system.

What contributed most to make him change his mind was a film about children learning Blissymbols: after he had seen it, he agreed to learn Blissymbols.

Sander was familiar with pictograms and had good comprehension of spoken language, so Blissymbols were taught explicitly in special Blissymbolics classes, in a similar way to that in which foreign languages were taught to the other children. The emphasis in these classes was on exploring how new Blissymbols could be extended with other elements to form new meanings and used in combination with other pictograms and Blissymbols to form sentences and complex meanings.

Vocabulary development

The first Blissymbols given to Sander was *EYE, NOSE, MOUTH, EAR, LEG* and *HAND*. The reason for this was that they could be used to demonstrate how he could use *ACTION*, for example to change *EYE* to *LOOK*, *NOSE* to *SMELL* and *EAR* to *HEAR*. Sander had already used the pictogram *EYE* for both 'eye' and 'look', and the focus on action markers was mainly for the benefit of the communication partners in the environment, who were not used to this way of using pictograms.

In this phase, Sander was very active in the selection of new vocabulary. When Blissymbols were introduced, he was most interested in getting Blissymbols that comprised meanings he did not have in pictograms, like *VISIT, BORROW, IMPORTANT, NOW, PAST-TIME* and *FUTURE-TIME*. He also asked the teacher to replace some of the pictograms with Blissymbols. By the end of second grade, at the age of 9;6, Sander had a communication board with 90 Blissymbols. During the next few months, this increased to 210 Blissymbols, and when he was 10;6 years old, his communication board contained 300 Blissymbols. Although the number of Blissymbols were lower than the number of Pictograms, the number of different lexical items he could produce with Blissymbols was much greater than with pictograms, which were more difficult to combine in a way that was understood by the communication partner.

The Blissymbols that contributed most to increase the range of meanings he could express were *OPPOSITE-MEANING, ALMOST-LIKE* and *PART-OF.* He combined *OPPOSITE-MEANING* with *LARGE* to say 'small', *ALMOST-LIKE* with *CASSETTE* to say 'CD', and *PART-OF* with *VIDEO-PLAYER* to say 'copy' (*COPY* is an element in *VIDEO-PLAYER*, see Figure 8.2). Two of these three Blissymbols represented new strategies, while Sander spontaneously had indicated parts of pictograms in order to communicate something he did not have a pictogram for on the board.

Sander had very few ready-made sentences on his communication board and most of them were instructions for his classroom assistant, like opening his book and writing something for him.

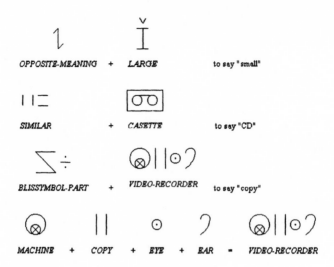

Figure 8.2. Examples of Blissymbols used by Sander.

When communicating at school, Sander often needed topic-related vocabulary that would have made his ordinary communication aid too large and slow to access. The teacher therefore made a large number of topic sheets related to different school subjects. These sheets were kept in a book that was accessible for Sander at all times, including outside the kind of classes that the sheets originally were made for. As the school work increasingly demanded written reports, the topic sheets formed the basis for making topical notes and reports, first in collections of individual Blissymbols and pictograms, later in the form of Blissymbol sentences. The teacher also translated texts from the textbooks into Blissymbols. In these texts, Sander would usually encounter Blissymbols that he had not seen before. As part of studying the text, he would analyse the new Blissymbol – if necessary with the help of the teacher who would also help him to analyse the letter combination of the written gloss.

These written notes, reports and texts made with Blissymbols and pictograms were important not only for Sander's accumulation of knowledge, but also for his language development. They increased his expressive vocabulary and made it possible for him to communicate about a wider array of topics.

Conversations and sentences

There was never a clear distinction between dialogues and sentence construction. A sentence was usually the result of several dialogue turns where Sander indicated several pictograms and Blissymbols, the communication partner interpreted their meaning and Sander acknowledged or rejected the interpretations. This could take a long time.

Most of the structured conversations that were part of his Blissymbol classes concerned music cassettes, books, personal belongings and everyday events. Music was Sander's great passion and he often initiated conversations about his latest purchase:

S: *I AND YOU LOOK THING.*
T: *What thing are we going to look at?*
S: *I HAVE THING LUGGAGE.*
T: *You have a lot of luggage today, cassette box, plastic bag and knapsack. Where is the thing we should look at?*
S: *LOOK.*

In this example, Sander had a new cassette that was in his knapsack. If he had indicated *CASSETTE* instead of *THING LUGGAGE*, the teacher would probably have looked in the cassette box and not found the cassette Sander actually wanted. This demonstrates subtle strategic choice of Blissymbols that was not always discovered by the communication partners.

In his first years as an aided communicator, his communication was very action oriented, he used language to get all the things done that he could not do himself. Because communication was slow and there were many things to do, he did not have much time for narratives. When he was ten years old, Sander began more often to take initiative to tell something. In the following dialogue the teacher tries to make Sander tell something from his holiday (age 10;1 years):

T: *What did you do in the winter holidays?*
S: *DO NOT KNOW.*
T: *Think carefully. I am sure you remember something. You don't have to tell everything.*
S: *YOU READ BOOK.*
T: *I know your mother usually writes in the message book, but she writes what she thinks. I would like to know whether you enjoyed it.*
S: *FAMILY TRAVEL.*
T: *Can you say more?*
S: *HUG GRANDMOTHER SAD.*
T: *Did grandmother hug you when you left?*
S: 'Yes' (mouth movements) (smiles).
T: *I guess she was happy when you came back.*
S: 'Yes' (mouth movements) (smiles).

In this small narrative he was 10;3 years old:

S: *I HAVE DOCTOR.*
T: *Have you been to the doctor?*
S: 'Yes' (mouth movements).

T: *How did it go?*
S: *I DOCTOR GET THING.*
T: *What kind of thing did you get?*
S: *LOOK KNAPSACK.*
T: *A golden pencil. Not bad. We have to try it.*
S: (Laughs).

In this dialogue, Sander used the Blissymbol *HAVE* instead of *PAST-TENSE*, a habit from his pictogram period when he used *HAVE* because there was no pictogram for 'past tense'.

Sander did not often communicate with other Blissymbol users, but there was a period around this time when he met with a girl (Anne) who used Blissymbols twice a week. They would discuss all kind of issues. In the following conversation, when Sander was 10;3 years old, he wanted to discuss religion, which did not interest her:

S: *I PRAY GOD.*
A: *I HAVE* w-i-s-h *BECOME* p-o-l-i-c-e.
S: *'I want to say something'* (attention device) *QUESTION YOU PRAY?*
A: 'No' (gesture).
S: *YOU MUST.*
A: 'No' (gesture).
S: I want to do something else (phrase on communication board).

In this dialogue, Sander disregarded Anne's topic change and used the attention device pragmatically to emphasize the importance of his question. He tried to convince her to pray, and when she refused, he terminated the conversation.

Script and narratives

Language is important for organizing experience and scripts are a form of representing everyday routines (Nelson, 1996). Sander's letter and other written productions often had a script-like structure and included both script-like descriptions of routine events and narratives about specific events experienced by himself or somebody else. This structure provided a framework in conversations that the conversation partner could use to ask questions in co-constructed narratives. Scripts thus represented a developmental continuation of the topic negotiations in earlier conversations. Because scripts were more elaborated, there was less need for negotiation of the basic event structure. This framework helped both Sander to communicate about events and the communication partner to elaborate in their joint construction. Figure 8.3 shows a full script produced in this way.

The texts with Blissymbols that were related to different school subjects did not comprise the vocabulary that Sander used in everyday communications. Therefore, orthographically written texts that described everyday

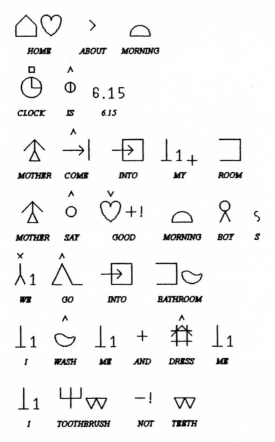

Figure 8.3. Morning script written by Sander. In the last line he says that he does not brush his teeth, because he does that after breakfast.

events – script-like texts – were translated to Blissymbols to give him access to a broader Blissymbol use. These were texts like *The Family Vik*, which described various activities and events of a typical Norwegian family. The same books were used by the other children in the class, and thus contributed to shared contexts.

Sander's work with scripts was shared by the other children, who wrote their own scripts with drawings and letters. Script knowledge was made explicit through the various scripts produced by Sander and his classmates with pictograms, Blissymbols, drawings and orthographic text. The children not only shared the content of these scripts, their script knowledge enabled them to share both personal experiences and experiences that were shared by all the children in the class. Through narration, discussion and role play of events, the children came to a shared understanding of the situations covered by the scripts. Sander's scripts, for example for birthday celebrations, were often compared with scripts of other children in the class. This led to conversations about similarities and differences between the children's scripts and lives. Through these conversations, Sander took part in ordinary exchanges of information, learned to see different perspectives and increased his social knowledge. The insight he got into his peers' perspectives through these conversations provided him with knowledge that is important for identity formation in adolescence (Kegan, 1980, 1982).

Scripts contain general everyday events, but they were often used as a basis to talk about specific events, often with a negative experience. In Figure 8.4, the dentist script has evolved into a narrative about a specific visit to the dentist. Figure 8.5 describes Sander's views about the music classes he participated in. Note that the interpretation is not obvious, and was written down only after clarifications from Sander. Through these narrative constructions, language became a tool for conflict management for Sander.

The script and narrative production was extending into essay writing. Sander began to write a book about routines and specific events. In the dialogue below, which took 20 minutes, Sander (age 12;6) took the initiative to write about a class excursion:

S: *BOOK WRITE* (looks at teacher).
T: *Which book?*
S: *BOOK BELONG ME.*
T: *Who should write in your book?*
S: *I.*
T: *What do you want to write about?*
S: *TRIP.*
T: *What trip do you want to write about?*
S: *LETTER-SHEET* s-k-v.
T: *Can you say something more to help me understand what you want to write about?*
S: *I CLASS TRIP.*
T: *Skurevik* (a place where the class had been on an excursion).
S: 'Yes' (mouth movements).
T: *You want to write about Skurevik in your book 'My day'.*
S: 'Yes' (mouth movements).
T: *Great, then we will have a new chapter in your book. Do you want 'Camp' as heading?*
S: 'No' (mouth movements) *FAMILY.*
T: *The family? I don't understand that, because they were not on the trip.*
S: *LETTER-BOARD* v.
T: *The Family Vik* (a book that is used in the class).
S: (Looks at teacher.)
T: *Should I try to find out what you mean?*
S: 'Yes' (mouth movements).
T: *Skurevik?*

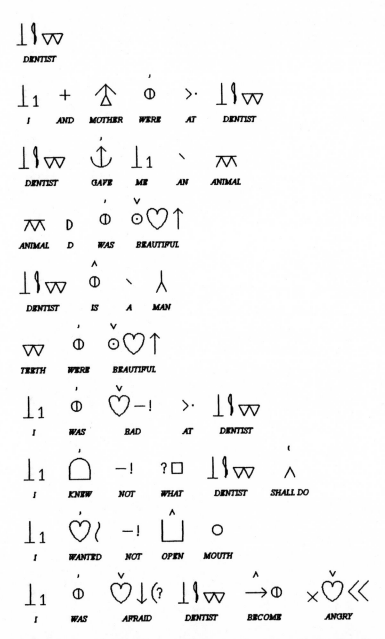

Figure 8.4. During the interpretation of the story, it became apparent that the reason Sander said he had a bad day was that he did not know what the dentist would be doing, and that he therefore refused to open his mouth. He was afraid the dentist would become angry (he did not), because then he would not have been able to open his mouth even if he wanted to. For Sander, the story was a way to talk about a situation he found emotionally difficult.

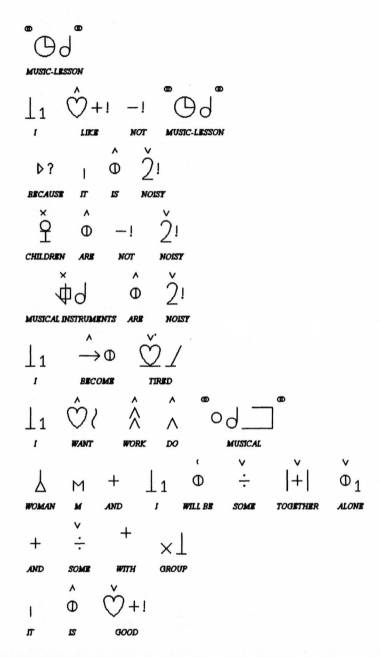

Figure 8.5. In his story about the exercises for a music play, which took several days to construct, Sander reflects on the dilemma that he wants to participate in the music but also gets tired of the noise. He wanted to take part in enough exercises to be part of the play, but not more than necessary because he became tired.

S: 'Yes' (mouth movements).
T: (Writes Skurevik as heading.)

The teacher did not repeat what he said unless she was uncertain about the interpretation. This increased the flow of the dialogue and emphasized the equality of his and her turns.

Reading

When Sander started with Blissymbols at the age of nine years his reading skills were limited. He could recognize some words, like <u>mor</u> (mother), <u>far</u> (father), <u>lese</u> (read) and <u>is</u> (ice), but he was unable to use phoneme–grapheme correspondences more generally and usually mixed up the order of letters in words. He would identify the first letter, but was unable to synthesize the rest of the letters. He spelled somewhat better than he read. Unlike other reading disordered children, he had particular problems with vowels. He had the Norwegian alphabet on the communication board, but did not use it much.

He knew the first letter of many words and used letters to indicate colours, for example *COLOUR-*<u>r</u> for 'rød' (red) and *COLOUR-*<u>b</u> for 'blå' (blue). However, in order to distinguish <u>grønn</u> (green) from <u>gul</u> (yellow), he had to go beyond the first letter. It was through this differentiation of Blissymbol meanings with letters that Sander started to develop better reading skills. Reading was no longer a meaningless academic activity for him, but a communicative strategy. He needed the letters to make his meanings clear.

When Sander was 11 years old, he could indicate all the letters of the alphabet. He used letters often with Blissymbols and developed his own orthographic strategies for expressing meanings he lacked vocabulary for, as in this dialogue when he was 12;6 years old:

S: *TRIP CLASS LOCATION* <u>a</u> *FAMILY* <u>v</u>.
T: *Class excursion to Aksvik.*
S: *PAST-TENSE DRIVE CAR* <u>t.</u>
T: *We drove taxi.*
S: *I AND TEACHER PAST-TENSE TRAVEL BOAT.*
T: *I and the teacher travelled by boat.*
S: *I SIT IN A* <u>s-a-c.</u>
T: *I was sitting in the saco sack* (sack-like 'chair').
S: *EAT* <u>s</u> *DRINK* <u>a-o-a</u> *AND* <u>w-t.</u>
T: *We ate sausages and drank Coca-Cola and water.*

This narrative demonstrates Sander's use of Blissymbols and letters. He spelled <u>a</u> and then said *FAMILY* <u>v</u> to refer to a book called *The Family Vik* to indicate that <u>a</u> and <u>vik</u> were elements in the name of the place he had been, Aksvik.

In order to facilitate the transition from Blissymbols to orthographic text, when a text had been written with Blissymbols and Sander had become familiar with it, it was printed out in large orthographic text only. Sander would scrutinize the text, which was also read aloud to him. After some time, Sander became increasingly able to read such familiar texts by himself.

When he was 12 years old, Sander spontaneously spelled words like <u>fest</u> (party), <u>sgole</u> (skole, school), <u>yse</u> (lyse, shine), <u>brs</u> (brus, pop), <u>biloek</u> (bibliotek, library) and <u>mus</u> (mouse). He could also spell other short words on dictation, but had problems with longer words.

Sander's lack of appropriate reading strategies was also evident when he was reading text with Blissymbols. Despite his experience with pictograms (page 186), in the beginning, he did not read the Blissymbols in a sequential order, but scanned the whole page and tried to understand the meaning of the text from the individual Blissymbols he recognized. He had to have explicit instruction on the sequential nature of texts, whether written ortho-graphically or with Blissymbols.

The language environment

A crucial part of facilitating Sander's expressive language development was to promote the use of graphic communication in ordinary interactions with adults and peers in the pre-school and school. The use of pictograms in new settings increased the number of potential communication partners and the language environment, but did not necessarily increase the number of different utterances, only the number of settings where the same meanings were expressed.

Pre-school age

In the pre-school, the staff were taught how to use pictograms when commu-nicating with Sander, but most of the communication consisted of yes/no questions. They used pictograms mainly in structured activities and when they felt that yes/no questions were insufficient to understand him. Much of the communication was spoken one-way information about what was happening and entertaining small-talk to which Sander usually reacted with smiling, eye contact and involuntary sounds. Because Sander could not ask for much information himself, great emphasis was put on providing information. However, except for the pictogram day schedule, information was given in spoken language only. This means that he got little help from the environment to develop means and strategies for expressing similar information himself.

The other children in the pre-school were taught pictograms as well and, in order to give status to Sander's communication form, many of the objects in the environment were marked with pictograms. That this worked to some extent is illustrated by one of the children saying: *Sander is lucky who can talk like this.*

As part of the education, the teacher introduced structured conversations. These were conversations about a particular topic where the teacher produced graphic sentences along with her spoken language. When the vocabulary allowed, the full spoken sentence was constructed with pictograms. These conversations were important also for the teacher. She had the main responsibility for adapting the strategies of the environment and for supporting Sander's ability to express himself, and the conversations provided her with information about the possibilities and limitations of both Sander and the potential communication partners in the environment. The conversations were important for Sander's vocabulary growth because they made the limitations of his vocabulary with regard to making sentences clear for the teacher, and her experience with true conversations was an important basis for the restructuring of the vocabulary throughout Sander's late pre-school and school age.

School age

Sander started at the age of 7;6 in an ordinary class in his neighbourhood school. It was an explicit scaffolding aim that Sander's communication form should not be 'private' but shared with as many people in his environment as possible. Both the teachers and his schoolmates were taught to communicate with pictograms. Before Blissymbols were introduced two years later, the children in Sander's class were invited to an introductory course by a person outside the school, and they received regular Blissymbol education throughout the school year. All the teachers of the class read the notes and reports Sander made with pictograms and asked the class questions Sander could answer without having to rely on yes/no questions only.

When Sander was given his first communication board with Blissymbols, all the children in the class made a copy for themselves, which they used in the class club (see below). Through this, Blissymbols became a part of the shared classroom culture. Every time a new topic was introduced in the class, the relevant Blissymbols were explained and Blissymbols were often used as headings on the blackboard and on posters that the children made in group work and hung on the wall.

Despite his classmates' competence in graphic communication, interaction between Sander and other children did not rely on spontaneous activities alone. A great deal of the child interaction was planned and formalized though the creation of a 'class club'. This was unique for this class and the children were proud of it. In the class club, two children were always together with Sander and an assistant. The speaking children changed every two weeks. The club activity varied, and included for example exchange of soccer cards and translation of jokes from spoken language to Blissymbols. Through the translations, which the children found very exciting, they discovered both how the Blissymbol system really worked and how difficult it was to translate something into Blissymbols and communicate it in another mode than speech. Sander was the expert and the other children had to ask him when they were uncertain about how to translate a word or phrase. These natural communication interactions also supported the development of phonological and other forms of linguistic awareness in the children. The class club continued throughout Sander's school years and contributed strongly to Sander gaining insight into the other children's lives, and they into his.

The language environment at school constituted a 'language acquisition support system' (see Bruner, 1983) even if the speaking adults and children in the surroundings did not use graphic communication when they interacted with Sander. The peers were probably very important for Sander's development of communication and language. Their knowledge of Blissymbolics and how the system works was important and the general use of Blissymbols in the classroom helped create a language environment of peers who shared a considerable part of Sander's knowledge about graphic communication, and made him to a greater extent part of the general 'community of learners', in which language plays such an important role.

Discussion

The present study illustrates the large differences between the typical development of spoken language and the acquisition of non-speech expressive means in a child with severe motor impairments. It has not been an aim to relate his expressive language to speech development, but rather to describe the skills and communicative strategies that emerge as the result of the means he has been given, the qualities of the language environment, his communicative experiences (of which many were planned), his reflections on these experiences, and teaching activities.

An environment that supports Sander's form of language acquisition does not seem to come naturally, and the language environment had to be planned to a great extent. Explicit teaching, which plays little or no role in typical development, was a significant environmental influence for Sander. This is probably also the case for other severely motor-impaired children who acquire aided language forms. The communications described here took place within educational settings, but still mainly represent interactions where Sander had true communicative responsibility. Although the aim of education is that children are guided to new knowledge by their teachers, Sander's communication with the teachers in school were not simple exercises where Sander was supposed to produce a predetermined sentence or find one particular answer decided by the teacher. The fact that they had to take part in true conversations made it necessary for the teachers also to investigate the untaught strategies that Sander applied.

There is reason to believe that the scaffolding provided by the special teacher in late pre-school and at school age was important for Sander's language development and that is was of a better quality than that of many children with similar motor impairments. Still, the teacher was also a learner and the communication in intervention activities represented true co-construction. There were no descriptions of the typical course of aided language development in children like Sander, which made it difficult for her to know what characteristics of the environment truly supported Sander's language development. Moreover, the teacher did not know the strategies that Sander applied and Sander needed the interpretation and insight of the teacher as a guide to how his messages were understood by others. He needed suggestions for new utterance constructions and strategies – the same function as conversations with adults have for typically developing children learning to speak. Through this process, both Sander and his teacher learned graphic communication in a 'native' manner. This is a process that is very different from both typical language development and ordinary school instruction.

The choice of systems

The choice of communication system is a planned element of alternative language development. There is no 'natural' process of selection of such systems. They are chosen by people who themselves are not native or even experienced users of such systems. When Sander was born, alternative communication systems were known, but not yet in common use. Direct speech training was still the usual approach in most educational environments in Norway. Moreover, because alternative communication intervention in this country had started with people with learning disability without motor impairments, manual signing was the most common form (von Tetzchner and Jensen, 1996). This explains why early attempts to enhance Sander's communication consisted of speech training and a few manual signs, in spite of the fact has he had little voluntary motor control. The late onset of appropriate means of expressive communication mirrors the findings in many studies in Norway and other countries (Calculator, 1997; Light, 1997; von Tetzchner, 1997).

The direct speech training and the manual signs were after some time abandoned for graphic communication, and the choice may have been influenced by the popularity of the systems rather than relevant characteristics of the systems. Blissymbols had been popular a few years earlier, but pictograms had become the most commonly used graphic system in Norway, and this was the graphic system that was first chosen for Sander. When he was nine years old, he started to learn Blissymbols. However, Sander's swift acquisition of pictograms and his good comprehension of spoken language indicate that he might have started much earlier with Blissymbols, quite possibly at the age when he started to learn pictograms.

The different systems provided to Sander demonstrate how core aspects of his and other communication aid users' language acquisition are decided by the beliefs that people in the environment have about different systems. The most important reason for Sander's late introduction to Blissymbols was probably the negative attitude of the professionals in the support agencies outside the school. They believed Blissymbols were too difficult for Sander to learn, and maintained that if he was able to learn Blissymbols he could just as well learn to read and write. These beliefs had a decisive influence on Sander's language development because they implied constraints on his access to expressive means of communication that went beyond what his motor impairment necessitated. The professionals' beliefs reflected limited understanding of the processes underlying the acquisition of alternative language systems and the interaction between planned and unplanned aspects of aided language development. The professionals were clearly ignorant, for example, of the significant problems many children with motor impairments experience in learning to read and write (see McNaughton, 1998; Sandberg and Hjelmqvist, 1997). Sander amply demonstrated such problems in his struggle with phoneme–grapheme correspondences. There is every reason to believe that the language development of children with the same kind of problem as Sander, who also depend on planned means and an adapted environment, will be influenced by similar beliefs.

Technology

For non-speaking children with severe motor impairments, technology, as well as the assumptions people in the environment hold about technology, may play a crucial role in their expressive language development. Technical solutions may allow functions not otherwise possible for the child, but a technological approach is essentially a matter of form, of how a message is presented, rather than of communicative intention. From early on, there was a strong focus on the possibilities new technology might hold for Sander, and technology was considered the solution to all his communication problems. He was given a computer when he was four years old and has been given several different communication aids based on computer technology throughout the years. However, although Sander did like the artificial voice output of computers and talking aids, these technological devices did not seem to enhance his communication development. Throughout his school years the computer-based technology never played an important role in his language development. One reason for this was that the focus of people in the environment was on independent operation – often requiring motor skills he was unable to perform – rather than on *language autonomy*, that is, on his ability to produce self-made language constructs. For Sander, the use of teaching methods inspired by behaviour analysis, with promises of rewards for motor acts which were not part of his potential motor repertoire, made the use of technical devices extremely frustrating. The strong focus on motor skills and independent mastery turned these devices into a succession of defeats, and the early attempts to make him use these aids may have hindered rather than promoted his development of expressive language. If the computer-based aids had been used in dependent mode (operated by an adult directed by Sander) instead of independent mode (directly operated by Sander), they might have enhanced his communicative repertoire (see von Tetzchner and Martinsen, 2000).

One might note that the type of difficulties described here are rarely reported in the international literature on aided communication. It is very unlikely that such problems in aided language acquisition exist only in Norway and the lack of such reports probably reflects a strong bias to report only positive experiences. This might imply inaccurate or even false descriptions of the language development of aided communicators, an underestimation of the developmental challenges of this group and hinder the adaptation of the language environment in such ways that gives optimal developmental outcomes. For example, when other children show difficulties in communication with technological devices for similar reasons, this may be attributed to weaknesses in the abilities of the individual rather than to the complex language learning situation. People in the environment may lower their expectations and provide the children with less than optimal communication options.

The language environment

Independent of variations in circumstances, language is always acquired through social interaction, and the social environment will have a decisive influence on children's language development. For most children acquiring alternative communication systems, the language situation is bimodal (Martinsen and von Tetzchner, 1996; Smith and Grove, 1999). Sander would express himself graphically and people in the environment would speak. In the pre-school, an attempt was made to indicate key word pictograms, but the adults found this form of communication slow and impractical, and the attempt lasted only a short time.

Although dialogues between young children and adults generally are steered by the adults (Dore, 1986; Snow, 1995), Sander had much less communicative autonomy than other children of his age. It is a common finding that adults in the environment of aided communicators are reluctant to take part in conversations with graphic communication and claim that they can communicate about anything with a child who is unable to speak, using yes/no questions. Also in Sander's early social environment, the pictograms that gave him a larger expressive repertoire were used mainly in structured activities. As has been described for other young aided communicators (Basil, 1992; Harris, 1982; Kraat, 1985; von Tetzchner and Martinsen, 1996), Sander's early communication was dominated by partners who often felt that the communication was going well because they received adequate answers to their yes/no questions.

These findings demonstrate how difficult it is to create a 'natural' environment of graphic communication, and emphasizes a need to plan language experiences that can support the language development of aided communicators. Due to the significance of the planned elements, the beliefs people have about a child's abilities will have a more decisive influence on a nonspeaking than on a typically developing child's development. Moreover, young non-speaking children are typically only allowed to express themselves in a restricted number of adapted situations.

Vocabulary growth

Much of the literature on aided communication has focused on vocabulary, especially on professionals' selection of vocabulary (Carlson, 1981; Fried-Oken and Moore, 1992; Grove and Walker, 1990; Yorkston et al., 1989). The expressive vocabulary of children who use graphic communication is much smaller than for speaking children, even if it is taken into consideration that one graphic sign may represent more than one spoken word, and will remain so until the children have acquired orthographic writing skills. The quality of the vocabulary is therefore decisive for their ability to express varied and complex meanings.

Sander's first vocabulary was 'yes' and 'no' (with facial gestures) and most of his early vocabulary was chosen in order to provide him with choices, usually with a maximum of seven items at a time. The vocabulary was object and activity driven rather than dialogue driven: when a food item or an activity was chosen there was not much more to talk about. This demonstrates the close relationship between language acquisition and the activities in which children take part. It may also be noted that in Sander's first years, he had no influence over vocabulary selection. It is not easy to find traces of Sander's life experiences or personal interests and favourites in the first vocabulary that was chosen for him. When the content of Sander's main vocabulary board is compared to the expressive vocabulary of normally speaking children of Sander's age, the difference appears enormous. In fact, only in a few settings would he have the means to say something meaningful beyond simple choices. Moreover, this early vocabulary did not create a foundation for expressing meanings with gradually increasing complexity and the development of language structure.

It is possible that the early vocabulary fulfilled an important function in Sander's early language development but it was only when the early vocabulary was totally revised, the number of situations where Sander expressed himself graphically increased and he became involved in vocabulary selection, that the vocabulary gradually expanded and allowed for more varied and complex meanings. It was also as an element of Sander's particular vocabulary development that he learned orthographic writing: he used letters in combination with Blissymbols to differentiate their meanings and thus increase the numbers of meanings that he could express. This means that the acquisition of spelling for many children with motor impairments and reading disorder initially is part of their vocabulary development and thus a part of a developmental process that is very different from typically developing children's acquisition of reading and writing as an academic skill (see McNaughton, 1998; Smith and Blischack, 1997).

Structure

Typically developing speaking or signing children start to put signs and words together in sentences when they have acquired around 15 to 50 words or signs (Bates et al., 1995). A similar relation between vocabulary size and structure was not apparent in Sander's utterances. He continued to use single-item utterances even when he had more than 200 pictograms on his communication board. There may be several reasons for this. In the preschool years, Sander was not encouraged to produce utterances with a structure, that is, utterances containing several semantic elements like agents, actions, objects and recipients (see Lyons, 1977). Moreover, the actions and objects in his pictogram vocabulary were quite difficult to combine. Even if his full vocabulary had been available at all times, the small number of pictograms representing actions were not easy to combine with his pictograms representing objects and states. This means that there were few natural affordances for creating utterances with an internal structure.

A similar lack of utterance structure has been observed in many other studies (for example, Smith and Grove, 1999; Sutton, 1999; von Tetzchner and Martinsen, 1996), and may be a result of a similar vocabulary structure or similar conversational strategies. However, when the communication partners were guided to give Sander more time before starting to guess or take over the communicative responsibility, there was an immediate explosion in multi-sign utterances. This suggests that the influence of the communication partners on the expressive development of young aided communicators is decisive and that an environment that supports graphic language acquisition does not evolve naturally.

Untaught strategies

Pictograms and PCS are usually interpreted literally, that is, according to their written gloss. The Rebus systems (van Oosterom and Devereux, 1985; Woodcock, Clark and Davies, 1969) have phonological strategies where the sound form of the written gloss under the Rebus sign is combined with letters to express the meaning of words unrelated in meaning to the Rebus sign, for example c-AT to say 'cat'. Some Blissymbols may be called 'strategies' because they not are part of the semantic structure of a Blissymbol, but elements used to direct the interpretation of the communication partner, for example ALMOST-SAME-AS and SOUND-LIKE. However, almost nothing is known about how children use such strategies. Language development is a generative and creative process, and both the typical use and the individual differences in the use of strategies may give insight into the aided language acquisition process.

From an early age, Sander used a number of communication strategies that were neither introduced nor elaborated by adults – for example, looking at objects in the room to communicate something about that object and looking at an object to communicate about something else than the object itself, for example, some object or event that is not present. A similar strategy was used by another young aided communicator, who looked at the door to his room to indicate 'I' when communicating with his father. This was much faster than directing his father to I in his communication book. Similar strategies have also been described for other communication aid users (for example, Collins, 1996; Smith, this volume). Typically developing speaking or signing children may look at or point to a desired object, but the symbolic use of gaze described above seems to be a strategy only found among aided communicators. It is a strategy that is not taught by speaking adults and thus seems to develop as a natural communicative means for motor-impaired children.

Sander also frequently used pictograms metaphorically to indicate meanings that were different from the literal interpretation of the gloss written under the pictogram, and details of the graphic representations to relay meanings not related to the total pictogram. It took some time before the strategies Sander attempted became functional, that is, before the communication partners discovered that he did not always intend the literal meaning of the gloss of the pictogram. The lack of awareness in the environment of the strategies Sander used probably hindered an optimal use of the available expressive means both by Sander and the people in the environment. As people in the environment learned the strategies Sander used, the quality of the 'communicative tool' they shared also increased. From a developmental perspective, it is very unusual that children develop a communication form that the parents and other adults do not master better than them. The children are in one sense constructing their own pidgin language (compare Bickerton, 1981). In addition, in these circumstances, adults may also fail to realize that there is more to know.

So little is written about the self-made strategies of young aided communicators that little is known about their prevalence and why some strategies are developed rather than others. Sander's strategies evolved out of a need to solve communicative problems, but within the limit of his cognitive and linguistic functioning. For example, he rarely used phonological strategies like *SOUND-LIKE*, which were used by the two children described by McNaughton (this volume) and Soto and Seligman-Wine (this volume). Sander also seemed to have more problems learning to read than these two children and differences in strategy use may reflect differences in phonological processing that influence reading acquisition.

Descriptions of the self-taught strategies used by Sander and other children in the process of becoming aided communicators are important because they show that children use the environment in a communicatively creative manner and spontaneously transcend the simple lexical meanings usually attributed to pictograms by speaking adults. Knowledge about such strategies may be used to guide and sustain the children's own creation of expressive language, as well as discovering and preventing problems that may appear in their language acquisition.

Scripts, narratives and conversations

Children's conversations are their most important opportunities for learning about themselves and others. Children learn about the social and physical world, about people and events, both fictional events and events in which they themselves have taken part (Dunn, 1999; Nelson, 1996). The passive role typical of children who use communication aids (Basil, 1992) is therefore likely to hinder their acquisition of language and knowledge in general. The majority of the communicative exchanges described in the literature on augmentative and alternative communication concerns how children express needs and wishes, ranging from simple choices of food items and activities to ordering hamburgers (Calculator, 1988; Light, 1988; von Tetzchner, 1984b). This was also true in Sander's early development. Most of the communicative means provided for him was assumed to be used for making choices. One reason for the lack of longer conversations is probably the slow speed that is typical of aided communicators, but also a limited focus on language use.

The co-construction that took part in the structured conversations with the special teacher contributed to cultural knowledge and a truly shared communication system. The focus on event knowledge and everyday events (see Nelson, 1985, 1996), rather than on teaching conventional syntactic constructions derived from spoken language, probably contributed to making the acquisition a more 'natural' process. Sander learned to express himself in real-life situations and conversations where he had true communicative responsibility, not in pretend games where the teacher always knew beforehand the utterance that should be produced. Importantly, the teacher became aware of the unplanned processes of aided language development and through this learned about the graphic systems and inherent possibilities that are not part of the ordinary educational repertoire. The result was increased competence in both Sander and the teacher.

The use of a script format was an important element in both structured conversation and Sander's communication about events with the children in the class. Scripts are mental representations that contain tacit, underlying knowledge that communication partners share and make it possible for them to understand the coherent meaning of sentences without the course of events being described in detail. They represent shortcuts in communication because it becomes redundant to negotiate the basic sequence of events (Hudson, 1993; Schank and Abelson, 1977). This makes conversations more efficient and prevents communication breakdowns.

Script representations are the basis of the most advanced forms of language use, and explicit knowledge about the shared knowledge implied in scripts may facilitate the acquisition of complex use of alternative language. However, within the field of alternative communication, script knowledge and other forms of cultural knowledge have received little attention. Although Sander had a relatively good comprehension of what other people said, language development is also dependent on 'talk to learn' (Clark, 1982), the possibilities of making oneself understood and having different positions when communicating with other people (see Goffman, 1981). For Sander, the script format represented a ready-made structure that he could use to supplement the communication board in narration. It thus filled some of the same functions as the pre-made text used by Jane and Anna (Waller and O'Mara, this volume).

Reading

Acquisition of reading is often slow in children with motor impairments and many of these children never become fluent readers in spite of good comprehension of spoken language and normal performance on non-verbal intelligence tests, although little is known about the bases of the individual differences in reading acquisition. As we have argued, for children who depend on graphic means to express themselves, like Sander, reading and spelling are integral parts of their language development. For them, delays and disorders of reading represent a double disability: their problems with ortho-graphic reading are not only related to reading texts but also hamper face-to-face communications. Sander acquired knowledge about orthographic writing through a communicative problem-solving process, rather than as a result of traditional reading instruction, which proved rather inefficient.

Sander also did not seem to be aware of reading as a sequential act. He developed a reading strategy where he searched for key elements of the meaning of the page, and then filled out details with the rest of the Blissymbols if he found it necessary. This may reflect that he did not have a clear element order when he made graphic sentences. However, this strategy was inefficient in narration and the reading and writing instruction with Blissymbols seemed to enhance his development of narrative skills. It is important to note that exposure to Blissymbols with written glosses was not sufficient for linking Blissymbols and orthographically written words. Similar observations have been made in other studies (Blischak and McDaniels, 1995; Gangkofer and von Tetzchner, 1996; McNaughton, 1998, this volume).

The problems experienced by many non-speaking children indicate that the ordinary instruction that supports the acquisition of reading in most children, may not always be applicable to this group of children, who bring a language basis to this developmental task that is very different from the language basis of typically developing children when they learn to read. Written language mirrors the spoken language and orthographic script may be conceived as an instruction to articulate. This is also evident in ordinary reading instruction (de Saussure, 1974; von Tetzchner, Martinsen and Ottem, 1983). An inability to articulate will influence a child's acquisition of written language and require other forms of educational strategies than for speaking children (McNaughton, 1998; Smith and Blischack, 1997; von Tetzchner, Rogne and Lilleeng, 1997) but such strategies seem rarely to be introduced in the curriculum of non-speaking children. Because the children use graphic communication for face-to-face interactions, orthographics may be most easily acquired as a communicative strategy, rather than as a tool for transferring text to spoken language and spoken language to text. In this way, reading skills are more closely linked with the language processes of the children, which may benefit both their language development and their acquisition of traditional literacy.

Implications for intervention

The present study provides evidence for the need to specifically plan some aspects of aided language development. These include traditional aspects of intervention like the provision of vocabulary items, direct teaching and adaptations of the language environment. The study also describes the unplanned aspects of aided language development, the communicative achievements and strategies that emerge naturally from the special communicative situation of children acquiring graphic language forms. However, the planned aspects of language development may both constrain and enhance the natural acquisition process. It becomes clear from the developmental path followed by Sander that intervention is not only a matter of giving children who use graphic communication more opportunities for choice and teaching a predetermined set of utterances. Interventionists will have to both guide the children's communicative problem solving and be guided by the way young aided communicators attempt to solve communicative challenges. This will imply establishing a variety of communicative situations where children who use communication aids have true communicative responsibility and the partners do not know what the children want to say. Only through observing the developmental achievements of the planned and unplanned aspects of language development will it be possible to provide intervention that leads the language acquisition of a child who uses aided communication towards an optimal developmental path.

Acknowledgement

We wish to thank Sander and his parents for their support of the research relating to Sander's development and his environment.

CHAPTER 9

Child-driven development of alternative communication: a case study

GLORIA SOTO AND JUDY SELIGMAN-WINE

Longitudinal studies are a prerequisite for gaining knowledge about typical and atypical developmental paths and for understanding their underlying processes. However, the number of detailed longitudinal studies of children who show atypical development is small. In particular, there is a dearth of long-term developmental studies of children with significant speech impairments who learn to use communication systems that presuppose alternative representational systems and alternative selection and transmission strategies. Consequently, neither the paths or the underlying processes are well known (see the introduction by von Tetzchner and Grove to this volume).

One aspect of the language-acquisition process that recently has received renewed attention is the question of what forces support the move from early pre-verbal communication to a linguistic system. For example, Bloom (1993) claims that it is intentionality that propels language learning: children acquire language because they have an inborn drive to understand and share thoughts, feelings and ideas with significant others who themselves have a vested interest in attending to the children's communicative acts and make themselves understood by the children, because of, for example, emotional attachment. Language development is thus a social venture (Bruner, 1983; Vygotsky, 1962). Adults often structure culturally significant events that routinize interaction, afford co-ordination of attention and assign specific roles to those involved (Schaffer, 1989). It is within such settings that children's language acquisition is best facilitated.

Bloom (1993) suggests that word learning is guided by three main principles: relevance, discrepancy and elaboration. The principle of relevance implies that children learn words that are relevant for their current interests. The principle of discrepancy implies that children learn words that enable them to describe events that are not known or evident to the listener. The principle of elaboration implies that as children's mental representations expand, they need to learn words that can express the complexity of the ideas that are represented.

The access to vocabulary is one of the most important issues in the study of augmentative and alternative communication development. The three principles suggested by Bloom are also applicable to the special characteristics of the language development of children who acquire augmentative and alternative communication strategies. For example, the principle of relevance indicates that the children must have access to a lexicon that is relevant for their interests and the meanings they want to share with others. The principle of discrepancy implies that there must be situations that afford language, situations where children with limited, if any, ability to speak have true communicative responsibility and opportunities to direct the attention of others, obtain wishes and co-construct and share information about people, events, ideas, and so forth. The principle of elaboration implies that, in the same way as other children, children with no or limited ability to speak must be guided towards culturally significant knowledge and personal experiences in order to conceptualize increasingly complex ideas to communicate about with others.

According to Burford and Trevarthen (1997), young children learn words that relate to persons, objects and events in which they are emotionally engaged. In order for communication about an 'object' (including people and animals) or an event to occur, the child must have personal involvement – that is, an active interest – in the object or event in question. This involvement may be termed 'communicative drive' and transcends simple instrumental communication where the communicative intention is to obtain an object or achieve a particular state of affairs, like play, sleep or access to food. It may be noted that the language teaching situations based on operant conditioning that are frequently used in the initial phases of augmentative and alternative communication intervention, for instance where children are provided with desired objects or activities contingent on the production of a particular communicative expression, are likely to fall short of creating the kind of shared communicative context that can foster children's active engagement and sustained interaction.

With the exception of children with autism, who tend to find human actions unpredictable and social interaction difficult to understand (Baron-Cohen, 1995), typically and atypically developing children alike enjoy social interaction and communication with more competent adults, even when they do not achieve anything apart from the communication itself. Thus, when children with severe speech and language disabilities sometimes seem unengaged and fail to sustain social interaction, it is not likely to be because they lack interest in communicating, but rather because their opportunities for communication are less than optimally adapted to their skills and interests and hence do not adhere to the principles of relevance, discrepancy and elaboration that afford language learning. As pointed out by von Tetzchner and Grove in the introduction to this volume, the 'communicative opportunities' provided for children who use manual or graphic signs often only allow children to use what they have already learned, instead of being natural occasions for acquiring new communicative skills. The communicative tasks of such often repetitive situations are within the children's autonomous mastery and thus below their zone of proximal development for language (Vygotsky, 1962). For children with severe motor impairments, when the meanings that can be expressed are limited in scope, the sheer physical effort required to produce a message without engagement may be so exhausting that a shorter message is constructed, or no message at all.

Moreover, the dependence on the beliefs and attitudes of professionals that characterizes the planned paths of alternative language development make non-speaking children vulnerable to learned passivity and helplessness (Basil, 1992; von Tetzchner, 1988; von Tetzchner and Martinsen, 2000). The limited knowledge of alternative language development that exists in the field until today may make optimal language acquisition dependent on the child's own ability to make people in the environment create situations that afford its language learning.

The present study describes the language development of Yehonatan who, at the time of writing, is 18 years old. He is motor impaired and lacks the ability to speak but has acquired non-vocal language skills that he uses for a variety of purposes, taking part in the same diversity of conversations as normally speaking children. The description is based on a review of the notes made over the years by Yehonatan's mother, his therapists and his teachers, and which are available today in a collection of personal notebooks that accompanied Yehonatan back and forth between school and home throughout his pre-school and school years, as well as on recent interviews with Yehonatan and his mother. The focus of the study is on Yehonatan's developmental achievements, from the early manual home signs, via a brief period of use of photographs and home drawn pictures, to the use of Blissymbols, a semantically based graphic system, through to the use of a multilingual and multimodal communication system, and on the significance and influence of his intervention programme on the acquisition process. The reciprocal influence of Yehonatan and his 'language planners' illustrates the transactional nature of the language acquisition process.

Yehonatan

Yehonatan is the only child in a single-parent family. He was born in August 1983, in the 29th week of pregnancy, weighing 800 g. He was on a respirator for eight days and on the fourth day he had several brain haemorrhages. He remained in the hospital until he was four months old. At the age of three months he had his first shunt operation. Through the years, Yehonatan has had a series of medical problems and has had 28 operations, of which 17 were related to his shunt.

Yehonatan has athetoid cerebral palsy with spasticity and severe speech impairment. At the age of 18, he is non-ambulatory and uses a powered wheelchair. He has limited use of his hands but is able at most times to point to a communication board. He has excellent vision and hearing. Yehonatan is a competent communicator who currently uses multimodal communication consisting of a combination of gestures, vocalizations for obtaining attention, a communication chart composed of the letters of the alphabet in both Hebrew and English and four pages of Blissymbols, digitized voice output, and a computer for written communication using traditional orthography.

Early development

Yehonatan did not develop spoken language and his first communicative means were gestures and manual signs. He was first assessed by a speech and language pathologist when he was 2;6 years old. At that time the use of pictures to request toys and activities was modelled for Yehonatan's mother. However, his gestures were understood well by his mother and a system of manual home signs had already developed between the two of them. 'Home signs' are signs used within a family or a small group which do not correspond to a conventional sign language or sign system (Lane, 1984). The home signs used by Yehonatan and his mother included, for instance, sticking out the tongue to say 'eat' and blinking to express that a particular food was sour or not good. Until he was three years old, Yehonatan continued to communicate, mainly through the use of these manual home signs and gestures.

The onset of graphic communication

At the time of Yehonatan's birth, the family lived in a small town in the south of Israel. When Yehonatan turned three, he and his mother moved to Jerusalem and he began to attend a special pre-school where he remained for four years, until he was nearly seven years old. It was in this pre-school that he first started to use graphic communication, at the beginning in the form of photographs and drawings of toys and other objects that were part of his everyday world, and photographs of himself in different situations, and later in the form of Blissymbolics (see Table 9.1).

Table 9.1. Yehonatan's early vocabulary

Age	
2;6	Photographs of toys and other objects from around the house.
3;0	Photographs of Yehonatan in different positions, such as watching television, standing in prone stander, lying in bed and playing on the floor.
3;6	Drawings of toys and different kinds of food, *YES* and *NO*. Photographs of family and staff at the preschool, and pictures that represented each child, for example a ball or a cat.
3;6–4;0	Drawings of many different kinds of food and class activities. Blissymbols *EAT* and *DRINK* and many other verbs, feelings, negative, prepositions, *PLEASE*, *THANK-YOU*, greetings, adjectives and adverbs, colour, shape and size, holidays and other special occasions, *OPPOSITE-MEANING*, *COMBINE*, *PAST-TENSE* and *PLURAL*.
4;0	*FUTURE-TENSE* and *POSSESSIVE*, *NO-SYMBOL* and *GUESS*, expansion of vocabulary with nouns, verbs, adjectives, prepositions and feelings, numbers 1 and 2. Sentence building according to Fitzgerald Key.
4;6	Questions, mathematical symbols, slang and words in fashion according to his choice, on-going expansion of all categories of vocabulary, the letters of the Hebrew alphabet.
5;0	Conjunctions, *THAT*, *WHICH* and numbers up to 10.

Even without formal assessment – which was difficult due to his motor impairments and a lack of appropriate assessment tools – the pre-school staff found Yehonatan's comprehension of spoken language appropriate for his age. He seemed to understand when they explained the use of the graphic signs to him, and they noted that he laughed and showed anger in accordance with the content of stories that were read to him. These observations provided the basis both for the communication aids the staff designed for him and for the choice of communicative activities in which he was encouraged to take part.

The importance that Yehonatan attributed to his new communicative tool was evident in his protective attitude towards his communication aid. He would protest strongly if anyone took the communication board away from him without a good reason.

Vocabulary growth

When Yehonatan started in the special pre-school, photographs and drawings of toys and other objects that were part of his everyday world, and photographs of himself in different situations, were used as part of intervention. At the age of 3;5 years, *YES* and *NO* in the form of drawings were added to his chart. Shortly thereafter, another manual communication board with line drawings replaced the photographs, and Yehonatan soon began to use it also in the pre-school environment to request toys and activities and to reject undesired ones (Table 9.1).

In the pre-school, each child had a picture that represented him or her. One child was a ball, another was a cat, and so forth. These pictures were used as the children's names on Yehonatan's communication chart. One of the children was represented by a ball, and several times Yehonatan also used this picture to indicate the concrete object 'ball'. Shortly thereafter (around age 4;0) he asked to have a separate representation for 'ball' to represent the actual object.

In the beginning, it was the speech-and-language pathologist and Yehonatan's mother who decided the content of the communication boards. The pre-school teacher was involved neither in the selection of graphic signs or in communicative interactions where Yehonatan used the communication board. It was Yehonatan's assertiveness and insistence on using his board and having his say in all pre-school situations that motivated his teacher to learn how to communicate with him using his communication board and to take part in vocabulary selection. Yehonatan also on his own initiative began to take his board to occupational therapy and physical therapy and vocabulary was added which was meaningful for use in these situations. He used *YES* and *NO* to take some control over what was happening to him, often in the meanings of 'want to' and 'do not want to', and also to direct the actions of others when he was playing with friends.

Yehonatan's participation in natural communicative settings and the observations of what Yehonatan was trying to communicate had a decisive impact on the staff's further elaboration of his communication aid. Under Yehonatan's 'guidance', the staff constructed a number of boards with photographs of his classmates, the pre-school staff, family members, and so forth. In the middle of his first year at pre-school, Yehonatan started using Blissymbols as his primary graphic tool. He learned Blissymbols quickly. On one occasion he verified for those around him his understanding of the logic of the system when he was shown individually the four Blissymbols *BOX*, *EAR*, *EYE* and *ELECTRICITY*. When presented with three pictures that could possibly represent the object indicated by the combination of these four Blissymbols, he correctly pointed to the picture of a television. Vocabulary selection moved from providing graphic signs for special situations and topics to finding lexical items that might be useful in many situations, as well as items that could be combined with other graphic signs.

The suggestions for vocabulary items came from three different sources: his mother, the pre-school teachers and therapy staff, and himself. As his vocabulary and communicative skills grew, Yehonatan would play an increasing role in vocabulary selection by demanding lexical items specific to his current conversational needs. He would indicate when he needed new graphic signs and provide clues as to what kind of lexical item he was looking for. He would, for example, write graphic sentences with one spot missing and indicate *NO-SYMBOL* (see below). He used this strategy frequently to indicate that he wanted to say something and did not have a way to say it. He would also circumscribe the intended meaning in order to make clear what he needed a word for. On one occasion when he wanted to tell about going to a wedding, he gave a string of Blissymbols: *PEOPLE, RABBI, FOOD, MUSIC, DANCE* and *CONGRAT-ULATIONS*, thus making it understood that he was talking about a wedding and wanted a Blissymbol for this. On another occasion he said *SOMETHING TO-CLEAN PAPER* when he wanted to ask for an eraser. Yehonatan seldom gave up and was almost always able to make himself understood.

As a result of his strong drive to solve communicative challenges, and his creativity in doing so, Yehonatan showed a real spurt in his vocabulary development during his early phase of graphic language use. By the end of his first year in pre-school, at the age of four, he had lexical items for names of many people, animals, objects, actions, emotions, prepositions and adverbs, and social comments, as well as attributes like colour, shape and size on his communication board. By this time he was also using Blissymbol strategies like *OPPOSITE-MEANING, COMBINE, PAST-TENSE* and *PLURAL*. He had begun to talk about feelings, for example *HURT ME*, and to make social comments like *GOOD-MORNING* and *THANK-YOU*. In fact, one of the characteristics that has remained with Yehonatan throughout the years is his use of social comments such as *PLEASE* and *THANK-YOU*.

By the age of 5;4 years, he had become a proficient communicator and used Blissymbols in all his everyday environments and in the same variety of ways as other children use spoken language: in play with his friends, in conversations with his mother, in directing story-reading activities (for example, *TURN PAGE*), to express food preferences, talk about emotional events and direct the behaviours and attitudes of others, like when at 5;2 years, he told someone who was feeding him to be patient. He was using a variety of strategies to expand his vocabulary to the greatest extent possible.

Sentences and narratives

Yehonatan's initial communication boards were designed for choosing food, toys and activities. Soon after he received his first communication board,

Yehonatan used it for conversations and for relaying information from pre-school to home and vice versa. The first narratives he told in the pre-school group were about what he had done on his holiday and on weekends, with the help of a special notebook made for that purpose.

Initially, Yehonatan would indicate a basic skeleton of graphic signs and then let the communication partner do the elaboration. For instance, he would start a conversation about a dress-up holiday by indicating *COSTUME*. Because his mother also described in a separate notebook the context of what Yehonatan was going to recount, the staff in the pre-school were able to support his narrations. Yehonatan, however, asked his mother not to write about him in the notebook. This gave him more communicative responsibility at the same time as it made the communication partner's task of understanding the narratives more difficult and created new communicative challenges. He learned to convey more information to facilitate the partner's comprehension, which in turn gave him true feedback as to when his communication was and was not sufficient for a naïve partner to understand what he wanted to say.

The conversation described below represents the first conversation Yehonatan had with his teacher in which the information was unknown to her. At this time, he was 3;7 years old:

T: *What did you do yesterday after school?*
Y: *TRIP STROLLER BATH PRONE STANDER* 'I went for a trip in my stroller, then had a bath and then stood in my prone stander'.

Following this conversation, the teacher would ask Yehonatan the same question every day. It became an ever-varying routine to talk about the events of the day before. At the age of 4;2 he relayed the following information:

Y: *STAND PRONE-STANDER SIT CHAIR PLAY MOTHER.*

A communication about a dress-up holiday at 4;6 included the following:

Y: *MAN WOMAN BOY GIRL NOISE NOT NOISE.*

When an assistant in the pre-school asked him to tell the other children the rather private information that he had made a movement in the potty, at the age of 4;9 years old, he chose to relay information he thought was more interesting:

Y: *GRANDFATHER BUY PAST-TENSE ME PANTS.*

An important characteristic of Yehonatan's 'communicative drive' seemed to be that he quickly put anything he learned in to general use. He was a very assertive and engaging communicator and needed no prompts from others to initiate or take part in conversations. His communication was truly multi-modal: he used vocalizations (to call for attention), facial expressions, a minimal amount of pictograms, Blissymbols, body gestures (for example, nodding and shaking the head to say 'yes' and 'no') and manual home signs and gestures (for example, a raised hand with fingers spread meant 'stop' or 'enough' and a hand to the forehead meant 'stupid').

During both structured and spontaneous conversations, Yehonatan consistently formulated multi-unit utterances, for example by pointing to the graphic sign for a body part (or the body part itself) together with *HURT*. The fact that he did this in a consistent manner enabled his communication partners to anticipate long strings of graphic signs plus graphic combinations to express new meaning. As a result, they would wait for a long utterance before starting to formulate the meaning in spoken language and obtaining his acknowledgement.

Yehonatan appeared eager to engage in role play with other children, such as storekeeping. He would be the sales clerk and give each child what they asked for when they came in to shop. He also seemed to enjoy telling stories at home and at pre-school – both true and invented ones – and to comment upon and retell stories narrated by an adult. Like many other children, Yehonatan liked to tell the other children in the group about himself. He had several activity-based communication boards for talking about specific topics and stories.

One of the benefits of graphic communication is the fact that there is no difference between the colloquial form and the written form. Towards the end of the pre-school period, Yehonatan started to write with Blissymbols on a computer and was able to read independently some books written in Blissymbols. He began to use the computer for summarizing stories and giving descriptions of his own activities in the pre-school and on field trips. He always became excited when he printed out these stories at the pre-school and took them home to show his mother.

At a somewhat later age than speaking children, but at a comparable phase of his late-onset expressive language development, Yehonatan started to use BECAUSE, thereby demonstrating causal reasoning in his narrative constructions (cf., Levy and Nelson, 1994). For example, he explained that he went to the local grocery store to buy cheese *BECAUSE NO AT HOME*. A friend stayed at home *BECAUSE SHE TO-BE SICK*. He had come to school in a taxi *BECAUSE MUMMY SLEEP* – his mother had overslept so he missed his usual transportation. It was in storytelling and personal narration that he began indicating the past and future tenses consistently when talking about events and using complete sentences, often with the help of phonological strategies (see below) and Blissymbol combinations to convey new concepts.

Language, although atypical in form, was Yehonatan's tool for all kinds of activities and investigations. He used it actively for investigating aspects of the world that are not visible, as well as a means to cope with stressful events. For instance, one day a rabbit was brought to his class.

Y: *RABBIT LITTLE AFRAID.*
T: *Maybe the rabbit is afraid because it cannot talk.*
Y: *I ALSO NOT TALK.*

On another occasion, Yehonatan was going to have an operation. Before the operation he told his mother that he was scared and asked her to sit with him in the operating room until he had fallen asleep. After the operation he requested that lexical items he needed for telling about this experience be added to his board, such as *TO-CLEAN, LIGHT, DARKNESS, BEFORE* and *AFTER.* Once these were available, he talked with everyone about the operation and all that went with it.

During the years in pre-school, Yehonatan's communication became gradually more independent. He frequently initiated conversations and once, at the age of 6;3 years, when the wheelchair tray on which his communication chart was attached was not mounted on his wheelchair, he turned his head in the direction of his communication board to indicate that he had something to say. He routinely sought out communication partners, sometimes signalling to them that he wanted to have an extended conversational turn to elaborate his narrative. He initiated conversations and questions and participated actively in group discussions in the pre-school. However, during recess, where communication was less structured than in group activities, it often happened that nobody took notice of his vocalizations and did not see that he was trying to point to his board. At the age of 6;5 years, he wrote with Blissymbols on his computer: *I WANT TO-TALK.* He explained the situation to his teacher, and as a result received one of the first single-message digitized speech communication aids available in Israel on which was recorded 'I want to say something'. Two of the children in his preschool group were responsible for making sure that someone would come when Yehonatan called out in this way.

Strategies

A limited number of lexical items is a characteristic of all non-orthographic communication aids. Yehonatan's first vocabulary was selected mainly to allow him to request toys and activities, but he soon began to use the photographs, pictures and then Blissymbols for directing his communication partner to talk about a particular topic. This means that, from the very start, Yehonatan did not use the graphic signs only for direct reference to persons, objects and events, but also for strategic purposes, that is, to direct the topic of the dialogue. He may not have had a vocabulary for saying much about a given topic, but it was his initial way of taking the floor, even if it was somebody else who did most of the talking. Similar strategies have been reported for other young aided communicators (for example, von Tetzchner and Martinsen, 1996).

Yehonatan also began early in pre-school to use a variety of strategies to communicate meanings that were not directly available to him through his repertoire of manual home signs and graphic signs. Probably related to his ongoing exposure to Blissymbol strategies, he spontaneously changed the word classes implied in the glosses written above the Blissymbols when he lacked graphic signs for what he wanted to say. For example he indicated *BED* to say that he was tired and EAT to say 'kitchen'. When he was 4;9 years he said *PLEASE ADA VISITOR,* telling Ada that he wanted her to visit him. A self-made semantic strategy was to use a specific graphic sign for expressing a wider category – for example, at the age of 4;0 indicating SLIDE to say that he wanted to play. Another semantic strategy was to indicate some character-istic of the topic he wanted to talk about. At 5;6 years, he indicated *CAR WITH MAN* to say 'taxi'. At 6;2 years, he vented his anger by telling the teacher *YOU LIKE DOG.*

At the age of 4;9 years, the strategies he used included the pragmatic strategy of starting imperative utterances with *PLEASE.* When using a topical strategy, he introduced a topic and then indicated *NO-SYMBOL* or *SYMBOL GUESS* to invite his communication partner to co-construct and express his own meaning in a more precise sentence. For example, he indicated *OPEN NO-SYMBOL* to tell the teacher to open a gift somebody had brought because he did not have a graphic sign for 'gift'.

He spontaneously started to apply a phonological strategy by indicating Blissymbols that sounded like the spoken word he was thinking of. For example, at 5;4 years he indicated *HIDE AND SINK* to say 'hide and seek'. Later it became clear that as a result of listening to rhymes and other forms of sound play, he had become aware of the initial sounds of spoken words. Towards the end of the pre-school period, an alphabet page was added to his communication chart; Yehonatan began to use the letters to provide phono-logical hints, thus developing yet another communicative strategy. Well before he learned to spell entire words, he indicated the initial letter of words he wanted to say as a clue to guide his communication partner in guessing and co-construction.

With the help of the above strategies, Yehonatan multiplied the meanings that he could express with his communication board compared with the meanings that could be expressed with the literal meanings of the glosses written above the Blissymbols.

For small talk in the pre-school, Yehonatan used a small electronic communication aid with digitized voice output. A small number of utterances were adapted to individual situations and events that Yehonatan wanted to relate to the other children, such as when he went to the dentist at the age of 4;4 years. One of Yehonatan's speaking peers would help record the utterances. Yehonatan was very critical about the tone and intonation of these utterances and would often ask for them to be recorded several times, until he indicated his satisfaction.

The school years

When Yehonatan started school at the age of seven, he was able to hold a conversation with another child, or an adult who was unfamiliar with aided communication, using his communication board without any adult assistance. He continued to be the leading force in his vocabulary selection, constantly discussing how to say things and the need for new vocabulary items with his mother and the educational staff. His phonological awareness was well developed as demonstrated by his enjoyment of rhymes and his ability to use phonological strategies to convey new meanings by indicating graphic signs with similar-sounding glosses.

Using both the Blissymbol and alphabet elements on his communication board, Yehonatan participated in literacy activities at grade level: he answered questions and did writing assignments. He also moved towards orthographic writing and, towards the end of his first year at school, he stopped using Blissymbols for written output. Like other first-graders, the main emphasis in his first few years in school was on literacy: to learn to read and write orthographic letters and to write and read in order to learn. He would use an alphabet board in combination with his Blissymbol board for conversations in the way he had started to do in pre-school, but his main communication form in school was Blissymbols. This was Yehonatan's choice as he found Blissymbols to be a much faster and motorically easier form of communication. He could express a whole word with one Blissymbol as opposed to pointing to letter after letter in order to spell out what he wanted to say, thus losing his audience and requiring great motor effort. For written compositions, he used a computer that he operated with two head switches to access the letters of the alphabet using an on-screen keyboard.

During his school years Yehonatan used a 128-message multilevel communication device with voice output. He used this device at school for participation in classroom subjects like mathematics, history, Bible studies, and so forth. He chose to not use the device outside of school as he preferred his communication board for interpersonal communication. However, Yehonatan has indicated that he would like to use Hebrew synthetic speech as an output form when it becomes commercially available, together with orthographically written communication.

Strategy development

As he developed in general understanding and ability to reason, Yehonatan continued to use the strategies he started to develop in pre-school but often with a more complex content. An example of phonological strategy use from this age is when he indicated *CD HEDER* to say 'CD ROM'. Heder means 'room' in Hebrew. Note that this is not only a phonological strategy but also a linguistic strategy related to his knowledge of the English language. When talking about a friend named Vardit, Yehonatan indicated *VERED,* which means 'rose'. Yehonatan told his mother: *NOT FORGET PUT DELET IN YOUR CAR.* He did not have *DELEK* ('gasoline' in Hebrew) and indicated *DELET* with a similarly sounding gloss, meaning 'door'. To talk about a man called Choomie, Yehonatan indicated *CHOOM,* which means 'brown' in Hebrew.

When applying a phonological strategy, Yehonatan often combined glosses with similar sounds and single letters. He indicated *WANT EAT* p *ITREOT* to tell his mother that he wanted mushrooms – *pitreot* in Hebrew. He used a single p and *ITREOT,* which means 'noodles'. When Yehonatan wanted to say that something is great, he chose to express the concept through the use of the word *mitamtame* in Hebrew, which means 'it can drive you crazy'. However he did not have this word on his communication board, so he expressed it by saying m *M'TUMTAM. M'tumtam* means stupid.

In early school age, his use of a metaphorical strategy became very inventive, like when he wanted mashed potatoes but didn't have a Blissymbol for 'mashed'. He asked his mother to make *FLOOR POTATOES,* using the flatness attribute of the floor to indicate a similar 'flat' attribute of the potatoes.

Second-language learning

Over the years Yehonatan had constant and ongoing exposure to many professionals and other people around him who spoke English. On three occasions he travelled with his mother to attend professional conferences in Stockholm, Maastricht and Dublin; on these occasions he freely interacted with numerous English-speaking people. In 1993, when Yehonatan was 10 years old, an English-speaking carer began to take responsibility for some of his physical care at home. His mother therefore added English glosses to the Hebrew glosses above the Blissymbols on his communication board. When Yehonatan and the carer were communicating, he would point to the Blissymbol on the board and the carer would read the English word. For her to communicate something to him, she had to find the English gloss and indicate the corresponding Blissymbol. At the age of 16, Yehonatan had one year of English instruction at school. At the time of writing, he demonstrates excellent understanding of spoken Hebrew and English. He is also literate in both written languages.

Yehonatan as a mature aided communicator

At the time of writing, Yehonatan is on the border of adulthood and is a mature aided communicator. His current communication aid was constructed by himself and his mother. It consists of four pages of Blissymbols, one page with the Hebrew alphabet and digits, and one page with the English alphabet. All his Blissymbols have glosses in both Hebrew and English. Although he can spell, he prefers to continue with the combination of Blissymbols and the alphabet for communication purposes, for reasons of speed and motor ease as indicated above.

There are a total of 252 Blissymbols on each page. The pages are divided into six blocks of 42 Blissymbols (6 × 7) that are arranged in a chequered manner with alternating white and yellow backgrounds. He prefers to directly point to the items on his chart for communication purposes – this arrangement enables Yehonatan to access his communication board through eye-pointing and partner-assisted scanning on those occasions when he is unable to hand-point accurately due to high muscle tone.

The first page of the communication chart contains Yehonatan's most frequently used Blissymbols: some verbs, names of people, social greetings, school-related items, feelings, grammatical markers and special Blissymbols like *COMBINATION-OF*, *OPPOSITE-TO*, *SIMILAR-TO*, *ACTION-OF* and *OBJECT-OF.* The second page contains colours, home and outdoor items, more verbs, animals, weather and seasons of the year. The third page comprises Blissymbols related to food and mealtimes. The fourth page includes months, days, holidays and miscellaneous. While his expressive vocabulary is still developing, more than 80% of the items are those which appeared on his board when he was six to seven years of age. Examples of recent additions to his board include *TRUTH, LIE, DEPRESSION, LUCK, SNAKE* and *PUDDLE.* He enjoys using slang and often asks for his communication board to be updated when new expressions become popular in his age group.

Yehonatan is socially active and communicative. Like speech for speaking young adults, graphic language is for him a tool for maintaining social relations and for participation in society. Yehonatan thinks about himself as a talking person and frequently says *DON'T YOU HEAR WHAT I TELL YOU?* One of his hobbies is writing letters on the computer and sending them to friends and family. He also writes to agencies and organizations advocating for his rights. He recently acted as a self-advocate by writing to a governmental agency to inquire about his rights to receive a computer. He also uses a computer for electronic mail and has just begun to browse the Internet.

Discussion

Language development entails acquiring shared meanings derived from communicative interaction in a variety of significant social and cultural activities. The literature on early language acquisition suggests that it is important for adults to follow the child's lead and label objects and events within their attentional focus, as well as to bring culturally significant objects and events to the child's attention, and to provide opportunities for communicative variation around familiar routines (Bruner, 1983; Nelson, 1996; Schaffer, 1989; Tomasello, 1999).

Language acquisition is by nature a transactional process. Yehonatan's mother and team of teachers and therapists were diligent in contingently responding to and co-constructing communicative productions within situations in which he had opportunities to generate new meanings, such as telling about his own experiences and retelling stories he had heard from others. They also seemed aware of the physical effort required for his communication and the need to create a language environment that afforded communicative autonomy. Their sensitivity and the adaptations they made may have contributed to leading him to new communicative challenges and to making him so diligent and insistent on solving them.

Still, as the title of this chapter indicates, Yehonatan was to a great extent the driving force in his own language development. Children's language acquisition has been called 'the guided reinvention of language' (Lock, 1980), but Yehonatan often developed new strategies before the 'guides' had become aware of them. Even before he turned four, and in spite of limited expressive means, he was an autonomous communicator. He sometimes needed physical support to access his communication board, but the meanings he produced were his.

Of particular interest for understanding graphic language development is his use of self-made strategies that significantly increased the number and scope of meanings he could express. They demonstrate that graphic language use is not a simple word-to-sign translation of spoken language but a generative production of utterances, as pointed out by earlier researchers (Gerber and Kraat, 1992; Smith, 1996; von Tetzchner, 1985). Similar strategies have been described in both developing and mature aided communicators (Brekke and von Tetzchner, this volume; Collins, 1996). One important task for future research will be to investigate the conceptual and linguistic bases of the strategies users of non-speech manual and graphic communication systems apply.

Yehonatan's interest in telling others about events he had been part of may have been a particularly significant factor in his communicative development. It was through the dialogical framework of his personal narrations that he first learned a wider use of action words. Single utterances used strategically to make others talk and fill in the information gave way to temporally ordered, causally coherent narrative sequences. His desire for personal narrative (talking about what happened in his own life) made him an apprentice to his own learning. Through narrative practice, he developed his social and moral reasoning and solved communicative challenges that transcended smalltalk related to what was going on in the immediate surroundings. In the beginning, it was the adults who elicited Yehonatan's personal narrative by questioning him about past events and his feelings about them, but in the same way as for speaking children, there was a gradual reduction in scaffolding (Bruner, 1983; Nelson, 1996; Schaffer, 1989). With increasing competence, his contributions became larger and more independent.

As Ochs and Capps (2001) have noted, apprenticeship is essential for development and learning, but does not guarantee a child's success as an apprentice. Motivation, talent and access to a setting in which more experienced persons clarify, highlight, repeat, intervene or otherwise accommodate to the child's individual learning style is equally critical for language development. Yehonatan did not have the role of a passive participant that is so often prominent in descriptions of both young and mature aided communicators (Basil, 1992; Harris, 1982; Kraat, 1985; von Tetzchner and Martinsen, 1996). He was active in his interactions with more competent communicators in socially organized activities that facilitated his competence. Through his active style, Yehonatan managed to influence the adults in his surroundings so that they provided him with opportunities and tools to learn and practice his language skills.

A final notable characteristic was Yehonatan's use of social comments or 'strategies' from a very early age. His insistence on using *PLEASE* and *THANK-YOU* had a positive effect on his communicative interactions. It was impossible for people to turn away from him or not stay to hear him out to the end when he opened his remarks in this way. Similarly, when he finished an utterance and his communication partner was about to walk away, he would suddenly add *THANK-YOU* to the end of the utterance, which would cause the communication partner to stay routed in his or her place – thus enabling more conversation to ensue. People often commented that they were impressed by his communicative abilities, frequently from their first contact with Yehonatan, which included *PLEASE* and *THANK-YOU.*

Implications for intervention

The developmental patterns described in this case study provide information that can be used to guide practitioners in the design of intervention programmes for children who need augmentative and alternative communication support. The three principles suggested by Bloom have implications for both the content of intervention programmes for children who need augmentative and alternative communication intervention and the settings in which the intervention takes place (Wetherby, Reichle and Pierce, 1998). First, the initial lexicon selected should reflect what attracts the child's attention and the meanings that the child strives to communicate to others. Second, the language-learning context must be such that there is true communicative responsibility, a real need to communicate, and opportunities to share new information. And third, it is important to work on broadening a child's world knowledge and personal experiences so that the child is motivated to communicate about increasingly more complex ideas. Only through participation in such situations is language learning possible.

The strategies developed by Yehonatan give important cues for intervention. One may note that phonological strategies are an inherent part of the Rebus system (Woodcock, Clark and Davies, 1969) but are rarely used in intervention with other graphic systems.

Yehonatan's narratives, from his early simple single and skeletal sign utterances to direct the communication partner to talk about something specific to the complex and coherent stories of later childhood and adolescence, appear to have played a major role in the formation of his communicative development. This points to the importance of using narratives not only as a target but as context for language intervention. Personal and other event narratives provide a rich opportunity for the use of complex language that extend beyond the here and now. Narrative interactions during book reading, 'show and tell', journal writing, and other school activities may promote the development of a cluster of language skills that are critical to further language and literacy development. Much of the first exposure of children to narrative language happens through early exposure to print. Early narrative discourse can help children learn what kind of information goes into a good story and how to organize a set of events in a specific sequence to get the narrative told clearly. Narrative discourse also gives them practice in comprehending the narratives of others and in negotiating the point of the story.

By providing opportunities for children who use augmentative communication to participate in story telling episodes relevant to their own lives, these children gain access to important narrative tools. As with typical children, narrative discourse provides the child with a linguistic means to make sense of past and present events, as well as to anticipate the shape of future events. Further research is needed to address the importance of narrative intervention in the development of language skills by those using augmentative and alternative communication strategies.

Acknowledgements

We would like to thank Ziva and Yehonatan Shvadron for their indispensable and significant contributions during the writing of this chapter. They provided us with the data and the inspiration that made this chapter possible.

CHAPTER 10

Narratives in manual sign by children with intellectual impairments

NICOLA GROVE AND SUKEY TUCKER

The ability to reconstruct an experience in a form that can be shared with others is fundamental to the development of human social identity. Typically, people do this in the form of a story or narrative, featuring themselves as protagonists in accounts of first-hand experience, and as spectators of events they have been related or witnessed. The act of storytelling involves complex cognitive, linguistic and social skills, which develop gradually from infancy to adulthood and which are important indicators of academic and personal achievement (Bishop and Edmundson, 1987; Greenhalgh and Hurwitz, 1999; McCabe and Rollins, 1994). Researchers have defined narratives in many different ways, some focusing on narratives as monologues (Owens, 1996) and others on narratives as collaborations between narrator and listener (Engel, 1995). Nelson (1998) identifies narrative as one of the three main categories of discourse, the others being conversational and expository.

Narratives can be subdivided into different genres: recounts of experience (accounts of specific personal or vicarious experiences) and fictional accounts with either real or imagined characters and events. Narratives can be either spontaneously generated or retold versions of stories presented in spoken language, manual or graphic sign, print or other media, oral, print or visual originals. Although there are many different approaches to the definition and analysis of narrative, all of them share certain key features. The emphasis is on the provision of information, which in its mature form is delivered over a stretch of discourse. The information consists of events linked in a structured sequence reflecting the meaning imposed on an experience, and the experience is one removed from the here and now: a real past or a fictional event.

Narratives have distinctive structural components, which mark them out from other types of discourse. Typically, narratives in both spoken and signed languages are introduced with particular devices signalling that a story is about to begin (for example, *Guess what?*; *A very long time ago . . .*; *The same thing happened to me once . . .*). Reference is made to the temporal or spatial setting of the action, to orientate the listener (for example, *We were in the garden . . .*; *It was last Tuesday . . .*). Actions and protagonists are described, and the events build up to a particular climax or problem and its resolution. Both linguistic and paralinguistic strategies are used to indicate the affective significance of the events to the narrator and the listeners: repetition; evaluative comments (for example, *It was awful . . .*); mention of the hopes, fears, desires and intentions of protagonists; prosodic markers such as stress, intonation, vowel elongation, pausing. Finally, closing devices may be used to signal the end of the narrative, either explicitly (for example, *So that was it, really*; *I just couldn't believe it*; *the end*) or implicitly, through body posture, head shakes, averting eye gaze and dropping the hands (Peterson and McCabe, 1991; Sutton-Spence and Woll, 1999).

Narratives in typical development

The ability to construct and share narratives begins early in childhood and continues to be refined even in adulthood. It takes a long time for children to develop competent classically structured narrative discourse which takes full account of the presuppositions and reactions of listeners. Only 50% of pre-school children can retell stories with complete episode structure (Stein and Glenn, 1982), and at 10, children are still discovering effective strategies for abstracting and conveying key information (Crais and Chapman, 1987). In adulthood, narrative skills can be further refined through professional training. Storytelling really does involve lifelong learning.

The origins of narrative may be regarded as a continuation of the use of proto-declaratives by infants in the pre-linguistic stage of communication. Whereas proto-imperatives involve relating to others in order to obtain desired objects or events, proto-declaratives involve the use of objects or events actions as a means of sharing experience with another person (Bates, 1976). Narrative opportunities are created when infants and their caregivers jointly focus on events in the immediate or distant past.

During the second year of life, children build on these opportunities by developing mini narratives that are heavily scaffolded by parents (Miller and Sperry, 1988). By 14 months, children are able both to talk about routine familiar events, for which they develop scripts, based on general event knowledge (Fivush, 1984, 1997; Hudson and Nelson, 1986; Nelson, 1996; Nelson and Gruendel, 1981), and they can also recall details of the unique individual events which form the basis of personal narratives (Hudson and Shapiro, 1991). However, under the age of three, children rely heavily on the cues provided by adults to help them construct their accounts. One or more child utterances describing a past event are produced, usually over several conversational turns similar to the vertical utterances described by Scollon (1979). Subsequently, children develop the ability to produce sequenced utterances relating to a single event within one turn. There is a close relationship between language skills and narrative skills, with a significant milestone in the achievement of a mean length utterance of around 2.5. Below this level, it seems to be difficult for children to make reference to more than one event, or more than one dimension of an event (Miller and Sperry, 1988). This is similar to what Gleitman and Wanner (1982) call the Goldlock hypothesis in children's early word learning, that one word initially covers one category, concept or idea. Sequenced utterances then progress from additive chains (for example, *He did this and then . . . and then . . .*) to complex structured patterns where the links are causal and or temporal (Westby, Dongen and Maggart, 1989).

Structural components of narratives begin to emerge at around three years. By 3;6, children are able to refer to place (where things happen), but are poor on person and time (who is involved and when) (Peterson and McCabe, 1983). Episodes become more complete as children get older. By four years, children are usually more likely to be including introductions, orientations, and actions that move the narrative forward, and by five years of age they begin to organize stories around conflict involving a progression of events. By age six, children can produce complete structured narratives, using the classic pattern featuring an event and its resolution (Peterson and McCabe, 1983). By the age of eight, they can shift between different narrative genres, creating classic stories from routine events, or personal experiences. A lot of affect is used in narrative by three-year-olds, but few explicit evaluative devices (Reilly, Klima and Bellugi, 1990). Five-year-olds can provide evaluative explanations, but make little reference to mental states unless prompted (Eaton, Collis and Lewis, 1999).

Narrative skills continue to develop in childhood, and the number of complete episodes increases up to the age of about 16. Between about eight and 12, children develop sophisticated linguistic skills for expressing the relationships between events, such as the marking of nominal and pronominal reference, embedding and textual cohesion. They also discover how to summarize stories appropriately, to draw inferences from events, and to provide explicit summative evaluations about the significance of a story for the characters (Botvin and Sutton-Smith, 1977; Crais and Chapman, 1987; Eaton et al., 1999; Liles, 1993).

Narratives by children with intellectual impairments

Learning-disabled children produce simpler stories, with fewer episodes and propositions than those of typically developing children (Roth and Spekman, 1986; Ripich and Griffith, 1988). Very little research has been carried out on the personal narrative skills of children with moderate to severe intellectual impairments. Although a wide range of abilities are seen within this population, the language skills of these children often fall below the level of the average five-year-old on formal assessments (Rondal and Edwards, 1997). They are likely to have difficulties in narrative recall because of cognitive impairments affecting attention and memory, and language delays and difficulties affecting communication skills. In addition to this general situation, certain impairments associated with learning disabilities may have particular consequences for the development of narrative. An example would be the fundamental problems with social cognition seen in children on the autistic spectrum (Lord, 1993). This impacts on their ability to take account of the perspectives of others, or to appreciate the emotional significance of events. Their narratives tend to lack emotional content, or reference to internal states and the context of the story (Capps, Losh and Thurber, 2000; Loveland and Tunali, 1993), and they seem to make little use of demonstrative gestures such as pointing or touching in order to enhance meaning (Loveland et al., 1990).

Different narrative profiles also appear to be associated with different genetic syndromes. Reilly and associates (1990) compared the use of narrative enrichment devices by children with Down syndrome and Williams syndrome and mild to moderate intellectual impairments. Children with Williams syndrome typically presented with advanced verbal skills relative to their non-verbal cognitive abilities, and produced narratives with rich and complex structures both in the referential and the affective domain. By contrast, the children with Down syndrome could reproduce some narrative detail, but they often seemed to miss the main point, included irrelevant information, and failed to make the sequence of events into a story. They were less likely to enrich their stories with either prosodic or linguistic affective devices (Fabbretti et al., 1997; Reilly et al., 1990). Boudreau and Chapman (2000) found that the retold stories of children with Down syndrome contained as many events and utterances as typically developing children who obtained similar age scores on intelligence tests, but were linguistically simpler.

Thus the findings of research on narrative development in children with intellectual impairment suggests that specific skills and difficulties may be associated with particular syndromes or disorders, but tells us little about the developmental course of narrative in these children, or about the settings which may facilitate or constrain its effective use.

Narratives in users of alternative communication systems

There has been remarkably little interest in the development of narrative within the field of augmentative and alternative communication, although there are several descriptions of shared interactions around storybooks (for example, Bedrosian, 1999; Light, Binger and Kelford-Smith, 1994), and many life-story accounts by users (see Brekke and von Tetzchner, this volume; von Tetzchner and Martinsen, 1996; and Waller and O'Mara, this volume, for examples of narratives produced by children using aided communication). Mature narrative construction involves the use of advanced language skills, and the ability to gain and maintain the attention of an audience. Research has shown that children who use graphic communication systems tend to take a passive, respondent role in communication, find it difficult to link phrases and sentences and may be limited by static vocabularies which are inadequate to meet their needs (Light, 1997; von Tetzchner and Martinsen, 1996). Children who rely on manual signs may have fewer problems initiating conversations than graphic language users, but their semantic and syntactic development also seem to be restricted (Grove et al., 1996; Grove and Dockrell, 2000). Studies of children who use manual sign in combination with speech suggest that they can participate effectively in conversations (Bray and Woolnough, 1988; Grove and McDougall, 1991) but there are as yet no investigations of their narrative competence.

A study of narrative accounts in manual sign by children with intellectual impairments

The present study was undertaken in order to explore the use of narratives in manual sign and speech by a group of children with moderate to severe intellectual impairments. The motivation for the study was to determine whether the children could construct personal and fictional narratives, and to compare the structure of their stories at two levels of narrative development.

The children

The 10 children in the study were selected from a survey of children attending special schools in the south east of England. All the children relied on manual signing as the main means of communication, with speech judged to be unintelligible by teachers, were able to sustain a brief conversation in sign over several turns with the researcher, and were observed to make reference to past events within the conversation.

The children presented with varying diagnoses including two children with Down syndrome, one child with spastic diplegia and one with Fragile X. Etiology was unknown for the remaining six children. Mean age scores, using the Snijders-Oomen Nonverbal Intelligence Scale, was 4;0 (sd 0;6, range 2;9–4;6). Language comprehension was assessed by a version of the Verbal Comprehension Scale from the British Ability Scales (Elliot, Murray and Pearson, 1983), as adapted by Harris and Beech (1995) to allow for the use of manual signs paired with speech. Vocabulary knowledge was assessed through checklists of the Makaton Vocabulary (Grove and Walker, 1990) completed by teachers and speech therapists. The mean number of signs reported receptively was 221 (sd 54.1, range 179-313). The mean number of signs reported expressively was 169 (sd 68.7, range 104-243). Teachers and therapists found it far more difficult to estimate receptive and expressive vocabularies in speech, and no records existed of receptive vocabularies in speech alone. There was considerable variation in the amount of speech used by the children. Six children could produce some intelligible words in conversation, three vocalized readily, but produced only the occasional word that could be understood, and one child never vocalized, either at home or at school. All the children were functionally very dependent on signs. Table 10.1 provides information on the language and communication scores for individual children.

Procedures

Language samples were collected in two settings: conversation with a teacher about a recent past event and a story recall task. The narratives of personal experience were collected in conversation with the child's teacher, who was asked to tell the researcher about recent significant events. In the story recall, the children watched a silent film on video that lasted for three minutes, which contained a novel climax: a girl gave a boy a 'spider sandwich' to eat, and he then chased her out of the room (see Appendix 10-A) (for more details, see Grove and Dockrell, 2000).

Transcription

Signed and spoken utterances by the children and teachers were transcribed using the Stokoe Notation System for British Sign Language, within the format outlined by Johnson and Rash (1990). Mean inter-rater agreements of over 90% were obtained for 10% of the data.

Coding narrative structure

Following the 'high point analysis' approach used by Miller and Sperry (1988) for analysing data spoken narratives from pre-school children, a protocol was formed for coding the transcribed narratives. These were analysed using Miller and Sperry's categories of: episode, event type, content, function, temporal structure, and discourse. Table 10.2 provides details of the coding framework, and the coding protocol is included in Appendix 10-B.

Expression of affect

As well as the coding for evaluations, non-linguistic expression of affect was coded following Ekman (1982). Three basic 'emotional categories' were selected that have been identified in early communication (Bloom, 1993):

Table 10.1. Description of participants

Child	Diagnosis	Age	SON Age score	BAS Age score	Signs Comp	Signs Prod	Spoken words
Pardeep	Unknown	14;11	4;6	2;6-2;8	243	243	>50
Jayesh	Down syndrome	16;10	3;11	2;6-2;8	265	217	>50
Asha	Unknown	14;5	4;3	2;6-2;8	211	211	Unknown
Jonathan	Unknown	13;10	2;9	2;6-2;8	Unknown		<10
Adam	Unknown	10;5	3;6	2;6-2;8	231	188	<10
Ana	Spastic diplegia	13;8	4;0	2;6-2;8	179	159	<10
Bina	Down syndrome	12;3	3;9	2;9-3;2	313	232	<50
Mark	Suspected Fragile X	13;1	4;6	2;6-2;8	193	104	>50
Louise	Chromosome abnorm.	12;9	4;9	3;0-3;9	207	130	<10
Matthew	Brain damage	14;8	3;5	2;6-2;11	114	35	Unknown

SON = Snijders-Oomen Nonverbal Intelligence Scale (Snijders and Snijders-Oomen, 1976).
BAS = British Ability Scales, Verbal Comprehension, Age equivalents.
Signs = manual signs reported comprehended and produced.
Words = reported expressive vocabulary in spoken words.

Table 10.2. Categories for analysis of narrative structure

Category	Definition or sub-category
Episode of talk	One or more child utterances on a subject
Type of event	Distant past Routine (habitual) Present or future Other or ambiguous
Content	Negative Positive Neutral Ambiguous
Function	Referential (information giving) Evaluative (conveying an attitude) Introductory or exiting Other (e.g., yes, no)
Temporal structure	Two or more temporally-ordered past acts within an episode
Discourse	Imitation Self-initiation

positive, negative and neutral, along with any change in intensity. Table 10.3 provides a definition of the categories of facial expression.

Inter-rater reliability was obtained on the complete set of data from one participant for all categories used in the analysis. This represented 11% of the data. Mean inter-rater agreement on these categories ranged from 93.1% to 98.4%.

Table 10.3. Categorization of facial expression

Category	Definition
Positive	Expresses pleasure, excitement. Mouth turns up at edges. Eyes narrow. Participant might laugh.
Negative	Expresses disgust, sadness, displeasure, fear. Mouth turns down at edges. Brow can be furrowed.
Neutral	Resting position. Does not appear to express any emotion.

Utterance length

Utterance length was calculated in terms of the number of lexical signs and words and deictic points which had clear and distinct referential function. Thus signs and spoken contributions were counted together with any overlap in content being discounted. Five children had MLUs in the range 1.28–1.79, and five were in the range 1.99–2.88.

Results and discussion

All the children were able to participate in both the conversation and the story recall. The range of child utterances in the conversation was from 22 to 57, with a mean of 37.4. In the story recall, number of turns ranged from 8 to 16, with a mean of 14.2. Table 10.4 contains the number of utterances, turns and the MLU for each child in each context.

Type of event

All episodes were analysed in terms of the type of event they represented. All of the video story episodes, by definition, related to past events. Out of a total of 85 episodes in the conversation, 34 were related to the past, and 16 concerned routine events. The difference can be seen in the distinction in a conversation between talk about what usually happens when the children went swimming (*the teacher says 'time to go' and then we get dressed*) (effectively a script) and what happened at one particular time (*I swam five lengths without armbands*) (effectively a personal event). Seven children

Table 10.4. Utterances, number of turns and MLU for each child in the two situations

Child	Conversation		Story recall		
	Total utterances	Total turns	Total utterances	Total turns	MLU
Pardeep	48	40	14	13	2.88
Jayesh	60	37	15	12	2.63
Asha	50	34	23	13	2.55
Jonathan	38	30	10	9	2.00
Adam	55	32	15	15	1.99
Ana	51	44	15	14	1.71
Bina	38	28	17	10	1.69
Mark	40	28	12	8	1.29
Louise	45	35	17	16	1.28
Matthew	22	21	10	8	1.37
Mean	44.7	32.9	14.8	11.8	1.93

made reference to past events in conversation (a range of 2–7 episodes). One child made no reference to routines and one made no references to the past and only discussed routines. There do not appear to be differences related to stage of linguistic development, as measured by MLU. The results therefore show that despite their communicative limitations, the children were capable of conversing about past events, but showed considerable individual variation in the type of event they described.

Content of talk about the past

The children made about equal reference to negative, positive and neutral events, with the exception of one child, who only talked about negative events. The data were also examined to see if there was a qualitative difference in content, depending on who initiated the episode. Of the episodes initiated by the children, 66% were negative, 28% positive and 6% ambiguous. A very different distribution was seen when the teacher initiated the episode with 3% negative, 32% positive, 61% neutral and three per cent ambiguous. The content of participant-initiated episodes was much more skewed in the negative direction when compared with other-initiated episodes. Miller and Sperry (1988) in their study of typically developing three- to five-year-olds found a similar pattern. Here, teachers may have predisposed the conversations to more positive scenarios.

Temporal structure

Miller and Sperry investigated the extent to which the typically developing children in their study children were able to express two or more temporally ordered past acts (first this happened, then that). They found that nearly a third of the children could not do this and all but one of them had an MLU greater than 2.5. A similar distribution was found for the present sample. No children with MLU below 1.99 produced any temporally ordered clauses, and four of the five children with MLU above this level produced one example each.

Function

Miller and Sperry found that children between the ages of three and five produce quite primitive narratives. They therefore concentrated on the basic distinction between the referential functions (conveying information) and evaluative functions (conveying attitude). They also coded the orientating introductory and exiting functions used to secure the listener's attention or to conclude the episode, ambiguous utterances and 'other' non-substantive utterances such as *yes*, *no* and *OK*. Introductory, exiting and ambiguous functions were not used at all by the children with intellectual impairments. They produced much higher levels of referential function than evaluative function. Table 10.5 shows the relationship between setting and narrative function.

The amount of referential language used is unaffected across the two conditions (whether they are conversing about past events or retelling the video story). The amount of evaluative language, however, shows a marked difference, with only 3% of utterances being evaluative during conversation, and 8% when retelling the video story. In Miller and Sperry's study, typically developing children with MLUs less than 2.5 evaluated 10% of their utterances. In relation to MLU stage, there is an overall trend for children with higher MLUs to produce more evaluative and other utterances in conversation. However, there are substantial individual differences, with Pardeep (the highest MLU scorer) producing only one evaluative utterance, and Ana, in the lower group, producing the highest number of other utterances.

Table 10.5. Functions of utterances produced in two settings

Child	Conversation Referential	Evaluative	Other	Story recall Referential	Evaluative	Other
Pardeep	35	1	9	16	0	1
Jayesh	34	3	3	9	2	3
Asha	32	3	6	11	4	2
Jonathan	29	3	10	9	2	0
Adam	29	0	7	13	0	2
Ana	34	0	12	15	0	1
Bina	26	0	2	9	2	1
Mark	26	2	4	7	0	1
Louise	39	0	0	14	0	2
Matthew	22	1	0	11	2	0
Mean	30.6	1.3	5.3	10.3	1.0	1.3

Expression of affect

Although the children in this study did not make much use of explicit evaluative strategies, it was possible that they might have been conveying their attitude to the events through displays of emotion. The data were examined to see whether displays of affect varied according to the timing, context and content of the narratives. Miller and Sperry (1988) found that pre-school children produced five times as many verbal evaluations when talking about the past than when talking about the present and future. However, in this study, neither temporal setting nor context of the event had a significant impact on the amount or type of facial affect expressed by the children. In both conversations and story recall, the children showed a neutral expression for just over 40% of the time, and detectable affect around 60% of the time, with no MLU related differences. There was no appreciable difference in demonstrations of affect when children were talking about the past as opposed to other temporal contexts.

Temporal context, then, did not seem to play a part in the children's use of facial affect. However, content might be assumed to have a more significant effect. If the children are using facial expression as a reflection of how they feel about the events they are talking about or, indeed, with deliberate communicative intent, one would expect the type of episode to have an effect. Most of the episodes came into the categories 'negative' (23%), 'positive' (34%), and 'neutral' (ordinary or routine such as helping a brother to get dressed) 38%. Overall, the children had a positive expression for 66% of positive events, 67% of neutral events and 38% of negative events. Negative facial expression was seldom used (3% of facial expressions whilst discussing negative events; none at all when discussing positive and neutral events). In the story recall tasks, despite its deliberate elicitation of a disgusting image (the spider in the sandwich), only two children expressed negative emotions (Jayesh and Asha). It should, however, be noted that the story was designed to be funny. Negative events are undeniably more reportable than neutral ones, but it could be that the emotions they excite are positive – such as excitement or humour. For example, in Asha's case, described in more detail below, an accident in the playground led to commendations for her prompt response. Some of the children showed significantly different affect depending on the type of event. Pardeep showed little affect when talking about positive or neutral past events (20% and 0%), but a much higher level of 64% when talking about past negative ones. Asha expressed affect when discussing 67% of positive events, but only 46% of neutral events. Adam discussed no positive events but expressed affect in 100% of the negative and only 38% of the neutral ones. All of these children used MLUs greater than 1.99, suggesting again that the ability to consistently combine two elements within an utterance is an important milestone in development.

In order to explore the effect of setting, utterances were therefore combined in order to indicate whether affect appeared neutral or marked (see Table 10.6). This showed that most of the children showed more marked affect in the story context. Again, individual differences were considerable. Jonathan and Matthew, for example, tended to smile indiscriminately throughout the interactions. The changing degree of expression was broadly more appropriate in the more developmentally advanced children, showing

Table 10.6. Marked and neutral facial affect in two settings. (Note that affect could be coded more than once per turn if it changed during a turn.)

Child	Conversation +Affect	Neutral	Story recall +Affect	Neutral
Pardeep	13	27	10	3
Jayesh	6	31	5	9
Asha	12	22	8	6
Jonathan	28	3	8	1
Adam	14	18	9	6
Ana	46	1	12	2
Bina	18	10	7	3
Matthew	0	23	0	13
Mark	16	12	7	1
Louise	30	5	8	8
Mean	18.3	15.2	7.3	5.2

complete appropriateness in the most advanced participant (Pardeep) through to being fairly inappropriate/meaningless in the least advanced children (12% from Mark and 33% from Louise). The three children with MLUs greater than 2.5 and some functional speech all used vocal intonation appropriately, which helped the listener to know how they felt about the subject matter. This was not seen in the children with the lower MLUs. All of the children with MLUs less than 2.5 showed high levels of smiling during the interactions, the majority of this behaviour appearing to be indiscriminate. Three children marked the high point of the video story with extra affect, but Pardeep (with the highest MLU) is the only one to mark the high point of more than 50% of all narrative episodes.

Despite some of the more developmentally advanced children showing appropriate facial expression, it seems to be more a reflexive manifestation of their internal state rather than a deliberate behaviour selected to produce an effect on others. Clearly, a mature and experienced narrator would be using affect to stress the important parts of the narrative, to let the listener know how they themselves feel about the event and also give information about the reactions of the people being talked about in the story. In turn, this information lets the listener know how they are expected to react. The experienced narrator would, therefore, be employing affective mechanisms such as facial expression to achieve this aim. Our participants are clearly not yet operating at this level.

Overall, although there are some specific differences between the two populations, possibly resulting from methodological issues, there are distinct similarities in the patterns of narrative elicited from typical two-year-olds, and children with intellectual impairments, using manual sign. Linguistic skill, as operationalized in length of utterance, does seem to contribute to the ability to narrate stories and personal experience. The final sections of this chapter explore the relationship between language skills and narrative structure in more detail.

Individual profiles

The two young people selected for profiling are Mark and Asha. Table 10.7 provides details of the narrative analysis for the two children and indicates that their skills were largely comparable. Although Asha's reported knowledge of signs is wider than Mark's, their profiles are similar in terms of the number of episodes involved, the number of utterances and the turns per episode. Asha used more utterances per turn and her MLU was higher than Mark's in both contexts. The youngsters also presented very differently. Mark, who has suspected Fragile-X had a short attention span and some obsessive behaviours. He often rose from his chair and wandered around the room. Asha was a more engaged participant, eager to volunteer information and to respond to the communication of others.

In the following transcripts, two episodes have been selected from the conversation, and the whole of the story recall transcript, to provide representative examples of the children's narratives. T represents the teacher and N the first author.

Mark, and his teacher and the first author are talking about the recent half-term holiday. She asks him what he did, and he tells her some of the activities. There is a vertically constructed utterance where, when asked what he did at the big house, he says that he walked to the fair.

Table 10.7. Narrative analysis for Mark and Asha

| | Mark | | Asha | |
	Conversation	Story recall	Conversation	Story recall
Episodes	4	1	5	1
Turns	28	8	34	13
Turns per episode	7.0	8.0	6.8	13.0
Utterances	40	12	50	23
Utterances per turn	1.4	1.5	1.5	1.8
Functions				
Referential	26	7	32	11
Evaluative	2	0	3	4
Other	4	1	6	2

T: *What did you do?*
M: SWIM. HOT.
T: *You went {SWIM swimming}? It was hot, was it? Hot weather?*
N: *Where was it?*
M: {HOUSE BIG *house big*}.
T: *You stayed in a big house?*
M: *Yes, house.*
T: *What did you do there?*
M: {WALK *walk*}.
T: *You went for long walks, did you? Where did you go?*
M: *Fair.*
T: *Went to the fair. Did you have lots of nice things to {EAT eat}?*
M: *Yes.*
T: {WHAT *what*} *did you have?*
M: *Sausages.*
T: *Sausages. What else?*
M: CAKE.
   CAKE *bubble bubble* (gestures blowing bubbles twice as he speaks).
T: *Cake? Bubbles?*
M: *Bubble.*
T: *Is that something to eat?*
M: 'Blow' (gestures blowing).
N: *Oh, like balloons.*
T: *Blow bubbles?*
M: *Yes.*
N: *Was that at the fair.*
M: *Yes.*

Mark now changes the topic to something he did more recently, namely going in an orange bus to visit a friend. However, he does not signal the topic change explicitly, leaving the teacher slightly lost.

T: *Did you go on the beach? {WHAT what} did you do?*
M: {ORANGE BUS *Orange bus*}.
T: *You went on an orange bus? On the beach?*
M: *???* (unintelligible utterance).
   {ORANGE BUS *Orange bus*}.
T: *You had a ride? Orange bus?* WHAT {WHERE *where*} *did the* {ORANGE BUS *Orange bus*} . . .?
M: {DINNER *dinner*}.
T: {DINNER *dinner*}?
M: G (hand alphabet).
T: *Gary?*
M: ME DINNER 'yes' (nodding).
T: *This was* {LAST *last*} *night? Went to West House on the* {ORANGE BUS *Orange bus*} *and you had* {DINNER *dinner*} *with Gary. What did you have to eat?*
M: *Pie.*

T: *Pie.*
M: 'Yes' (nodding).

Here is the transcript of Mark's story recall.

M: SANDWICH BREAD.
N: *There was some bread, that's right, it was a sandwich. What happened next?*
M: SPIDER (claps hands and rubs them together).
   EAT.
N: *Yes, that's right. And what happened?*
M: DRINK. CAKE. CAKE CAKE.
N: *Then what? Do you remember the beginning of the story? There was a boy.*
   What did he do?
M: *Running.*
N: *Yes, but before that?*
M: {RUN *run*}.
N: *They were running, you're quite right. But that happened at the end. But at*
   the beginning, Mark, what was the boy doing? He was watching TV, wasn't
   he? Then what happened?
M: BROTHER
T: BROTHER? *And then what happened?*
M: RUN.
   {LADY *lady*} CRY. *Run.*

In both situations Mark introduced information about events and individuals but was very dependent on adult scaffolding. He initiated topics of his own (the trip to Gary's house), but did not signal the change of topic, making it difficult for the adults to follow his train of thought. The narrative function of most utterances was referential, but he provides two examples of what are coded as evaluation because qualitative judgements are provided about the weather (HOT) and the house (BIG). Affect was positive throughout the interchanges – he maintained a smiling face – but as he never altered his expression, this was not regarded as meaningful communication of attitude towards the events he is describing.

The two episodes illustrate how a narrative account can be constructed across turns. Mark temporally ordered the information in the second, where it is obvious that he went on the bus and then had dinner. Interestingly, this is the topic he initiated himself. In the two other episodes, no temporal structure can be discerned – the events are enumerated, but not sequenced.

Turning to the interaction between the partners in this dialogue, it is evident how his teacher effectively scaffolds the story with him. She often recapitulated what he said with a questioning intonation. For Mark, this seems to be a very successful strategy, perhaps because it helps him hold the information in memory. It is noticeable that he often follows repetition by the teacher with a new piece of information. For example, when the teacher repeats DINNER, he signs G, the first sound in the name of the person he had dinner with. Open questions, like *Where was it?* and *What did you do?* also seemed to help him recall details. There is only one guess by the teacher (*On the beach?*) and this is ignored by Mark. Finally, the teacher provides a complete recapitulation for Mark of the story so far at the end of the first dialogue extract. The story has been jointly constructed, with Mark providing the individual events, and the teacher integrating them into a coherent whole.

In the following dialogue, Asha is talking to her teacher (S) and the researcher (N) about an accident in the playground:

S: LOOK *at Nicola, and tell Nicola all about Rashid.*
A: {SICK *a fit*} (index finger point downwards) *a fit* {ILL *sick*} {ILL *sick*}.
S: *Who was sick?*
A: R.
S: *Rashid?*
A: R.
S: {R *Rashid*} *was* {ILL *ill*}?
A: {ILL *sick*} 'there' (point upwards).
A: {GOOD *good*} {ME *me*} {GOOD *good*}.
    {LOOK *me watch*} {COME *help*}.
S: *That's right. You* {LOOK *looked*} *at* {R *Rashid*}. *You* {LOOK saw} *that he was* {SICK *sick*}.
A: R.
A: {ILL *sick*}.
S: *Who did you go and see?*
A: {R *Rita*}.
R: {R *Rita*}.
S: {R *Rita*}. *You went to see* {R *Rita*}? *And Rosemary – and what did you say?*
A: {GOOD *good*}.
S: *You didn't say good! They said you were* {GOOD *good*} *What did you say?*
A: {HELP *help*}.
S: *Yes, you said* {HELP *help*}. {ILL *What was*} *the matter with* {R *Rashid*}?
A: {ILL sick}.
S: *What was happening?*
A: {Index finger point downwards *fit*}.
S: *He was having a fit, wasn't he?*
A: *Yes.*
S: *But Asha was very* {GOOD *sensible*}.

In the final episode, Asha describes getting her brother (who also has learning difficulties) ready for school in the morning.

A: {HELP *help*}.
S: *Who do you help?*
A: BROTHER {index finger point clothes} {GET UP *up*} {GET UP *help*} {BROTHER brother} {GET UP *help*} *yes.*

S: *Have we* {FINISHED *finished*} *with* {SWIMMING *swimming*}? You want to {TALK *talk*} *about something else? Do you want to talk about something else?*

A: {BED *bed*} {GET UP *up*} 'phew!' (her body slumps) BROTHER {SLEEP *sleep*}.

S: *Yes, your* BROTHER {SLEEP *sleep*} *was very* {SLEEP *tired*}{BED *tired*} *wasn't he?*

A: {SLEEP *sleep*} GET UP BROTHER.

A: *Yes yes* SCHOOL {GET UP *up*} (point to clothes).

S: *He was still in bed and you had to get him* {UP *up*} *for* {SCHOOL *school*} *and get him dressed, didn't you?*

Here is the transcript of Asha's story recall

A: SANDWICH SPIDER (mouth open wide) {SANDWICH *Sandwich*} {SPIDER *ooh*} {DINNER *Eat*}. {BOY *Boy*} *on* SPIDER {GIRL *girl*}. {DINNER *Eat*} {SPIDER *urgh!*}.

S: *A spider.*

A: SPIDER *Yeah.*

S: *Really. Oh it wasn't really?*

A: SICK *Aargh!*

S: *Did you feel sick?*

A: *Yeah.* GOOD FILM THAT FILM THAT *good.* {SWEET *sweet*}. {BOY *boy*}.

N: *That's right. There was a* BOY. (Pause). *What was he doing at the beginning?*

A: DINNER.

N: *He was sitting down. And then what happened?*

A: {DRINK *drink*} {CAKE *cake*}.
   {DINNER *eat*} {SWEET *sweet*}.

S: *Eating sweets was he?*

A: SPIDER.

S: *The spider came along did it?*

A: SICK (tongue out). SANDWICH GRAB {SWEET *sweet*}.

S: *Picked it up? What did she do with it?*

A: SANDWICH.

S: *Put it in the sandwich?*

A: {DINNER *eat*}. SICK

S: *Oh no – she put it inside the sandwich?*

A: {SANDWICH DINNER *eat it*} {BOY *boy*}. RUN {ROUND *round*}.

Asha seemed to have more idea than Mark that events can be constructed as a story to interest an audience. Although it is the teacher who initiated the topic at the beginning of the conversation, Asha conveyed her own interest through body posture, settling in her chair, turning to S and beginning the story in an animated way. She demonstrated temporal sequencing both within utterances like in LOOK *me watch* COME help in the dialogue about Rashid and SLEEP GET UP BROTHER in the dialogue about her brother, and across turns, with prompts from the teacher.

Her recall of the spider story followed the sequence of the film quite faithfully, and although there were several adult interpolations, these were mostly confirmations of what she is saying, rather than prompts. There were only two prompts. After she paused for some time in the middle of the story recall, N asked what he was doing and then one turn later, asked again what happened. Asha showed far more ability to evaluate events in the story than Mark. She conveyed an affective stance towards the event through vocalizations, facial expressions and body posture. For example, in the beginning of the story she slumps her body to say 'phew!' A couple of turns later she keeps her mouth wide open while signing SPIDER, and towards the end of the story, she signs SICK with her tongue out. She also evaluated events linguistically, notably at when expressing that the spider film was good. In the Rashid dialogue she says GOOD ME GOOD. There was a non-verbal evaluation when she placed emphasis on {ILL *sick*} in that dialogue. The range of evaluations was also varied – conveying pride, disgust, amusement and exhaustion.

Compared to the conversation, there were more evaluations in the spider story, where almost one in every four utterances was evaluative, illustrating her awareness of its significance. Asha was one of the only children to mark the high point of the story (the boy eating the sandwich), which she did through emphasis in her signing and by its appropriate placement at the end of the sequence of events, followed by the coda in the next turn. Affectively, Asha demonstrated contrastive emotions, looking neutral and serious when conveying information, and showing positive or negative affect to mark particular events, like slumping the body to say 'phew!' and keeping the mouth wide open when telling about a spider in the sandwich, and sticking the tongue out or saying *argh* when signing SICK. Note that evaluative utterances were not always accompanied by distinctive affect. As Asha describes the spider sandwich story, she made a face of disgust (SICK *argh*), followed by a smile as she corroborated that she felt sick watching it (*yeah*), and then reverted to neutral, serious expression as she conveyed an overall judgement about the film (GOOD FILM THAT FILM GOOD).

With regard to input by the teacher, there were many examples of explicit narrative scaffolding. She directed Asha's attention to her naïve listener (N), and asked very specific questions to elicit details – particularly the protagonists involved. She started with encouraging Asha to tell N about Rashid, and then asked more direct *Who has sick?* in the next turn. Other examples of scaffolding are *What did you say?* and *Who did you help?* towards the end of the same dialogue. The teacher also repeated for confirmation several times and paraphrased to provide a conclusion in her last turn. She contributed evaluative information which represented her perspective on the accident in the playground (*But Asha was very good*). The teacher also provided a highly satisfactory audience for Asha in the spider sandwich story, expressing incredulity (*Really. Oh wasn't it really?*), surprise and disgust (for example, *Did you feel sick?* and *Oh no – she put it inside the sandwich?*). Again, the stories were constructed jointly, with most of the information coming from Asha, but the teacher helping to clarify and move the story forward.

General discussion

Overall, despite their cognitive and linguistic limitations, the children's strategies for story construction appear similar to those identified in typical early child language. They communicated about routine events, probably using scripts. However, they produced fewer verbal evaluations than might be expected and they are constrained in the provision of information by their lack of awareness of word order rules. Analysis of the narratives produced by children at different stages of language development suggest that, in general, children who can produce longer utterances, whether in sign or speech, are more aware of narrative structure and the needs of the audience than those who only use one or two signs or words per utterance. The nature of this relationship is not clear. It is possible that working memory may be involved, as proposed by Bates, Bretherton and Snyder (1988), because telling stories places particularly challenging demands on communication. Children must recall and sequence the relevant events, convey their own attitude to them, and monitor the interest of the listener. This will be easier once they have attained a certain fluency in language. It is apparent that the ability to narrate successfully goes beyond the basic requirements of available vocabulary, and the ability to string lexical constituents together. Without a rule-governed system for expressing relationships between constituents, it is difficult for children to construct logically coherent narratives which make explicit who is actor, who is patient or recipient, and the temporal order of events.

The problem may be related to the children's cognitive limitations. Perhaps they are not consciously reflecting on and encoding the causal and temporal events they perceive happening. In the absence of relevant information it is impossible to tell, although the fact that they are scoring on tests of non-verbal cognition at age-equivalents of between three and five suggests that they should be capable of these insights. The literature indicates that the ability to talk about an event at the time is related to the ability to tell about it later (Bauer and Werkera, 1995, 1997). The ability to reconstruct and retell a story appears to be closely related to the quality of talk about the event as it is ongoing (Nelson, 1994). Some adults may take opportunities to discuss events with a child, whereas others do not. Longitudinal studies are obviously needed to investigate the relationship between discourse related to ongoing and past events.

Another possibility is that children receive relatively little exposure to extended opportunities to engage in narrative dialogue. In the home situation, typically developing children get hours of exposure, both to scaffolded narratives with their parents, and overhearing the narratives of others (Miller and Sperry, 1988; Preece, 1987). Children with intellectual impairments may well overhear similar dialogues, but it is not clear how often they actively participate in them. They may be less able to pick up on the incidental talk around them, and thus be disadvantaged in acquiring both the vocabulary to construct narratives and narrative conventions.

It is clear that part of the problem for the children in constructing narratives is linguistic and that it seems to be particularly associated with reliance on sets of manual or graphic signs (see Smith and Grove, 1999). The process of language development becomes constrained by the limitations of the available expressive system. It has been argued elsewhere (Grove and Dockrell, 2000; Grove et al., 1996) that this may be a problem relating to input rather than a deficit within the children because they receive so little modelling of contrastive word order in graphic or manual modalities. The children were using a basic topic–comment structure (see Martinsen and von Tetzchner, 1989; von Tetzchner and Martinsen, 1996), which provided the kernel of a narrative. However, they needed support to extend and elaborate their stories, and had difficulty signalling who were actors, patients and recipients.

Implications for intervention

Effective intervention to support narrative development needs to be multifaceted, focusing on the provision of opportunities and experience (environmental engineering), appropriate listener responses, and support for the children's own recruitment of a range of linguistic and communicative devices to structure and elaborate information.

Firstly, children need experience of events that are interesting enough to talk about, and the vocabulary to support discussion of these events (see Tavares and Peixoto, this volume). Secondly, listeners can facilitate or inhibit the development of narrative, depending on the way that they respond to the children's contributions. In a longitudinal study of parental interaction styles with young children McCabe and Peterson (1991) found that effective parental scaffolding started with open-ended 'tell me your story', then specific questions 'what was the dog doing?' then yes–no questions. Young children gave more information, and more accurate information in response to the closed and specific questions, but more complete and longer narratives in response to general questions. Parents who asked too many or too few questions end up discouraging narratives in their children. The following strategies appeared to encourage narrative with young speaking children and are also applicable to co-constructed narration with children using augmentative and alternative communication.

- Modelling – tell the children a story in sign yourself: 'once I had this awful injection . . .' and then ask for a similar personal experience from them.
- Topic extensions – those which help children to follow up their own narrative: 'What happened then?' or 'How did you feel?'.
- Repetition – for example, 'you fell down?' with expectant intonation.
- Expansions – repeating what the child says and adding further information: 'you fell down, and you hurt your knee!'
- Communicative attention – show that you are attending keenly, with feedback and reactions, positive engagement.
- Clarifying questions directing the child to provide orientations and evaluations.
- Persistence – keep prompting the child to participate in the dialogue, by offering your own contributions, responding to what the child is telling.
- Prompts for unshared experience – that is, a genuine motivation for the child to tell about something unknown to the communication partner.
- Information-rich feedback.

Other approaches actually seemed to discourage the production of narrative. These included:

- Topic switching – suddenly and abruptly asking about another event, when the child is still focused on a previous topic.
- Over-use of closed or specific questions, which turn the interaction into an interrogation.
- Inattention – failing to react contingently to what the child communicates.
- Direct correction – for example: 'no, that's wrong, say it like this.'
- Drilling – getting children to fill in the blanks: 'we went to the . . . and we got wet because it was . . .'
- Over prompts for shared experience, when the child knows that the parent knows the answer and there is little motivation to construct a new and interesting account.
- Repetitious feedback, with no expansion.

Another consideration in the scaffolding of narratives is the way in which different modalities may have particular affordances for aspects of narrative construction. The work of Brekke and von Tetzchner (this volume) and Waller and O'Mara (this volume) suggests that the provision of explicit models may help children to organize and communicate their accounts of experiences in graphic and written forms. Graphic representations, being static, provide useful cues for the recall of events. Manual signs and gestures are dynamic and offer opportunities for communicating information about action and space. A positive feature of the children's sign output, however, is their spontaneous recruitment of gestural morphology to indicate the size and shape of objects and the direction of actions (Grove and Dockrell, 2000; Grove et al., 1996; Launonen and Grove, this volume). This appears to be another example of an untaught strategy (see Brekke and von Tetzchner, this volume), which provides them with the resources to elaborate specific features of events, objects and actions. Such elaborations make different contributions to aspects of narrative structure. Information about the size of objects handed to the boy in the story would count as specific referential content, enhancing description. Incorporation of direction of an action (for example, the sign GIVE inflected to show that the action is from the girl to the boy) specifies relationships between actor and recipient, which helps to clarify the roles of the protagonists.

An example of this was provided by Andy, a man with no functional speech, describing how his bag was stolen on a bus. He mimed how he failed to notice the thief as he sat facing forward, and signed LOOK BUS-DRIVER. He displaced the sign for BUS-DRIVER forward in space so that it was coterminous with the end point of the sign LOOK. This was glossed by the staff member to whom he was speaking as 'You were looking at the bus-driver'. She therefore picked up the significance of the inflection, which gave precise information about what he was doing.

Fox (1993) suggests that unless narratives are enriched with evaluations that convey emotional significance, they amount to no more than shopping lists of events. Many of the story grammar frameworks currently used in narrative research focus exclusively on logical coherence and linguistic cohesion. For example, Stein and Albro (1997, p. 6) characterize the purpose of narrative as:

> to communicate an understandable account of events experienced by a protagonist with respect to the ways in which the protagonist's world changed as a result of experiencing certain events . . . Maintaining causal connections among these elements is essential in ensuring that a narrative be perceived as coherent and understandable.

However, the coherence and comprehensibility of a narrative is not an inevitable guarantee of its interest for an audience. Reilly (1992), for example, found that the stories of three-year-olds were less complex and coherent, but more affectively enriched and exciting than those of seven-year-olds. This suggests that as well as paying attention to sequence and structure, it is necessary to help children convey affective information. The children in this study did have access to a range of resources for elaborating information – by drawing on non-verbal means of communication such as mime, vocalization and facial expression. For example, Bina conveyed stealth and caution as she mimicked the girl holding the spider, hunching her shoulders and moving her feet quietly and slowly. However, it was noticeable that those who provided the most evaluations and came over as the best storytellers were the ones who were able to draw on vocal prosody, using stress and intonation to convey feelings. This suggests that even with children who have limited verbal skills, it might be useful to encourage vocal play and the use of contrastive facial expressions, for example in drama and role play. Encouraging the use of mime and gesture to represent affective dynamic and spatial information may compensate to some extent for limitations in narrative coherence. The ability to express one's own feelings and respond to that of others is also fundamental to the development of social and moral cognition (Dunn, 1988; Hobson, 1993).

These findings suggest that a total communication approach to narrative scaffolding, which recognizes the contribution of different modalities in effective communication, is extremely important. Interactive partners need to be sensitive and alert to the creative strategies that children introduce to communicate information. In particular, no one modality should be privileged over another.

Storytellers are made, rather than born, for storytelling is highly culture specific, and learned through participation in socially valued experience. It is necessary to consider not only the individual resources of the child, but the support and modelling that the child receives from others. Repeated natural experiences of sharing storytelling may provide effective models of what information needs to be included and ways of engaging and maintaining listener's attention. The interaction is dynamic, with both partners influencing each other as tellers and audience. The more skilled partner identifies the level at which the child can contribute, and intuitively adapts to this by offering the appropriate level of support. Gradually, as the child demonstrates increased competence, it comes to take over more responsibility for the narration. An interactionist perspective on narrative makes it apparent that both partners share responsibility for constructing an effective account, which becomes more complete and satisfying when both sets of contributions are considered. The emphasis is on how people make the story an interesting one together, and what each partner has to offer, rather than on the limitations of one of the participants. The story itself becomes the goal, rather than the means for the development of particular skills. This story-centred focus may help to increase the motivation of participants to elaborate information, through the range of available modalities. Total communication is the seedbed for the nurturing of storytelling skills.

Appendix 10-A: Story recall

Prior to showing the film, still photographs were used to check the children knew the sign vocabulary for the following items: GIRL, BOY, CAKE, SWEET, DRINK (noun), SANDWICH, SPIDER, LOOK, EAT, DRINK (verb), WALK and RUN.

The two participants in the story are G (girl) and S (boy). Slashes indicate where the film was paused, during the second showing.

1. S is watching television/
2. G enters, carrying a tray, which she puts down on the table. Close up shows tray contents/
3. G chooses cake, sits down and unwraps it. She holds it to her mouth/
4. S puts his hand out. G hands it to him/
5. G looks fed up/
6. S eats the cake/
7. G gets up, goes to tray and takes a sweet, sits down, and holds it to her mouth/
8. S puts out his hand. G gives him the sweet/
9. S eats the sweet/
10. G gets up, goes to tray and gets a drink, sits down and holds it to her mouth.
11. S puts out his hand, G gives him the drink/
12. S drinks/
13. G looks down on the floor, and expresses shock/
14. Close up of large spider, jumping up and down/
15. G picks up the spider/
16. G tiptoes to the tray/
17. Close up of sandwich, G putting spider into it/
18. G holds up sandwich with gleeful expression/
19. G sits down, holds sandwich to her mouth/
20. S puts out his hand/
21. G hands him the sandwich/
22. S eats the sandwich – close up of his horrified expression with the spider in his mouth/
23. S chases G around the room/

Instructions used in story recall:

Make sure that if one teacher is involved with two children, single signers are filmed first. Do not amplify on what children do. 'WE are going to WATCH a VIDEO on TV. We'll WATCH it THREE times. YOU've got to TRY and REMEMBER it to TELL (teacher's name). OK?'

If child is inattentive: 'LOOK CAREFULLY.' If child responds too fast: 'NO, WAIT a minute.' During the second showing of the film, when the film is paused: 'WHAT's happening? WHAT's he/she/they DOing?'

When teacher comes in: 'OK, can YOU TELL- (teacher's name) about the VIDEO. Wait five seconds. WHAT HAPPENed on the TV? Wait five secs. It was a STORY about a SANDWICH. Can YOU REMEMBER how it STARTed? There was a BOY and a GIRL. WHAT did they DO? Wait five seconds.'

Teacher is asked to give enough time to the child to tell the story, but to ask questions until she or he understands what happened, as appropriate.

At the end: 'THANK YOU. YOU REMEMBERED that REALLY WELL (or, for children who found the task very difficult) YOU REMEMBERED X and X. That's REALLY GOOD.'

Appendix 10-B: Coding protocol for narrative structure

Episodes

An episode of talk was defined as one or more utterances during an exchange on a particular topic. The episode was coded as being over if there was a change of subject matter. Episodes were also coded into the number of turns taken by both the children and adults. If, during the episode, there was a time where adults exchanged comments that did not promote any reciprocal input, such adult turns were not counted. The data within each episode were looked at in terms of:

Type of event

The timing of each episode was coded in the categories:

- distant past – an event that happened before the taping session;
- routine event – talk about habitual events and routines;
- present – conversation about the present;
- future – conversation about the future;
- other – ambiguous episodes.

A single episode could contain more than one type of event, but events are exclusive.

Content

The subject matter of each utterance was categorized as:

- negative (to include physical harm, emotional harm and damage to property);

- positive (to include material and emotional gain);
- reportable (not positive or negative, but reportable in terms of being unusual or surprising, such as seeing a funny-looking baby);
- neutral (not reportable, ordinary or routine, such as helping the child to get dressed);
- ambiguous (uncodeable – doubt as to which category was appropriate).

The coding of content was based purely on the signs and words used. Even in cases where it may have been clear that to the children it was something they enjoyed or hated, if the language used was purely 'referential' information giving, it had to be coded as neutral.

Function

Each utterance was coded by function:

- referential – when the utterance gives objective information about the event;
- evaluative – when the utterance also conveys an attitude towards the event;
- introductory and exiting – to secure and maintain the listener's attention or to conclude the episode;
- other – non-substantive utterances such as yes, no and OK.

The evaluative category includes both lexically encoded devices that refer to the narrator's reaction to the story (for example, 'I was scared' or 'that was good'), narrative enrichment that indicates the significance of an event (repetition: 'he did it again and again', or intensification: 'it was really awful') and paralinguistic devices such as affective prosody expressed through pitch changes, vocalic lengthening and modifications in volume.

Temporal structure

This count measured the extent to which the children were able to express two or more temporally ordered past acts within an episode. As the teachers gave such a high level of input, the children were only credited with this structure if it occurred within an utterance as opposed to across utterances.

Discourse

This provided a measure of a participant's ability to take an active and independent role when communicating about the past:

- imitation – where an utterance repeated words from a preceding adult utterance without changing the order of the words or adding new information;
- self-initiation of episodes – and its relationship with content.

CHAPTER 11

Aided communication and the development of personal story telling

ANNALU WALLER AND DAVID A. O'MARA

One of the many stumbling blocks for individuals who use communication aids is that of initiating and maintaining a conversation. A stark reminder of this came in this conversation where Kelly, a 12-year-old Blissymbol user, is talking to Alice (an adult visitor to the special school). Kelly points to Blissymbols on a board. Alice knows that Kelly has just returned from a holiday in France.

> A: *Hello Kelly how's it?*
> K: (Smiles).
> A: *I hear you've been away?*
> K: 'Yes' (nods).
> A: *Where did you go?*
> K: COUNTRY F.
> A: *How did you get there?*
> K: AEROPLANE.

The conversation continued in a similar vein with Kelly simply responding to the dominant conversation partner. At no time did she initiate or take any control of the story about her visit to France, despite many opportunities and the cognitive and linguistic abilities to make appropriate use of available vocabulary. This episode is sadly common, problems with initiation and the use of closed questioning being acknowledged in much of the literature on aided communication.

Although some individuals who use communication aids do use narrative within conversation, many more tend to use one-word or short sentence responses to questions rather than taking the lead when relating personal experience (Alm and Newell, 1996; Light, 1988; von Tetzchner and Martinsen, 1996; Waller et al., 2001). This passive style of interaction may be a result of the initial introduction of aided communication to enable users to experience the power of communication without elaboration. The reduction in communication rate and the increase in communication breakdown mean that aided communicators rarely move beyond questions and answers. This in turn limits the development of more complex communication skills. The focus on questions and answers is also reflected in the use of computer-based communication aids that offer access to single words and phrases – composing longer utterances takes time and physical effort.

This chapter discusses issues of narrative skill development that have arisen as part of research conducted into the design of communication aids to fully support individuals in their acquisition of communication skills. In particular, data gathered from two young people newly introduced to a story based communication aid will be contrasted with the narrative progression of typically developing speakers.

Acquisition of narrative competence

Social interaction is achieved using various types of discourse, but the bulk of interaction can be identified as narrative (Cheepen, 1988). Narrative is a complex type of discourse requiring participation in topic initiation and change, turn taking, communication breakdown and repair, elaboration and an agreed conclusion.

Labov (1972, p. ix) defines a narrative as 'one method of recapitulating past experience by matching a verbal sequence of clauses to the sequence of events which (it is inferred) actually occurred'. Eaton, Collis and Lewis (1999) describe narratives as usually comprising of event clauses that describe what happened and contextualizing clauses identifying the setting and characters and why the event may have occurred.

Some types of structured narrative, like question-and-answer-type jokes, adhere to a strict turn-taking convention. Narratives can also be told as a monologue, for example in a lecture or relating a tale. In these instances, the narrator speaks with little or no interruption from the audience. However, conversational narrative is usually co-constructed and allows evaluations to be exchanged and matched during the interaction. Although storytelling as a monologue can be found in illiterate cultures, much of 'storytelling' in literate cultures is co-constructed (Cheepen, 1988).

Narrating personal experience is one of the primary dimensions of discourse development in the pre-school years (Meng, 1992). Real and fictional events are related by children as young as two years of age (Eisenberg, 1985; Hudson and Shapiro, 1991; Miller and Sperry, 1988; Sachs, 1983). Children are known to relate experiences before they have acquired full verbal communication, for example through pantomime (Goodman et al., 1990). Waller (1992) tells about an 18-month-old who used single words, gesture and body posture to tell his father how his balloon had popped when it had landed on the grass. The child relayed the exact sequence of the experience and responded appropriately to interjections from the father requesting clarification and elaboration.

Studies show that children's story structures develop initially with much help from an adult (Meng, 1992; Reilly, 1992). When children are young, the adult scaffolds the telling of a narrative by providing a framework in which the narrative is developed. The adult is the dominant conversational partner, eliciting the content of the narrative by prompting the child. Meng (1992) found that three-year-olds would seldom expand on an experience themselves, even though they would initiate an interaction. The initiation of a story in the early stages may involve simply telling the punchline with adults prompting for elaboration (Schober-Peterson and Johnson, 1991). By 4;6 years of age, the children in Meng's study would initiate and expand on an experience they wished to relate. By the age of six years, the majority of children have developed their narrative skills to such an extent that they are able to initiate, maintain and conclude a narrative (Peterson and McCabe, 1983).

Scaffolding narratives

The dialogue extract below demonstrates how an adult provides the scaffolding needed to enable a typically developing child to take control of the interaction, while maintaining the participation of the other communication partner. This scaffolding is provided through encouraging the boy to elaborate on what he has to say. Christopher, a typically developing child (aged 4;3), was listening to his father, Jack, and Sheila, an adult friend, talking about what they had been doing recently:

J: *Thursday?*
S: *I went to see Harry Potter on Thursday.*
S: *When?*
C: *???* (unintelligible speech). *Lion King* (attempts to be heard). I get I just get (attempts to be heard).
J: *Best time to see films like that.*
S: *When I should have been working.*
C: *The Lion King.*
S: *Do you like the Lion King?*
C: *Yes the Lion King.*
S: *What happened to the Lion King.*
C: (Time elapsed, 3 seconds.) *???* (unintelligible speech) *got hyenas.*
S: *Hyenas I don't like hyenas.*
C: *I don't either. Simba doesn't either they just scare him.*
S: *Uh uh.*
J: *What do they do to him.*
C: *They just scare him but but her but but Simba's father gets dead.*

The dialogue extract illustrates initiation by Christopher, prompting from adults and then elaboration by Christopher. Christopher is persistent in his wish to talk about The Lion King, interrupting while the adults are still speaking. Sheila eventually acknowledges the boy's initiation (*Do you like the Lion King?*) but has to prompt the child to expand further: *What happened to the Lion King?* Christopher takes a short time to answer *Hyenas* and responds again with some elaboration. The father prompts saying *What do they do to him?* and Christopher responds with more elaboration.

Although the adults use questions to elicit information from Christopher, this interaction differs from the first dialogue extract in which Kelly restricts her answers to 'yes' and one-word utterances. Christopher, on the other hand, initiates the topic of the Lion King. The adult partners then use questions to scaffold a discussion about the film. Christopher responds by elaborating on what he has already said – something that Kelly does not do.

Kelly illustrates the tendency of aided communicators to rely on yes/no and one-word answers, while Christopher uses longer sentences in his elaborations. The following example from von Tetzchner and Martinsen (1996, p. 69) shows an aided interaction which shows a similar use of closed questions to those found in Kelly's extract on page 256. Father (F) and Henri (aged 8;4), using a communication book containing 145 PIC signs, are talking about Henri's school day.

F: *Did you learn about any particular animals today or which animals did you learn about? It is in your book, so I know about it. Which animal did you learn about in school today?*
H: *DOG.*
F: *Yes. Dog. Yes. Did anyone bring a dog to school today? Who was it? Who brought a dog to school today?*
H: (Looks at the table and smiles.)
F: *Was it Mary?*
H: 'No' (head movement).
F: *Was it Joan who brought a dog?*
H: 'Yes' (head movement).
F: *Yes, it was in your book that Joan brought the dog.*

Despite the four-year age difference between Kelly and Henri, both conversations were initiated and directed by the speaking adult communicators with the aided communicators using yes/no and one-word answers. Neither Kelly nor Henri took any initiative in attempting to expand on their responses. The adults in all three conversations knew about the incidents being reported. However, it is only Christopher who demonstrates the ability to make novel contributions to the conversation when he says that hyenas scare the Lion King.

Co-constructing narratives

The dialogue extract below introduces a further development in the acquisition of conversational skills. It shows an example of co-construction whereby both father and son contribute to the unfolding of the story. It also provides an example of the progression from scaffolding into the use of more sophisticated conversational devices, for example posing a question to introduce suspense.

Mary (mother), Doug (father) and John (aged 5;0) are talking while having their evening meal.

> M: *Yea and before that?*
> D: *Before that we did. We.*
> J: *We played casino.*
> M: *Casino (laughs). Yes, John is going to be a gambler when he grows up are you. Who won that game by the way? Who had the most money at the end? Did you really?*
> D: *John had the most money.*
> M: *Wha. Did you manage to win with or without cheating John?*
> J: (Time elapsed, two seconds.) *Without cheating.*
> D: *He won without cheating but he um. He did sort of shuffle a bit in the bank though didn't he half way through.*
> M: (Laughs.)
> J: *I put it on. Um any colour and then do you know what?*
> M: *What?*
> J: *It didn't do th the colour. I think eve a berserk was being made in that spinner.*
> M: (Laughs) *Why why do you think he he went bersekas in the spinner?*
> J: *Because it always um it always does wrong colour.*
> M: *It always the wrong colour. So do you think he went berserk? What what do you think he's doing to make it do that?*
> J: *He's not pressing the right buttons.*
> M: (Laughs) *Ah yes.* (Laughs) *Ah you're probably right John. Well just make sure when you're grown up and you play in a casino that you go to one ?????* (unintelligible speech) *and berserk isn't.*

The conversation is co-constructed – both John and Doug are contributing to sharing their experience with Mary. John responds to his father's suggestion of cheating by explaining what the roulette wheel did with the coloured discs. John then controls the conversation by discussing why the wheel did not stop at the desired colour. In response to Mary's question regarding winning with and without cheating, both John and Doug reply, with John continuing to explain what actually happened by posing a question to his mother before telling her why he thinks the wheel was being controlled.

A different type of co-construction is used extensively when attempting to expand on the limited communication from an aided partner. This occurs when the speaking partner suggests an elaboration to a one-word utterance by the aided communicator. In contrast with the use of question prompts in Kelly's and Henri's dialogue extracts, the following interaction from von Tetzchner and Martinsen (1996, pp. 81–2) illustrates how an aided partner's communication can be co-constructed using suggestions and confirmation requests from the speaking partner.

Eva (aged 5;4) was sitting in the living room together with her mother, communicating about a visit to an aunt. Eva uses direct selection and a communication book with 285 PIC signs and photographs.

M: *When we went to Aunt Kari, what did you bring?*
E: *BICYCLE.*
M: *You brought that bicycle when we went to Aunt Kari.*
E: *BICYCLE. (TO) BICYCLE (lifts arm up and down, which is a manual home sign for 'to bicycle').*
M: *Yes, you did bicycle there.*
M: *Hm?*
E: *SANDBOX.*
M: *Were you also in the sandbox?*
E: 'Yes' (nods).
M: *Hm.*
E: *SWING.*
M: *And then you used the swing.*
E: 'Yes' (nods).
M: *Hm.*
E: *SWITCHBACK.*
M: *And the switchback was there. Eva was in the playground when we visited Aunt Kari?*

Eva's mother only prompts once, at the beginning of the interaction, to elicit the story about Eva's visit to her aunt. Eva then takes control of the conversation with her mother expanding on Eva's interaction. The mother does not initiate as in Kelly's and Henri's extracts, but rather expands on the young aided communicator's initiations. Von Tetzchner and Martinsen (1996) refer to this use of graphic signs as *directive* in that the aided communicator is directing the speaking partner to fill in the detail.

Some comparisons can be made with the interaction in the extract in which John's father expanded on John's *Without cheating* by saying *He won without cheating but he um. He did sort of shuffle a bit in the bank though didn't he half way through.*

Two types of co-construction will be used in this chapter. *Directed* co-construction will refer to interactions in which speaking partners elaborate on the aided communication. *Mutual* co-construction will refer to conversations where both partners contribute to the unfolding of a story. This may involve questions, but is different to scaffolding where questions are used to frame a story.

The development of narrative in aided conversations

Even though aided users may develop the skill to introduce new topics into a conversation, few move from using one-word or short utterances within conversation.

Two young people aged 9:6 and 17:0 who used aided communication took part in a year-long study to investigate how their use of personal stories within conversation would evolve when they were available in a narrative-based communication device (Waller et al., 2001). The software program used in this study allowed the communication-aid user to edit, add and select appropriate text whilst engaged in interactive conversation (Figure 11.1). Unlike conventional storage-based devices the user can control the delivery (narration) of a story by 'speaking' selected parts via the speech synthesizer. Text can also be edited during a conversation using word-prediction software when required.

Anne was 9;6 years old when she joined the study. She was born with some dysmorphic features and congenital abnormalities. Anne was ambulatory. Her speech was telegrammatic and unintelligible due to articulatory dyspraxia. She had most difficulty expressing her thoughts and ideas about

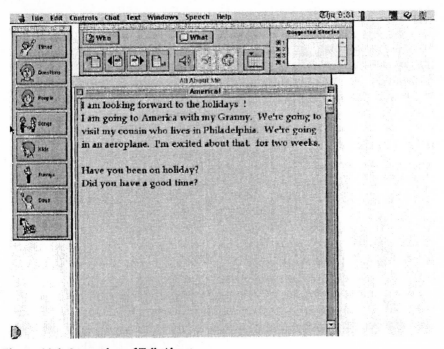

Figure 11.1. Screenshot of Talk:About.

issues outside of the immediate situation. This sometimes caused frustration for her but generally she was quite passive in communication and offered little spontaneous expression. Anne was introduced to manual signs from the Makaton vocabulary while at nursery but did not use them effectively. A voice output communication device that stores digitized speech units was first introduced when she was 5:0 years old. The digitized speech units were retrieved by pressing squares with pictures. This device was followed by a PC-based communication software package that combined picture retrieval of synthesized speech units with an on-screen keyboard. Anne only used these systems to respond to others. She began to locate and type individual letters prior to the study. She was unable to spell words correctly but was able to select words with some help using word-prediction software.

Jane was 17;0 years old when she joined the study. She had spastic cerebral palsy and used a powered wheelchair. She could not speak and used some manual signs which were understood by those who knew her well. She used a dedicated code-based voice output communication aid, using codes for proper names, some verbs and small words such as conjunctions and prepositions. However, her preferred method of communication was to type letter by letter. Each letter was spoken by the speech synthesizer as it was typed, as was the message once it was complete.

A research speech and language therapist and a research special education teacher spent an average of two hours per week during the school term working with the participants creating story texts and supporting the use of the story-based communication aid. The participants were videotaped regularly during the year. The videos recorded conversations between the participants and two adults: Helen (the research speech and language therapist) and Paula (a university staff member with no previous contact with aided communicators).

Scaffolding using closed questions

Neither Anne nor Jane were able to maintain an active role in a conversation before they joined the study. Both participants would answer closed questions, leaving the control of the conversation with the speaking partner. Here are Anne (aged 9;8) and Helen in conversation:

H: *How do you get to school?*
A: *By the bus* (speech approximation).
H: *Oh right. And does it come right to your house?*
A: *Ye.*
H: *Who else is on the bus?*
A: (Time elapsed, six seconds.) 'No' (shakes head).
H: *Nobody?*
A: 'No' (shakes head).

H: *A whole big giant enormous double decker bus.* (Spreads arms wide.) *With one one driver and one Jane* (holds up one finger).

A: 'No' (shakes head).

H: *Really?*

A: 'No' (shakes head).

H: *Cor blimey you must be a queen.*

A: (Laughs.)

H: *Wow. Oh my goodness that's that's just wonderful.*

A: (Laughs.)

H: *A whole bus to yourself. Mm.* (Smiles) *And and I believe that.*

A: (Laughs.)

H: *Ok how long does it take to come to school. There's lots and lots of time ???* (unintelligible speech).

A: *???* (unintelligible speech).

H: *Mm.* 'Yes' (nods). *And tell me about your class. Who's in your class?*

A: (Time elapsed, four seconds.) *???* (unintelligible speech).

H: *Good.* (Time elapsed, six seconds.) *And.*

A: (Time elapsed, four seconds.) *???* (unintelligible speech).

H: (Nods) *Mm and.*

A: (Time elapsed, 11 seconds. Rubbing hands, looking down.) *???* (unintelligible speech).

H: *Is she one of the children in your class?*

A: 'No' (shakes head).

H: *Who is she?* (Time elapsed, seven seconds.) *Who is she?*

A: (Time elapsed, six seconds.) *I don't know* (speech approximation).

The transcription shows Anne being involved in the interaction, but in a passive, responsive mode. Anne would answer closed questions like *Does it come right to your house?* and *Is it one of the children in your class?* but had great difficulty when questions invited a more complex reply, such as *Who else is on the bus?* Anne listed children in her class after the question *Who's in your class,* but took time to think of the answers. Helen was able to understand who Anne was speaking about because of her knowledge of the class, but the observer was not able to transcribe the names of the children. Conversation breakdowns were difficult to repair. At the end of the dialogue excerpt there seems to be an attempt to elaborate but with no success. Helen tried to engage Anne in a story about getting to school and while both seemed to enjoy this interaction, it was Helen who maintained the conversation by asking questions. Helen was providing the scaffolding so that Anne's answers would contribute to the interaction, a characteristic of early narrative development.

Jane's initial story telling depended on the communication aid in use. Jane who was 17;0 years old, exhibited more developed skills than Anne (aged 9;6) when she had access to word prediction. An early example of a story told by Jane illustrates how she would summarize an event by giving the punchline – a characteristic of story telling in very young children.

Jane was using the story-based communication aid in a conversation with Sheila:

S:	*What have you been doing lately?*
J:	(Time elapsed, 30 seconds. Using word-prediction.) *'The mirror broke'* (laughter).

Jane burst into laughter after typing the sentence and did not attempt to elaborate on what transpired to be the punch line of the story. Sheila spent the next 15 minutes helping Jane to articulate the beginning (*my dad was putting a mirror up in the bathroom while I was in the living room*), the middle (*suddenly there was a crash – we went through and found Dad looking sheepish and a broken mirror on the floor*) and the end (*Dad had stuck the mirror up with adhesive tape instead of drilling holes for the screws*).

Although Jane developed story telling skills as she gained experience in using the story-based communication aid, she exhibited similar problems in initiation and elaboration to Anne whenever she used her regular communication aid.

Jane (aged 17:6) using her regular communication aid in a conversation with Paula about education:

P:	*Do you enjoy being at this school?*
J:	(Time elapsed, eight seconds. Prepares to use keyboard.) *'y-e-s'* (looks at Paula).
P:	*And what's your favourite um sport?*
J:	(Time elapsed, seven seconds. Prepares to use keyboard.) *'S-w-i-m-m-i-n-g swimming'* (looks at Paula).
P:	*Ah right how often do you go swimming Paula?*
J:	(Time elapsed, 13 seconds. Prepares to use keyboard.) *'O-n-e-c-e-a-w-e-e-k once a week'* (looks at Paula).
P:	*You must be very fit are you?*
J:	(Time elapsed, 10 seconds. Prepares to use keyboard.) *'y-e-s yes'* (looks at Paula).
P:	*Do you like do you like any other studies at school? Do you like writing do you like writing stories?*
J:	*'Yes'* (looks at Paula).
P:	*What sort of stories do you write?*
J:	(Time elapsed, eight seconds. Looks up and then at keyboard.)
P:	*What was the last story you wrote about?*
J:	(Time elapsed, 20 seconds. Prepares to use keyboard.) *'c-i-o-l-h'* . (Time elapsed, 21 seconds. Prepares to use keyboard.) *'c-o-l-l-e'*. (Time elapsed, 12 seconds. Prepares to use keyboard.) *'e-g-e college'*. (looks at Paula).
P:	*Ooh what's happening at college.*
J:	(Time elapsed, 11 seconds. Prepares to use keyboard.) *'I-e-h-i-s-e period'*. (Time elapsed, 19 seconds. Prepares to use keyboard.) *'i-a-m-g-o-n-i-n-g-t-o-c-h-e-c-o-l-l-e-g'*.
P:	*College, where where are you going and what?*

Jane did not use acceleration techniques when using the communication aid, but typed words letter by letter. Her spasticity made typing slow and laborious as can be seen in her first turn where it took eight seconds before she was able to position her arm for typing. The resulting conversation is one-sided with Paula initiating questions and Jane responding to them. Jane was able to respond well to closed questions that required one-word answers but did not expand on the discussion in any way. Christopher, in the second conversation extract in this chapter, answered Jack's question as to what the hyenas did to the Lion King and then added unsolicited information that Simba's father died. Jane only answered questions and at no stage takes the initiative to expand on the topic Paula introduced.

Viewing the videotape it was evident that Jane was finding it difficult to decide what she wanted to say before she began to prepare herself to physically access the communication aid. Jane's spelling limitations also affected her ability to respond. Paula tried to encourage Jane to answer a general question about the stories Jane writes but needed to narrow it down to *What was the last story you wrote about?* and then it took some time for Jane to begin typing an answer.

In conversations between equal partners there tends to be a balance of conversational control (Cheepen, 1988). This balance changes gradually in development. This was not the case with Anne and Jane, where all control lay with the speaking partner, as in much younger typically developing speaking children. The partners were responsible for initiating and controlling the conversation, attempting to elicit elaborations from Anne and Jane where possible. The need for the speaking partner to encourage elaborations compares with Christopher's dialogue extract. However, Christopher (aged 4;3) responded to minimal prompting with some elaboration. He even redirected the conversation from hyenas to the death of Simba's father. The ability of John, in the third dialogue extract, to use questioning to introduce intrigue into the conversation illustrates conversational skills beyond the abilities of either Anne or Jane.

Adults usually frame or scaffold children's narratives early in their development by using prompts to elicit elaboration. This can be seen with Christopher's conversation. This scaffolding lessens as children take more control in telling a story. John had a more active role as he elaborated without prompting and even used questions to highlight a part of the story. The adults in the conversations with Anne and Jane used prompting to elicit elaboration, but little or no elaboration was forthcoming.

Taking full control

After the introduction of the narrative-based communication aid and structured dialogues about past events a more active role was evident. As soon as the girls had mastered the operational demands of the communication aid (approximately a month into the study) both took more control of the conversation, often to the exclusion of the speaking partner. Initial observations of Anne and Jane using the communication aid show how they would retrieve and tell a story in its entirety without responding to the partner's interaction.

In the following dialogue, Anne (aged 10;1) is using the narrative-based communication aid in conversation with Paula:

A: *'My birthday is on the twenty-first of June'* (smiles, eyes raised from computer, looks down to work with trackball).
P: *How old will you be?*
A: *'This year I was ten.'*
P: *Ten.*
A: *'I got a telly tubby called Laa Laa.'*
P: (Giggles).
A: *'She's yellow with a blue sparkly patch. She says laa when you press her sparkly patch.'* (Smiles, raises eyes from computer, looks down to work with trackball.) *'I got clothes for me going to America on holiday.'*
P: *Oh you're going to America whereabouts?*
A: *'My grannies and aunties and cousins came for a barbecue.'*

The conversation above seems to flow naturally. Anne initiates the story about her birthday. She responds appropriately to Paula's question as to her age. In reality, Anne had already clicked the button to speak *'This year I was ten'* as Paula asked the question. Anne was running through the text with little interaction with Paula and the appropriateness of the conversation here was coincidental. (It does, however, illustrate the predictability of some interactions.) Although Anne raised her eyes from the screen, she never looked at Paula. Paula's question about where Anne was going was completely ignored as Anne stepped through the text sentence by sentence without responding to Paula, without hesitation telling that her grannies, aunties and cousins were coming for barbecue. In comparison with the dialogue extract recorded six months earlier, Anne has control of the interaction and is elaborating using full sentences in this extract.

Jane also told some stories as a monologue when she was first introduced to the story-based communication aid, but this did not last long.

Co-constructing narrative

A conversation recorded six months into Anne's use of the story-based communication aid illustrates the development of a more equal sharing of control. Here Anne (aged 10;1) is using the narrative-based communication aid in conversation with Paula:

A: *'Sometimes when Mary comes to see me at home. Funny things happen.'*

P: (Laughs) *Such as?*

A: *'When ???'* (unintelligible synthetic speech). *'The hamster was out of his cage mum put him in his ball'* (laughter). *'Mum throws the ball across the floor and then he was terrified he was going to ???'* (unintelligible synthetic speech). (Laughter) *'He was so silly'* (laughter) *'???'* (unintelligible synthetic speech) *'upon the table he was very very stupid'* (laughter) *'???'* (unintelligible synthetic speech) *'on the floor now'.*

P: (Laughs.)

A: *'I have a new hamster now.'*

P: *Whats his name? What do you call him?*

A: *'My hamster is called Cher.'*

P: *Cher after the singer. Why is it called Cher? Is it a he or a she? A she presumably.*
Why did you call her Cher? (laughs).

A: *Look. 'Sonny.'*

P: *Sonny and Cher. Do you know who they were? You won't remember. They were pop singers. I think Sonny is dead now. I think he died last year. Cher is still alive singing away.*

Anne has a pre-stored story about her hamster which she initiates when talking to Paula. Anne and Paula interact with laughter as Anne tells the bulk of the story. Anne then initiates the story about her new hamster, responding to Paula's query about the hamster's name by using a pre-stored utterance. The following question as to why the hamster is called Cher, necessitates a novel answer from Anne who types and 'speaks' the word *'Sonny'* after vocalizing *Look*. Anne is not directing the story as Eva did in the dialogue extract about her visit to her aunt but is initiating, elaborating and responding to her partner appropriately. The small monologue about the hamster in the ball has a beginning (*'Funny things happen'*), a middle and an end (*'on the floor now'*). There is also a topic shift introducing her new hamster. Anne and Paula are engaging in mutual co-construction as they share the hamster story.

The two types of co-construction (directed and mutual) can be identified in two of Jane's conversations below. Jane began to use directed co-construction early into her use of the story-based communication aid. Here is Jane (aged 17;3) using the story-based communication aid in a conversation with Helen:

H: *And you were going to tell me something I have not heard.*

J: (Vocalizes, works on computer.)

H: *Tell me something about yourself.*

J: (Works on computer, time elapsed, 21 seconds.) *'I live in the country'* (looks at Helen).

H: *That's really nice. You've just moved there haven't you?*

J: (Vocalizes, works on computer.)

H: *Yeh do you like.*

J: *'Ever since July.'*

H: *Right* (nods).

J: *'It is a very big house'* (glances at Helen).

H: *That's lovely.*

J: *'The garden is very big. It is on the flat'* (continues to look at Helen).

H: That's good for having your chair isn't it Jane? That must mean *you've got lots of space to move around. And you've got big enough spaces to move in* (gestures 'wide' with arms while speaking). *That's really good and you can can you move all around the house.*

J: (Vocalizes, time elapsed, 17 seconds.) *'Yes'.*

Helen initiated a topic in the first turn of the dialogue extract by asking Jane a question. Jane spends some time locating a story and then begins the story. This reflects a major development when compared to Jane's use of a punchline in her earlier dialogue extracts above, when she was unable to initiate a more specific topic about her stories without help. Jane responds appropriately to Helen's comment about her having moved to her house recently, adding an elaboration that she lived there since July. Helen was not expecting this elaboration and had already begun to ask another question in the previous turn. Jane retains control and elaborates further by telling about the size of the house and the garden before Helen in turn expands on Jane's comments about the house. Helen has helped to co-construct the conversation by expanding on Jane's communication. The balance of conversational control has shifted back and forth between both communication partners instead of residing with one or the other.

Here is Jane (aged 17;6) using the story-based communication aid in a conversation with Helen:

J: (Works on computer) *'I was a little bit frightened but very happy to be coming to this college but I was a little bit sad about leaving home and my family.'* (Looks at Paula.)

P: *I bet you are but you enjoying are you enjoying college?*

J: (Time elapsed, 22 seconds, works on computer.) *'Yes'* (looks at Paula).

P: *So what di you tell me a little bit about what you have been doing down there can you?*

J: (Time elapsed, 38 seconds, works on computer.) *'My classes is very good.'*

P: *And what are you studying?*

J: (Time elapsed, 66 seconds, continues to work on computer.) *???* (unintelligible synthetic speech.) (Time elapsed, 44 seconds, works on computer.) *'I am working hard at computers'* (looks at Paula).

The story that Jane had accessed is about college. Instead of speaking all the sentences, Jane used a narration toolbar to skip sentences until she found an appropriate answer to Paula's question about what Jane had been doing down there (the story had additional sentences between *'leaving home and my family'* and *'my classes is very good'*). This only took 38 seconds – the length of the answer is very different to the one-word utterance *'college'* in her earlier dialogue about education with Paula, which took 53 seconds. Moreover, Jane entered new text into the story in her last turn of that dialogue. Jane's development has progressed from using the punchline of a story to using a combination of pre-stored and novel text in mutually co-constructing a story.

Conclusion

Narratives comprise topic initiation and change, turn taking, communication breakdown and repair, elaboration and conclusion, requiring a complex set of skills. This is an interactive experience but aided communication does not easily allow for conversational interactivity and aided communicators generally do not experience the typical development of narrative skills. Both Anne and Jane took a passive role in conversations at the beginning of the study. The dialogue extracts illustrate how the girls progressed from being passive communication partners to being co-constructors of interactions.

Anne began to use the story-based communication aid to take full control of conversations before she developed turn-taking skills. There is evidence that she progressed from being scaffolded through narratives to mutual co-construction with the communication partner. Anne later became more confident in using her speech but elected to retain the aid for situations where she was communicating with unfamiliar people (Waller et al., 2001).

A similar development was evident in Jane's narrative skills although she continued to use aided communication. Jane's inability to initially expand within a conversation could be attributed to two things. Either Jane was not prepared to spend the physical resources to type an expanded answer (this can be seen in the fact she took so long to type out individual words) or she lacked the pragmatic knowledge to do so. Jane's use of a punchline to tell a story suggests that she had never learned how to tell a story and her narrative development was similar to what would be expected of a much younger person. Having the opportunity to control the delivery of a narration and lead a conversation allowed for a more typical experience to take place. Jane's story-telling skills developed to the level where she became a communicator who used mutual co-construction rather than being a passive communicator.

The girls' telling of stories as monologues also reflects their lack of knowledge coming from experience with telling a story. Jane and Anne were initially able to access whole stories, but did not yet have the pragmatic knowledge required for effective, interactive conversation. The observations suggest that the opportunity to manipulate narrative, and the positive experience of telling their stories, helped the girls to become more active communication partners. It seems crucial, in terms of intervention, that the development of narrative skills as outlined above is experienced as close to typical development as possible. These skills can only be developed through experience and it is crucial that communication partners facilitate a shift of control if aided communicators are to become true conversationalists.

Acknowledgements

This research is funded by the Engineering and Physical Science Research Council. We are indebted to Anne and Jane, their parents, teachers and speech therapists for participating in this study.

CHAPTER 12

Late development of independent conversation skills with manual and graphic signs through joint activities

LOURDES TAVARES AND ANA PEIXOTO

In the study of typical language development there is a strong focus on parent-child interaction and the early phases of language acquisition (compare Fletcher and MacWhinney, 1995). A similar emphasis is apparent in studies of augmentative and alternative communication. Most of them describe the first years of intervention and are relatively short term. However, descriptions of child–professional interaction have to some extent replaced descriptions of parent–child interaction. In our clinical experience, alternative modes of communication are used mainly with professionals during training and in some cases with close family members (but often only as a last resort).

One consequence of these biases is that many individuals who use manual and graphic signs have a limited expressive repertoire and sometimes there is also little use in the environment of the communication form that they can understand. They have experience with only a small number of conversation partners, and receive limited support in the more advanced phases of language development, such as during the changes in language and communication that characterize the transition from childhood to adolescence. In Portugal and other countries there is currently a tendency for specialist habilitation services to direct their resources at early intervention - unfortunately at the expense of adolescents and adults. Language plays an important role throughout development, although its nature and function changes over time. The biological and social changes of adolescence will have profound influence on patterns of language use.

During late childhood and early adolescence, conversations replace play as the most time-consuming activity. From the ages of 10 to 15, the average time typically developing adolescents spend talking with each other increases from 1.3 to 2.5 hours per day, or from 9% to 18% of their waking time (Alsaker and Flammer, 1999). An important function of these conversations is to communicate about oneself and others – in particular, the self-disclosure that is typical of adolescence (Rotenberg, 1995). According to Derlega and Grzelak (1979), self-disclosure functions to validate the individual's attitudes, to achieve acceptance from family and friends, and to become aware of which ideas and attitudes that are acceptable and which are not. Both self-disclosure and validated attitudes are social constructions in the sense that they are results of a dialogic collaboration. Self-disclosure is also an important aspect of mature friendships. While 12-year-olds rarely say that they share emotions and personal problems when asked about their relations with friend, these aspects of friendship are typical of the descriptions of those who are a little older. Friends play a pivotal role in young people's construction of identity and their adaptation of new values and attitudes.

Adolescence poses new challenges for the adaptation of the language environment of people who use alternative means of communication. Early provision often focuses on choice-making and the communication of 'needs', issues that are not central to the communication of adolescents, except for those who are severely intellectually impaired. The interpersonal and social skills previously acquired in restricted family and school environments will have to be extended to less familiar settings. Adolescents are expected gradually to gain personal autonomy and independence from their parents through their relationship with peers and joint activities. They look actively for new forms of information and interaction outside the family (Sampaio, 2000).

It may not be the presence or lack of a particular skill that is decisive for communication, but rather how individuals use their skills for communicative purposes in various social situations (Martinsen and von Tetzchner, 1996). Most adolescents who use alternative communication systems have little communicative autonomy – that is, they do not have sufficient means to express their own ideas, opinions and attitudes. They may lack both the appropriate vocabulary and pragmatic skills. At an age when the social network is typically both changing and increasing, and mature relationships are started, most alternative language users have difficulties communicating with speaking people who are not used to their mode of communication. Typically developing eight- to 12-year-olds usually have 40 or more regular communication partners, and no trouble gaining new ones. On average, children in the same age group who use alternative communication have seven interlocutors at the most who can actually understand them (Sweeney, 1999). Moreover, their greatest difficulties usually occur in communicating with other users of alternative communication forms. They are likely to need a speaking person who will interpret between them and relay the content from one communicator to another.

Young users of alternative communication systems face a series of barriers that make it difficult for them to participate in age-typical activities (Beukelman and Mirenda, 1998). They are thus rarely involved in activities such as going to sports events, concerts and cinemas, doing joint activities with a group and sharing holidays, thereby losing a core source of cultural knowledge (Basil, 2001; von Tetzchner, 2001e). Moreover, co-operation involving negotiation of conflicts and disagreements between peers is considered important for social and moral development in adolescence (Juvonen, 1997; Piaget, 1932, 1965; Sampaio, 2001). Limited access to this kind of social encounter may also limit the development of mature communication and language skills, which in turn will make participation in joint activities more difficult and reinforce social and communicative passivity (Alm and Newell, 1996; Basil, 1992).

Unlike typically developing adolescents, the acquisition of new communication skills by young people who use alternative communication will to a great extent depend on the communicative means and experiences provided by professionals. Intervention has typically focused on the individual child and its communication with speaking partners, even in classrooms with more than one user of alternative communication. By contrast, the creation of a community of alternative language users within the greater group of speaking people may increase opportunities for joint activities and for acquiring the values and norms of society and facilitate the development of reciprocal relationships and the acquisition of advanced communication and language skills. This in turn may promote greater autonomy and the construction of identity based on relationships with peers.

The present chapter describes the late development of independent conversation skills with manual and graphic signs in a group of six adolescents, through joint activities and scaffolding by professionals over a period of three years (1998–2001). The examples include only some of the activities that took place in that period of time. The main focus is on the interaction within the group, rather than on individual achievements, but the examples illustrate changes both within the group and in individual adolescents.

Method

The group

The group consisted of four boys and two girls with cerebral palsy who were 10–15 years old when the study began: Pedro, Paulo, João, Helder, Carina and Daniela. They were selected for the study because of similarities in communicative characteristics and learning needs expressed by their families. They lived in the metropolitan area of Porto and attended different schools near their own homes, some of them in regular classes and some in special classes. Five of them had mild motor impairments and could walk, while Pedro used a walking aid due to severe athetosis. All had difficulties with chewing, swallowing and controlling drooling. Pedro also had a severe hearing loss.

All six had severe dysarthria and were unable to express themselves intelligibly in speech. João was unable to produce sounds even to gain the attention of others. They had learning disabilities, but there was little systematic information about their cognitive development. Their comprehension of spoken language was low compared to typically developing peers. Language assessment was carried out with the Bankson Language Screening Test (1977), which is commonly used in Portugal for assessing adolescents with intellectual impairment and limited speech, and informal evaluation. Taken into consideration that norms should be applied with caution, the understanding of language by these young people seemed comparable to that of typically developing children aged three to five years. Comprehension was better than expression, even when allowance was made for the adolescents' use of alternative communication modes, including manual signs, points of objects and graphic representations. However, observation suggested that their everyday comprehension was better than would be predicted from their scores on the Bankson Test. Similar discrepancies between test results and everyday function have been noted by other authors (Soto, 1999; von Tetzchner and Martinsen, 2000). None of the six adolescents were able to read and write, but most could recognize their first name, and some could write it. The children had been taught alternative communication in the form of Picture Communication Symbols (PCS, Johnson, 1981, 1985, 1992) and manual signs adapted from the Portuguese sign language, but they rarely used these in spontaneous communication (see Table 12.1). Due to the motor impairments, many manual signs were performed in an idiosyncratic manner.

Procedures

The adolescents met with the professionals one afternoon every week at the Cerebral Palsy Centre. This was the starting point for joint activities within and outside the Centre. Activities were generally planned for the whole school, and the aim was to facilitate the development of conversational skills and social relations.

Questionnaires were used to investigate the parents' expectations and opinions about their children's development during the study. Meetings with parents were arranged for discussing the adolescents' development at home and in the group activities and to influence the language environments at home. The meetings were also used to teach manual signs to the parents,

Table 12.1. Manual and graphic vocabulary among the adolescents in the group

	Age	MLU	Preferred mode	Graphic signs	Graphic signs spontaneous	Manual signs comprehended	Used
Daniela	12	1–2	Manual signs	290	70	120	?
Paulo	10	2–3	Gestures and vocalization	138	0	?	0
Pedro	13	2–3	Manual and graphic signs	324	120	?	45
João	12	2	Manual signs	228	0	?	50
Carina	15	1–2	Gestures and vocalizations	156	80	?	30
Helder	10	1–2	Gestures and vocalizations	158	50	?	20

discuss new vocabulary and pragmatic goals, and to let the parents share personal experiences with their children's communication. Based on opinions expressed in the initial questionnaire, parent meetings were arranged every two months. After six months, the parents decided to meet every month. They also started to bring other relatives and friends of the family to the meetings.

Video recordings were made every second month in order to assess communicative skills related to the activities. The communicative behaviours observed in the recordings were used to define new communication goals and strategies. The videos were also sometimes presented at the parent meetings, as a basis for the parents' discussion of the group's communication and as communicative models for the parents.

Dependency

A shared characteristic of the adolescents in the group is that they were dependent on an 'interpreter' (typically the mother) to communicate with other people. The problems related to this dependency were expressed throughout the individual family sessions. The mothers said they had to play a double role: on one hand, they were responsible for helping their children to produce more conventional and elaborated utterances than they could express with alternative communication; on the other hand, they had to accept their children's idiosyncratic productions. This concern was related to the different settings in which their children functioned. For example, the mothers were usually interpreters in conversations between fathers and sons, and not always with the desired effect. Challenging behaviours were common among the adolescents and their parents experienced frustration when communicating with them.

The parents' concern at home was transferred to the school, where the parents feared that their children lacked the necessary abilities for making friends. Despite their use of manual and graphic signs, the adolescents were not autonomous communicators. At school, they were dependent on the ability and motivation of others to communicate. The fact that the adolescents often showed challenging behaviours made it difficult for them to establish any kind of positive relationships with their peers, not to mention friendship. Potential conversation partners were wary of their behaviour problems and tended to avoid social and communicative contact. The adolescents therefore had limited conversational skills and usually showed a passive style of communication. They seldom initiated a conversation or changed topics and they never asked any questions. They revealed little ability to organize a message, most of the time appealing to the interlocutor's ability to foresee the content of the message and fill the information gaps. They would stop trying to convey a message if they were not understood at the first attempt.

The apprehension expressed by the adolescents' parents before the group was established was related to all areas of social functioning: communication, enculturation, relationship and autonomy. The adolescents were severely socially dependent in everyday activities. Although five of them had the motor abilities required for physical independence and mobility, they had little experience with social participation and gatherings with peers.

The first group gathering

The group was primarily established to facilitate conversational skills and interaction with peers, but it was assumed that this would influence the adolescents' social and communicative autonomy and their ability to express complex meanings in general. The passivity and social dependence was well illustrated at the first gathering of the group in November 1998:

> Each of the adolescents were shown a picture and produced the corresponding manual sign, which the others in the group should 'guess' the meaning of by indicating the corresponding PCS on their communication board. After having done this several times, until the adolescents seemingly understood the 'game', the professionals went out of the room and the adolescents were left to continue the game by themselves (with the video camera recording). For about five minutes nothing happened. They looked at each other, the cards, the table and the door, until Paulo opened the door and called the professionals.

The inability of the group of adolescents to continue a simple game independently – or engage in some other joint activity – demonstrates that social engagement and positive communicative experiences within the group did not arise spontaneously. There was an evident need for scaffolding both their conversational skills and their communicative autonomy. As a result of this observation a range of activities were targeted to stimulate their use of alternative communication skills in ordinary community settings. The situations and activities included, changed somewhat over the three-year period, from more specific communication situations like buying tickets and shopping in the first year, to more interactive group activities in the third year, like chatting and parties. In addition to expanding the adolescents' communicative experiences by decreasing their level of support, it was also decided to address more formal aspects of alternative communication use through explicit instruction. These formal aspects included learning the conventional form of manual signs, the structure of the vocabulary, the production of multi-sign utterances, and the temporal organization of narratives and longer messages.

Activities and settings

The group took part in a wide range of joint activities during the three-year period. These included making and 'writing' Christmas cards, shopping for clothes and other 'teenage accessories', having snacks in restaurants, going to cinemas, theatres, exhibitions, birthday parties and public parties like San Martinho and San João, and going camping. However, the main activity became chatting.

All the activities were prepared in the weekly sessions with the approval of the adolescents as well as their parents. The adolescents were guided to foresee any challenges they might face in the activities and to become aware of the vocabulary they might need. They said they felt more confident in outdoor activities when they were together, supported each other and shared the same enjoyment and fear related to the activities. If one of them had difficulties in communication, the others would provide help and at the end congratulate him or her with the success of the task. Communication difficulties did not always reside with the adolescents. Unfamiliar communication partners also learned through interaction with them, as in this visit to the cinema:

When Helder as the first of the group opened his communication board and started to order tickets using PCS, the lady behind the glass in the ticket box stared at the professionals that accompanied the group, clearly asking for help. She was just told to read the glosses above each graphic sign. Helder was also looking at the professionals, and looked like he was going to give up, but was encouraged to repeat his message by pointing at the signs again. Slowly Helder started to do so. On the other side of the glass, the lady was reading aloud, gloss-by-gloss and then asked Helder: *Do you want a ticket to the film at seven o'clock?* Helder nodded affirmatively, gave her the money and took the change and the ticket, with a victorious look in his eyes. He then signed THANK-YOU, forgetting that the ticket lady did not understand manual signs. When he saw the look of surprise on the lady's face, he opened the communication board once again and indicated *THANK-YOU*. The lady answered: *You're welcome.*

When Carina as the next one in the queue arrived at the counter, the lady was no longer staring at the professionals, but looked at Carina and read aloud the glosses of the PCS signs to which Carina was pointing. After the lady had sold tickets to four of the six members of the group, understanding between her and the adolescents was well established. When Daniela needed to ask for her ticket, she got lost in her request at one point. Graciously, the ticket lady showed Daniela the PCS sign she was supposed to point at next. So Daniela managed to buy her own ticket like the others.

In the example above, the success of Helder in meeting the communicative challenge of buying a ticket contributed to making the speaking woman a more competent communication partner. She was able to understand the graphic communication, and in fact took a supportive role with Daniela, with no prior knowledge of aided communication. This demonstrates that not only do aided communicators change through more varied communicative experience but their language environment also changes through their use of communication aids.

Each time the group went out, the professionals had decided beforehand the amount of scaffolding that would be provided if difficulties arise. As a rule, the adolescents and their interlocutors were supposed to solve familiar problems that arose. The professionals functioned as a safety net, and help was usually given only in new situations, in unforeseen circumstances and if severe breakdowns of communication occurred. If help was requested by the adolescents, the lowest functional level of help was given. As the adolescents became more used to handle new communicative challenges, requests for help became fewer. They learned to be aware of the skills of their communication partners and to use graphic rather than manual signs when they addressed unfamiliar communication partners. In fact, their communicative confidence is illustrated by the fact that they would tease people who did not know manual signs, as in this example where they were buying stamps for Christmas cards:

> Paulo was the first in line and used manual signs to ask for stamps. The lady in the shop just stared at him. Turning to the others in the group he signed: SHE DUMB! SHE NOT TALK HANDS! They all laughed and Paulo brought the communication board to ask for stamps.

As manual signs were not in common use in Portugal, the adolescents were often asked to show signs that corresponded to certain spoken words. For example, when the group was camping, the electricity failed, the adolescents had to go to the reception to ask for candles. The man in the reception showed great interest in manual signing and asked them to teach him a lot of signs. The adolescents were usually proud when asked to teach manual signs to others, and this kind of reaction from speaking people gave status to manual signing and promoted its use.

The increase in social and communicative autonomy of the group may be illustrated by the gradual decrease in the numbers of professionals needed on the annual camping trips. In the first year, there were six adults and six adolescents. In the second year, there were five adults, and in the third year, there were three adults and the camping trip lasted one day longer.

Talking about the past: narratives

All the members of the group had difficulties relating personal and fictional events in a coherent and comprehensible manner and making themselves understood by others who did not share the same knowledge. In November 1999, each family was asked to select a significant social event in the family to be told to the group in the weekly sessions. The focus was on facilitating the development of narrative skills, but this home task became a joint family project that involved the parents in the alternative communication forms used by their children. The parents' concern was that their children should be able to make themselves understood and relay the significant event to the others. The family tended to rehearse the story, focusing more on whether the group would understand than on the comprehension of the family members. For example, they started to reject idiosyncratic 'home' signs, which they had previously accepted at home in favour of conventional manual signs understood by everybody in the group. The adolescents knew each other prior to the study, but had not been used to communicate directly with each other and did not always understand each other's home signs. Instead of accepting just one sign as representing the idea or event that should be expressed, and which they later might end up explaining, the parents began to demand simple sentences, usually with the word order of spoken Portuguese. As a result of this joint activity, the parents used more manual signs in conversations with their children, asked professionals to teach them new signs, and provided the children with help when they became lost in attempts to relay the information. In this process, the parents in fact scaffolded the children's narratives in the same way as parents of younger typically developing children do (Pan and Snow, 1999). Through this, they increased the communicative autonomy of their children.

In spite of the families' efforts, at the group meetings, the adolescents still had difficulties relating events in the correct order. However, they would ask for help only when they were totally unable to proceed with the idea or event they wanted to relay. The personal narratives were always unknown to the others and usually elicited many questions and comments, which to some extent also functioned as scaffolding during narration. The process allowed the adolescents to learn about themselves and the others and provided the members of the group with more shared knowledge. In February 2000, the personal narrative was established as a routine of the weekly meetings.

A special narrative: the black light theatre

The ability to reflect the actual sequence of events in a narrative retelling remained a major problem for the adolescents in the group. Stories and drama have been demonstrated to enhance the communication skills of children using alternative communication (Grove, 1998; Grove and Park, 2000), and as a means to facilitate narrative skills, a suggestion for performing a play was made. The format of the black light theatre was chosen, that is, a stage where only elements painted with fluorescent light are visible.

However, narration was not the only reason for presenting a play. The first group gathering had demonstrated the adolescents' inability to use language to create joint activities independently. While the personal narratives were communicated individually – with some help from the family and the audience – the play required collaboration and teamwork. A traditional folktale was used because it was known and would be understood by nearly everybody. The sequence of the play and the inherently consistent text made it easy for the adolescents to memorize their parts and help each other. However, there were still significant disagreements and even conflicts in the negotiation of roles and tasks. There were several attempts at joint construction of the play – with quick alternations between consensus and disagreement – before the final version was ready. Errors and mistakes were not always well accepted by all. The limitations in expressive means made these discussions and the group work complicated, while at the same time providing the group members with serious and meaningful communicative interactions.

In the course of the shared work, the group evolved from mainly being helped by adults (parents and professionals) to helping and supporting each other. The help they gave each other replaced the verbal and physical assistance of the adults, and they gradually took increasing responsibility for the performance of the play. Thus, when the play was shown in May 2000 to a group invited by the adolescents, for the parents it was the attainment of their children's autonomy. For the adolescents, to present a signed play had a significant effect on their self-esteem. The fact that in most of the play only six pairs of white, fluorescent hands were visible emphasized the function of manual signs and gave prominence to their communication. (One year after the first performance, the group was still asked to present the play in various public and private institutions.)

More important, however, was the effect that the teamwork had on the adolescents' ability to solve disagreements and conflicts through negotiations using language. This is illustrated by the change in Daniela's behaviour. When the group was established, she often showed challenging behaviour. The behaviour often occurred unexpectedly and it was not always easy to understand the reasons for it. It happened when she was understood and when she was not, when she was happy or bored, scared or angry, when she had to wait for her turn and when she was anxious, but it seemed particularly frequent when she was in unfamiliar settings and when she was frustrated. Her parents always made sure nobody was near their daughter when they arrived somewhere, because Daniela would pull the hair of anybody nearby. In the first rehearsal Daniela would pull somebody's hair when it went dark and when there was a sudden sound. As the group work proceeded, Daniela stopped being wary of the adults during the play. She knew not only that the play had to be performed in the dark but also that there would be loud music every now and then. It seemed as though the control of the situation gained through her discussions about the play helped her regulate her emotional reactions. The behaviour problems thus gradually disappeared as her communicative skills increased and her understanding of the world around her enabled her to predict what was going to happen and adjust to the demands of the environment.

Talking about the future: planning as communication

The communicative dependency shown by the members of the group when the study was initiated also implied a general dependency and lack of personal autonomy. In May 1999, six months after the beginning of the group's activities, it was suggested to the parents that the group should go on a two-day camping trip. The parents were not used to their children being away, and hence there was one indisputable condition linked to it: the trip was only for the adolescents with no parents allowed. The trip was planned for July and the two to three months prior to this were used to plan the camping trip, both in the weekly sessions where the adolescents were alone and in the sessions when the parents were present.

When planning the first trip, the primary objective was to provide all the members of the group with vocabulary items that they would need for the discussion, as well as new vocabulary that might be needed during the camping trip, for example related to setting up tents, finding services, asking questions about how, where, who, how many, what, and so forth. It was assumed that discussion about weather and clothing might arise. Manual signs related to clothing were reviewed in the group, and each of them had to make a list with PCS signs containing the clothes they planned to bring along, and which they could use when they were packing. The vocabulary was thus expanded both through a domain-oriented strategy (adding new manual and graphic signs belonging to an activity or a topic) and through surface-oriented strategies (adding signs for new activities and topics) (von Tetzchner and Martinsen, 2000).

When a similar camping trip was planned the following year, a number of new topics were discussed, based on the group's experiences on the first trip. One central topic was the rules that everybody would have to obey during the trip. The professionals did not introduce certain rules, but left it to the group to agree on rules and discuss the reasons for particular rights and duties. There was usually swift agreement about the negative consequences of someone starting to make noise when others wanted to sleep, or of someone putting rubbish in a place where others wanted to play cards. In these planned 'intervention sessions', the role of alternative communication changed. The focus of the discussions was no longer primarily on the alternative communication but rather on the rules within the group and in society in general. Although the expressive means of all the members of the group were limited, the group had moved from mainly using activities to learn language to using language to plan activities and to discuss issues that were important for the adolescents.

Language is at the same time an instrument for and the outcome of enculturation. The increased communicative autonomy seemed to contribute to changes in independence and autonomy in general. Parallel to the group discussions, there were also discussions about independence and autonomy in the parent meetings. For example, through discussion it had become known that João never bathed alone, and did not put on his shoes or got dressed by himself, despite the fact that he did not have a motor impairment that would have prevented him from doing so (and in fact he did it when he was at the camp). When his parents were asked about the reasons for this, they answered: *Simply because he isn't used to it and always asks his mother to do it.* The passivity learned over many years thus went far beyond the domain of communication.

Through the group gatherings, the adolescents had also started to chat, talk about this and that without any particular purpose except talking. The pleasure of chatting can only be learned through chatting, and as the vocabulary and conversational skills increased, chatting had become a favourite pastime, as it is for typically developing adolescents. During the camping trip, with the possibility of staying up late without any parents making them go to bed early, the group started to go for a cup of coffee at the café in the park, which is also a culturally significant activity of adolescence and adulthood in Portugal.

Discussion

The present study demonstrates that significant achievements in language acquisition are possible in late childhood and adolescence, even when alternative communication has been implemented relatively early in life. The adolescents described here seemed to have a developmental potential that had not been realized due to lack of scaffolding. Their conversational skills at the start of the study were much lower than that of their peers. Although this was also related to their cognitive and linguistic impairments, it is probable that conversational skills would have developed earlier had scaffolding by adults been more skilled. The early focus on choice making, communication to obtain things and interaction with caregivers seemed to have persisted into late childhood and adolescence. Commenting on a similar situation, Basil and Soro-Camats (1996) write: 'This means that in some cases where progress appears satisfactory, more ambitious goals and more advanced intervention strategies should be introduced' (p. 271). As users of alternative communication get older, the planning of their language environment should also change, always focusing on communication within settings and activities that are meaningful for them in the different phases of development. In late childhood and adolescence, the conversational skills needed for interacting with peers would be a natural target for intervention.

The intervention described here was truly 'functional' in the sense that it emerged from age-typical activities instead of some predetermined goal. The use of joint activities seems to have been critical in the intervention and is underpinned by the recognition that adolescents with disabilities should be allowed to do what other adolescents do and, importantly, that constraints on functions may not lie solely in the individual's impairment but also in the quality of adaptations of the environment. A common definition of disability is that it is the gap between the demands of society and the abilities of the individual. If the demands are lowered or the abilities increase, the gap will be narrowed (Frederiksen et al., 1991). The adolescents in the present study became less disabled due to both their improved communication skills and the change in the language environment.

Joint activities ensured that the focus was on functional use of language and on group participation as a force of change. Another critical factor was the scaffolding approach used in the present study, supporting the adolescents in creating solutions to their own communicative challenges. While dependency characterized their communication at the start, they appeared much more autonomous at the end of the study. This was mainly achieved by scaffolding communicative situations that the members of the group had never experienced before, partly by giving them access to relevant vocabulary and the opportunity to plan conversations, and partly through support to overcome many years of learned helplessness and passivity. Although their vocabulary increased, the most important development was their greater assertiveness in its use.

One important consequence of the adolescents becoming more independent communicators was increased use of alternative communication by their parents. Over the three years, the parents used more manual signs in conversations with their children, asked professionals to teach them new signs more frequently, and scaffolded their children's communication but provided them with gradually less visual and manual help. The effect of the adolescents on their parents thus led to the parents having a positive influence on their children, and so on, in a positive transactional chain (see

Sameroff, 1987). However, it was probably the increase in peer interaction that was the most significant in effecting change. Many authors have pointed out the importance of horizontal relations (between equal partners) in the acquisition of cultural knowledge and morals (see Bukowski, Newcomb and Hartup, 1996, Dunn, 1999). The group members showed more co-operative and helping attitudes towards each other, attentiveness and responsibility. This change is also a fundamental aspect of communication development and enculturation.

In Portugal, as in many other countries, there are significant barriers to the social participation of people who use alternative means of communication (compare Beukelman and Mirenda, 1998). Group membership not only increased conversations with familiar communication partners but gave better access to the society at large, and thus to the process of enculturation in general. The implication for interventionists is that it is autonomy and social participation in meaningful local activities and in society in general that should guide professionals working for people acquiring alternative means of communication.

CHAPTER 13

Supporting the development of alternative communication through culturally significant activities in shared educational settings

GLORIA SOTO AND STEPHEN VON TETZCHNER

The critical environments for the acquisition of communicative and linguistic competence comprise three major activity settings: the home, the nursery or school, and the environment of unstructured and structured leisure activities. Each has its different demands and influences. However, for children who acquire alternative means of communication, the quality of the environments and the type of influence they have on the children's communication and language development may differ significantly from that of normally speaking children.

As identified by a number of researchers (see Soto, 1999 for a detailed description), language learning for children using alternative communication forms might be influenced by factors that are not usually at issue in typical language learning environments and that might interact in ways that are not yet fully understood. Some of these factors relate to the multi-modal representation of linguistic elements, the asymmetry of input mode (primarily auditory) and output mode (primarily visual) and the acquisition settings. What Bruner (1983) calls the 'language acquisition support system' - the environmental support provided by more competent children and adults - may be very different for speaking children and children using alternative communication systems. In addition to the exploratory and interactive restrictions associated to their disabilities and the transactional effects of their limited initiations, most children who use alternative modes of communication have no access to proficient alternative communicators. As Brekke and von Tetzchner describe (this volume), the children's most significant communication partners may have only marginally higher – or even lower – alternative language competence than the children. This is likely to lead to very few interactions with competent users of their own communication form and as such hinder the children's development of communicative skills. Moreover, most children who need alternative communication forms do not begin to use them until they start their schooling experience. As such, the educational environment is a critical setting for the acquisition of communication and language skills for children who use alternative communication systems.

Typically, the educational environment of children and adolescents has a set of requirements that differ from those of most other settings of which children are part. It is a relatively predictable setting in which children spend hundreds of hours in the forming years in interaction with significant adults and peers. Shared or 'inclusive' education of children with diverse skills and abilities is based on the postulate that it is the responsibility of society to meet the educational needs of all children regardless of their ability levels, national origin and linguistic, cultural and family background, and that all children have the fundamental right to be educated with their peers in age-appropriate heterogeneous classrooms in their neighbourhood schools (Thousand and Villa, 1992). A growing body of research documents that children who use alternative forms of communication can receive appropriate education within ordinary classrooms along with their typically developing peers, and that this in fact may lead to higher academic achievement than in secluded settings (e.g., Hunt et al., 2002; Soto et al., 2001).

The present chapter is not concerned with ordinary educational goals and academic achievement but with the role of educational settings as language environments for children who use alternative communication forms. Although education is important for participation in society and quality of life in general for most individuals, the focus of this chapter is on communication and language and the most optimal conditions for their development.

The school environment will influence vocabulary growth and other aspects of language development in all children in different ways explicitly through literacy education, explanations of words and the teaching of grammatical analysis; and implicitly through the teacher's and the students' conversations about various topics. In addition, children take part in a great variety of peer conversations, some within group work and other forms of educational activities, but most outside instructional activities. For children who use alternative forms of communication, the influence of educational settings on language acquisition may be even larger than for typically developing children because explicit teaching may also comprise the meaning and use of manual and graphic signs. There may also be implicit influences through adaptations of the environment in order to enhance ordinary conversations within and outside the classroom. However, little is known about the interactions in which children who use alternative communication systems are part in nursery and school – that is, about the changes in their language environments and the 'natural' course of these children's language development.

Guided participation

In social-constructivist theories of development, children acquire language and other 'cultural tools' through interaction with their caregivers and other adults and children. In these interactions, those who are more competent, 'guide', 'assist' or 'scaffold' the performance of those who are less competent (Renner, this volume; Rogoff et al., 2001; Vygotsky 1962, 1978). According to Vygotsky, individual development is the result of joint problem solving with others who are more skilled and competent in the use of relevant cultural skills and tools. In order for a child to acquire new skills and knowledge, this co-construction must be within the child's 'zone of proximal development', that is, the child must understand the nature of the 'task', for example a communicative challenge, but is unable to solve it without the help of others.

Rogoff has supplemented Vygotsky's notion of zone of proximal development with the concept of 'guided participation'. This concept refers to the process of involvement of children with other children and adults as they communicate and engage in shared endeavours (Rogoff, 1993). It is through engagement in social interactions that children are attempting to understand and interpret other people's communicative intentions so as to make sense of situations and events (Nelson, 1985; Tomasello, 1999). For instance, few words are learned through simply naming and pointing. When attempting to comprehend the use of novel linguistic symbols, children use all kinds of interpretative strategies based on the assumption that the novel linguistic symbol is somehow relevant to the ongoing action and interaction (see Akhtar and Tomasello 1996; Bloom, 1993, Tomasello and Akhtar, 1995; Tomasello and Barton, 1994). However, guided participation is not limited to the kind of dyadic interactions that often have been the focus of developmental research. Rather, it promotes a focus on systems of relationships – including present and distant partners, groups and institutions – that must be described in terms of local implicit developmental achievements rather than on 'ideal' milestones of development.

Throughout development, the amount and quality of guidance change with the unfolding of new child competence. What constitutes optimal support at a particular point in time depends on the prior developmental achievements of the individual child. This implies that a child's communication partners must have appropriate understanding of its competence and at least an implicit understanding of the kind of adaptations that may promote the child's communication and language development. Physical and social guidance and adaptations that support the acquisition of alternative language forms afford true communicative co-constructions within the child's particular zone of proximal development in the area of communication and language.

Development through activity

According to activity theory, which belongs to the social-constructivist tradition, children's development is situated in their participation in activities that are specific to the social and cultural settings that comprise their culture. The culture encompasses the range and type of the settings and activities that together constitute the immediate ecology of children. In Western communities, many early communicative interactions are related to the variety of activities that takes place within everyday routines. Play is one pivotal activity in which learning takes place, although learning is not an objective of play. In fact, the only definitional characteristic of play is that it has no other purpose than itself. Teaching may be fun, interesting and positively challenging, but it is never play. As children develop, they participate in an increasing range of physical and social settings, and the complexity and variety of the activities increase. In this process, the 'communities of learners' that are tied to didactic schooling play an increasingly important role – first in the nursery, later in school (Brown and Campione, 1994; Elkonin, 1988; Rogoff, 1993).

Within the framework of activity theory, 'activity' is not just any set of individual actions or social interactions, but a stable and complex system of purposeful actions and interactions that children gradually take part in as they get older and more competent. The internalization of the culture's activities is an essential part of children's cognitive and linguistic development. Vygotsky and Elkonin describe six stages in the development of activities in children (Table 13.1). In the fourth stage, beginning around the age of seven years, instructional activities start to play an important role in children's development of thinking.

One important implication of the internalization framework of activity theory is that there are two aspects of development: 'external' and 'internal'. The activities in which children take part comprise their external thinking, where they are guided by more competent members of society. External thinking precedes children's internal thinking and contributes to create internal thinking through a process of internalization. It may be noted that the external and hence the internal thinking will be influenced by historical changes, for example in technology, that may determine the significant activities of the culture.

Table 13.1. Vygotsky and Elkonin describe six stages in the development of activities (Thomas, 1996, p. 288–289)

---

1 *Intuitive and emotional contact between child and adults (birth to age 1)*
   The basic types of development produced by this contact include feeling a need for interacting with other people, expressing emotional attitudes towards them, learning to grasp things and displaying a variety of perceptual actions.

2 *Object-manipulation activity (ages 1–3)*
   Children adopt socially accepted ways of handling things, and through interaction with adults they develop speech and visual-perception thinking (memory images).

3 *Game-playing activity (ages 3–7)*
   Children engage in symbolic activities and creative play. They now have some comprehension of how to cooperate together in group endeavours.

4 *Learning activity (ages 7–11)*
   Children develop theoretical approaches to the world of things, a function that involves their considering objective laws of reality and beginning to comprehend psychological preconditions for abstract theoretical thought (intentional mental operations, mental schemes for problem solving, reflective thinking).

5 *Social-communications activity (ages 11–15)*
   Adolescents gain skills in initiating types of communication needed for solving life's problems, in understanding other people's motives and in consciously submitting to group norms.

6 *Vocational-learning activity (ages 15–17)*
   Older adolescents develop new cognitive and vocational interests, grasp elements of research work and attempt life projects.

Inclusive education as an appropriate cultural setting

Educational environments comprise a particular set of activities instituted by society for providing children with valued knowledge and skills. From a language perspective, nurseries and schools typically provide social and cultural settings that afford the transition from everyday communication and language to both literacy and communication about complex academic issues like mathematics and science. Educational inclusion means that children with atypical language development participate in ordinary educational activities in physical and social settings shared with typically developing children, and are guided towards language and other forms of shared cultural knowledge through the adaptation of activities and settings to the developmental achievements and skills of these children. Thus, true inclusion depends on appropriate guidance from adults and more competent peers. However, even within a structured environment like a school, in most cases, adapted guidance does not seem to evolve naturally. In order for shared participation to take place, interactions with more competent peers may have to be supported or 'scaffolded' by adults (see von Tetzchner and Grove, this volume), for example by staging enticing settings for peer interaction and guiding typically developing children to adapt their style of interaction to the developmental achievements of children using alternative means of communication (Hunt et al., 2002; Schuler and Wolfberg, 2000). The main objective of scaffolding is to make links between children's already established knowledge and new knowledge. Language development is not a process whereby linguistic knowledge is delivered in appropriate 'packages' by more competent language users to less competent children. Inherent in the process of alternative language development are the shared efforts by children who use alternative communication and speaking adults and peers in establishing joint understanding on which they base interaction and co-construction of knowledge. All participants are active.

The present chapter describes some strategies that have been used to support communication and language development of children who use alternative communication in general education classrooms. These strategies are related to class–teacher interaction, group activities, conversations and play, and include the use of narratives and scripts, the adaptation of settings to promote shared participation and facilitation of peer mediation and support, such as peer tutoring, conversation books, play groups and circles of friends. Most of the strategies have been investigated over the last few years.

Peer interaction

When children who use alternative communication are included in a general education classroom, both they and the other children in the class may need some support to interact successfully. The function of the support is to facilitate the children's initiation and maintenance of interaction. The types of support that are applied will depend on the age and developmental achievements of both the speaking children and the children using manual and/or graphic signs, as well as the activities in which the children are engaged. For instance, during the pre-school years a substantial part of peer interaction occurs in play activities. For school-age children, peer interaction in the classroom is constrained within group work and other activities involving co-operative learning. Outside the classroom, children form groups that are involved in various forms of interaction. Membership in these groups is related to popularity and peer acceptance, but close friendships may exist both inside and outside the wider groups (George and Hartmann, 1996; Parker and Asher, 1993).

The nursery unit and classroom are essential parts of children's language environment and a shared means of communication is a necessary foundation for interaction between peers within and outside the unit or classroom. It is a characteristic of children who use alternative communication that they are unable to speak or speak so unintelligibly that speech cannot function as their main form of communication. This implies that a shared form of communication depends on speaking children becoming competent in the alternative form. Even if a child using manual signs understands spoken language, it is not true inclusion if the speaking children in the class only understand a few signs and communicate mainly by asking yes/no questions. Joint participation implies at least some degree of communicative autonomy, of equality in taking the floor and having one's say. Inclusion thus requires the creation of a shared language environment and the most important role of the interventionist may in fact be to teach alternative communication to the speaking children and ensure that they have enough competence to expand their manual or graphic communication in natural settings involving group interactions and child–child conversations without support of adults. This means that the alternative communication forms become part of the everyday communication in the unit or class. This may be illustrated with the description by Brekke and von Tetzchner (this volume) of how Pictograms and Blissymbols were taught to the whole class and used in group work by all the children, not only by the group that the child who used graphic signs for expressive communication was part of. With shared communicative competence, all kinds of joint activities and conversations became possible.

Nurseries

Research suggests that play activities and materials may have an effect on the amount of communicative interaction in nurseries. Opportunities for social interaction occur frequently in activities that require co-operative or shared play, such as blocks, trains, dolls and stores. Highly structured and predictable routines with clear roles that require co-operation seem especially appropriate to foster social interaction, such as doctor and shop play. The same qualities seem to affect social interaction among children in inclusive environments. Social interaction also increases when children with disabilities use highly preferred toys because typically developing peers try to negotiate access to those toys (Guralnick, 2001; Odom and Bailey, 2001).

Play is a language-affording activity. For children using alternative communication, the planned aspects of their language environment in the nursery may include adults establishing groups around pretend play with a familiar outline and allocation of specific roles to the children involved. For example, during storekeeping play, one or two children may be vendors and the others customers, and the roles may change during play. Communicative scaffolding may include a communication aid with voice output which the storekeepers can use to ask the customers 'What would you like?' or 'Who is next?' and so forth. However, the children may negotiate roles and other elements of the play without much interference from adults, depending on the age and cognitive functioning of the children.

Scaffolded play groups thus offer children who use alternative communication opportunities for playing and communicating with speaking peers. The various forms of support are directed at both the speaking children and the children using alternative communication. Scaffolding corresponds with the principle of guided participation – that is, that children develop while participating actively in culturally valued activities with the guidance, support and challenge of children and adults who vary in skill and status (Rogoff, 1993; Schuler and Wolfberg, 2000; Vygotsky, 1978). There are opportunities for 'novice' and 'expert' users of alternative communication to co-ordinate play, and experts may challenge other players to produce increasingly complex meanings with alternative communication forms. Adults may entice the players to discover common ground on which they can collaborate in mutually enjoyable activities. Initially, most speaking children will require some assistance while acquiring the competence needed to use alternative communication in various forms of play. This may entail supporting speaking children in recognizing and responding to utterances in an alternative form of communication, and maintaining and expanding interactions between children in already established play routines. As all the children become increasingly competent in interacting with alternative communication forms, the degree of scaffolding is naturally reduced. However, as in nursery interaction in general, adult support may be needed if communication breaks down or conflicts arise.

Schools

When children start school, they become members of the school community and especially their classrooms. They participate in school events and instructional routines. Communication activities include participation in classroom conversations, following teacher directions, answering questions and requesting clarifications, as well as understanding the teacher's explanations and descriptions. In inclusive settings, the communication forms children bring to school and the ways in which they use language to make sense of ideas and information are the bases for interactions with teachers and peers. As discussed above, how the alternative communication functions as a shared cultural tool will depend on the alternative language competence of the teacher and the other children in the class.

Within the classroom setting, co-operative learning activities in groups usually constitute good opportunities for peer communication. There may be a small group of children with varying language means and skills, who work together to complete a common task related to a school topic. This learning model requires that children help and support each other as they complete tasks (Merritt and Culatta, 1998). Hence, co-operative strategies are interactive, language-based didactic structures that may support the acquisition of conversational skills and social skills in general, both for speaking children and children using alternative means of communication. During co-operation children may provide or request information, recount past events, comment or clarify on some idea, event or state of affair, resolve conflicts and elaborate on others' ideas. As students acquire new competence in interacting with each other, they become partners within instructional exchanges with the opportunity to learn from and teach each other (Damon and Phelps, 1989). Co-operative learning has been recognized as a scaffolding environment for heterogeneous groups of children, including those who use augmentative communication systems. During co-operative learning, the complexity of the task and the corresponding communicative activities with different possible executions and outcomes are related to the spoken and alternative language skills of all the children within the group. If the alternative language competence in the environment is poor, this is likely to limit what Valsiner (1987) calls children's 'zone of freedom of movement' in learning. Co-operative learning strategies have also been found related to positive interaction and interchange between children (see Hunt et al., 2002; Rogoff et al., 2001).

In a recent study, Hunt and her colleagues (2002) found that co-operative learning in classroom activities increased the number of communicative opportunities available to children who used alternative communication and their level of engagement. Three young aided communicators in ordinary nursery, first grade and fifth grade received various communication supports to promote classroom participation, including communication boards for commenting to classmates, voice-output communication devices to support participation in classroom discussions and a bell to indicate the desire to ask or answer questions. They received social supports, including partner systems, social facilitation by adults, small group instruction and learning centres, to increase their interaction with peers. Communication and social supports were also established to decrease periods of non-engagement in classroom activities and increase the children's possibilities for initiating communicative interactions and ask questions, make comments and answer questions within instructional activities, and increase interactions between the aided communicators and their classmates.

Observations and interviews with parents and professionals showed that after 25 weeks with scaffolding in the form of social and communication supports, the share of time spent in interaction with peers increased for the three aided communicators from an average of 2%, 5.2% and 8.7%, respectively, to 40.8%, 35.7% and 37%, which is a degree of interaction comparable to their peers (see Hunt et al., 2002). In addition to the significant increases in interactions with classmates, the amount of time spent without engagement in classroom activities decreased to levels consistent with those of their classmates. According to interviews with the professionals, the three children using communication aids had become more eager to participate in class activities and discussions, and more confident, assertive and independent in conversations in general.

Increases in communicative interactions and decreases in time without engagement in classroom activities may have been due, at least in part, to participation in interactive, collaborative activities with adaptations and support from peer partners. True participation – as opposed to opportunities for being a spectator only – was scaffolded by the provision of vocabulary that was relevant to the co-operative task, in this case dissecting a frog and discussing the process and the findings. This activity was also organized so that one speaking child worked together with one child using alternative communication. Other interactive activities that may serve as the basis for reciprocal exchanges can range from educational activities like storybook reading, journal writing, interactive mathematics and art projects to recreational activities like doing games and gossiping or telling jokes.

As children grow older, leisure-time play is substituted with other joint activities, in particular conversations. Thus, among school-age children, play groups gradually grow into cliques and adolescent groups and groupings related to interests and ethnic background (von Tetzchner, 2001a). For children acquiring alternative language forms, organized 'circles of friends' may be part of the planned language environment. These organized groups may meet regularly around a common interest, such as movies, books or music, after school or during lunch break or recess (Forest, Pearpoint and O'Brien, 1996).

When circles of friends meet regularly and consistently, they become an important social setting for the development of conversational skills for children who use alternative communication as they negotiate the topics of each meeting, and for enhancing the competence in alternative communication among the speaking children. For older children and adolescents, circles of friends may become natural environments for sharing age-related experiences and for the self-disclosure conversations that seem to be so important in identity formation (Rotenberg, 1995).

A scaffolding strategy related to circles of friends is that of 'peer buddy systems'. Speaking classmates may support children who use alternative communication through the educational activities of the school day and joint child activities before, during and after school. Buddies are communication partners and may assist children who use alternative communication when communicative challenges arise (Hunt et al., 1996). The communicative and social supports provided by buddies can vary from being social company during transitions to working collaboratively or having lunch together in the student cafeteria (Villa and Thousand, 1996).

The buddy system is usually organized as one peer partner for the day. It is our experience that this is a very popular role. Usually each child is allowed to be buddy for a day every five weeks, depending on class size and number of children using alternative communication system. The function of the buddy is to collaborate with the alternative communication user in the participation of ordinary school days. The partners complete their work for the day and follow the same routines as the other children in the class. Some of the children are motor impaired and may need physical assistance in some activities in addition to communicative scaffolding. However, the role of the buddy is not primarily to be a helper, but to be an equal companion, even if the companionship is planned. The buddy system may apply to users of manual signs and of graphic communication.

Narration

Supports that have been used to sustain communication include conversation books, peer-buddy systems, interactive media and book reading (for example, Hunt et al., 2002). 'Conversation books' contain photographs of objects, places, activities and people that interest the children. Conversation books serve as a topic menu for initiating conversational exchanges. Both the speaking children and the children using alternative communication are guided to use the book as a shared basis for communication in accordance with their communication and language skills and abilities and interests in general. For children with intellectual disability, scaffolding may comprise teaching them specific comments related to the photographs, for example: *JACK DOG MINE*. Speaking peers may be guided to ask questions that the vocabulary of the child using alternative communication allows to answer. They may also be told to give the alternative communication user enough time to initiate and reply, and prolong the dialogue by making new comments (compare Hunt, Alwell and Goetz, 1991).

However, in this kind of scaffolded interaction between speaking children and children using alternative communication systems, the speaking children may take the role of teachers rather than peers, as in this dialogue between

an aided communicator (A) and a naturally speaking peer (N) described by
Romski and Sevcik (1996, p. 98):

    N: *Hi there. What are you eating?*
    A: *???* (unintelligible speech).
    N: *Pizza. Is it good?*
    A: *'Good.'*
    N: *What do you need to eat with?*
    A: *'Fork.'*
    N: *Good, fork. OK, let's eat.*

Although it often happens that more competent peers adapt their style of
communication to a perceived less competent communication partner, the
language environment becomes 'normalized' as the speaking children take
the role of ordinary conversation partners on an equal footing.

Conversations around books that include personal photographs have
been used to facilitate children's joint construction of personal narratives. In
typical development, early narratives are usually scaffolded by parents or
other adults (Fivush and Hammond, 1990; Pan and Snow, 1999). Together
with adults, children describe events and actions they have been involved in,
such as taking a trip to the zoo or an amusement park. This also introduces
children to conventionalized discourse practices.

Narration is a central means of enculturation in school and other settings.
Adults' true and fictional stories serve to establish cultural values and guide
children's understanding of self and others (Fivush, 1991; Snow, 1995). Early
co-constructed narratives may become mental schemata for perceiving and
interpreting events. With personal photographs and the same kind of
guidance from adults and peers as other children, although adapted to their
communicative means and skills, children using alternative communication
may learn to talk about important events in their lives (see Brekke and von
Tetzchner, this volume).

Conclusion

Children in segregated environments do not have the same opportunities for
social discourse with a heterogeneous group of peers as children in ordinary
nursery and school settings. Children who use alternative communication
forms are more dependent on the educational environment than speaking
children, so the social constraints typically associated with segregated
settings may have a greater negative impact on them than on speaking
children. They may have less access to age-typical and culturally significant
knowledge, as well as pragmatic and conversational experiences of significance for the further advancement of language and communication skills.

Inclusive educational settings can be optimal linguistic environments for children who use alternative communication, even if such environments, to some extent, may be organized and scaffolded in more elaborate ways than for typically developing children.

The introduction of conversation books, peer buddy systems and interactive activities has been found to be positively related to increases in communicative interaction between children and true communicative responsibility for children using alternative communication modes, in particular for children using communication aids (Hunt et al., 1991, 1996, 2002). However, the strategies described in this chapter tend to be teacher oriented and focus mainly on the helping role of peers. A truly inclusive educational setting would imply that the children in some way belonged to the same community of learners regardless of their diverse level of abilities. This would not necessarily imply a shared or even overlapping curriculum; there are usually large differences between children belonging to the same class. The main feature needed for inclusive educational settings to become culturally appropriate is that peer conversations are on an 'equal footing' (see Goffman, 1963). From an interventionist perspective, this implies a change of focus from the communicative roles of teacher and helper to partnership in communicative co-construction and guided participation. Otherwise, all conversations may become exercises in teaching and learning. For this change of focus to appear, there must be changes in professional attitudes and practices. However, this does not imply a reduction of the importance of professionals for children acquiring alternative communication forms, even if the professionals may become less prominent in the children's language environment. On the contrary, the changes in practice needed for scaffolding communicatively heterogeneous groups of children in nurseries and schools will imply the innovation of a larger and more complex set of professional strategies. And if this work is successful, the result will not only be more true inclusion in school, but a greater shared participation later in life.

CHAPTER 14

Patterns of language use in Hindi speaking children with cerebral palsy: natural speakers and aided communicators

SUDHA KAUL

In the study of augmentative and alternative communication, there has been considerable debate about the importance of grammatical structure or linguistic competence for augmenting communication skills (Harris, 1978; Light, 1988, 1989; Sevcik, Romski and Wilkinson, 1991; Soto, 1999; Tager-Flusberg, 1994). Perhaps in reaction to an over-prescriptive insistence on the development of language structure at the expense of functional communication, the focus in traditional child language research shifted towards the development of effective pragmatic strategies to promote communication (Bates, 1976; Dunst, 1978; Hymes, 1971; Slobin, 1967). More recently, however, there has been a revival of interest in the extent to which children acquire the grammar of their native or primary languages, with a recognition of the connections between language and literacy, and the role of both in enabling children to fulfil their potential.

The questions at issue are firstly whether children using augmentative and alternative communication do acquire grammatical competence; secondly, the nature of the processes that underpin either typical or atypical paths in acquisition; and thirdly, what are the optimal ways of supporting grammatical development (that is, the development of a rule governed system for expressing meaning). The content, form and use of a language are greatly influenced by the particular communicative situation or environment in which an interaction takes place, and the skills of the interactive partner. Languages also vary in their structure, and cross-linguistic studies suggest that age of acquisition of morphosyntax is partly affected by the complexity of particular structures (Leonard, 1992; Slobin, 1985b). To date there have been no published studies of language acquisition by children using aided communication in the context of Asian languages.

300

Augmentative and alternative communication and grammatical competence

As described by Smith and Grove (1996, 2001), there is an asymmetry in the modalities of input and output for users who rely on augmentative or alternative modalities. The input language is spoken, but the output must be realized through the visual-motor forms of graphic representations or manual signs. Sutton (1997) points out that there are several reasons why, a priori, it might be expected that the development of morphology and syntax would be affected: the vocabulary for expressing these structures may not be available; pragmatic and physical constraints may mean that content or functions are prioritized over form, leading to a topic–comment or telegraphic structure (see von Tetzchner, 1985); and children may devise highly individual solutions to the problem of expressing complex meanings through the somewhat simplified systems of communication (such as key-word signing or pictorial representations) with which they are often provided.

In answer to the first question – whether children do in fact acquire grammatical competence – there is growing evidence that for some children, at least, acquisition of expressive morphology and syntax is more problematic than would be expected given their intellectual abilities and the potential of the communication systems they are using. Word order is a particular example. Languages differ in the extent to which they use fixed constituent order or inflectional morphology to denote contrasts in meaning (Siewierska, 1988; Tomlin, 1986). English, for example, has a relatively limited morphology, and relatively fixed word order, whereas sign languages are rich in morphology and word order is relatively free (Brennan, 1994). In graphic systems of communication and manual sign systems, which lack the possibility of realizing meaning through morphology, constituent order is one of the only devices available for signalling the argument structure of sentences. Evidence from children with physical and/or learning disabilities who are reliant on augmentative and alternative communication for expressive purposes, suggests that they may not use the word order of the spoken language of their environment when constructing sequences through graphic representations (Smith, 1996; Soto, 1999; van Balkom and Donker-Gimbrère, 1996). Soto and Toro-Zambara (1995) report that Spanish non-speaking children used graphic signs in multiple positions when forming multi-sign utterances, thereby changing the sign order. Soto (1997a) queried whether non-speaking children using graphic communication systems would apply syntactic rules governing speech to their expressive graphic output. Smith (1996) and Sutton and Morford (1998) show that even typically developing children sequence constituents in an order that differs from that of their spoken language when required to construct sentences by pointing to one picture after another. They suggest that the syntactic order of English is not naturally transferred to boards with pictures or graphic signs, and that additional skills may be required to translate from one system to another. Lack of systematic word order by users of alternative communication has been observed cross linguistically, in Irish, English, Spanish and Dutch, and does not seem confined to those using graphic representations because atypical word order also appears in sequences of manual signs produced by hearing children (Fenn and Rowe, 1975; Grove and Dockrell, 2000; Iacono, 1994; Light, Watson and Remington, 1990). This might not be a problem if the children developed a systematic and rule-governed approach to signalling meaning contrasts as, for example, did the group of deaf children using home sign studied by Goldin-Meadow and her colleagues (Goldin Meadow and Feldman, 1975), and adult English speakers using picture displays in experimental tasks (Sutton et al., 2000). Grove's participants did appear to place subjects before verbs, possibly using the principle of animacy (Siewierska, 1988) but were inconsistent in the placing of objects. Moreover, atypical word order occurred not only in signs, but also in the accompanying speech, for children who produced both modalities simultaneously.

Sutton and Gallagher (1993) point out that although children might produce utterances with a limited grammar, it cannot be presumed that their comprehension of linguistic structure is adversely affected. It appears that children can develop good receptive understanding of grammatical distinctions despite these limitations, although individuals may show particular weaknesses (Redmond and Johnston, 2001). For example, the four children in the study of Sutton and Gallagher, all of whom had cerebral palsy and no functional speech and used graphic representations to communicate, were able to make appropriate judgements of the grammaticality of spoken sentences, although they did have problems detecting tense marking errors on regular verbs (for example, *she open the box* versus *she opened the box*). Smith and Grove (2001) suggest that it is the lack of compatibility between receptive and expressive grammatical systems that creates a need for employing the metalinguistic skill of translation even when, in theory, it should be possible to use the template available in the input language as the basis for constructing output. It is possible that lack of structured output may be a transitory stage for many individuals, perhaps resolved as they develop the metalinguistic skills to translate from the receptive to the expressive mode of communication, or as more grammatical structures are made available.

In a cross-linguistic study, Nakamura and associates (1998) found that adults communicating through picture board sequences usually (though not always) followed the word order of their native languages, Japanese and English. The adult speakers studied by Sutton and her colleagues (2000) used a range of strategies to convey complex syntactic relationships. However, as yet there is a lack of longitudinal data to illustrate the processes whereby children acquire the grammatical structures of the input language. Moreover, the studies quoted rely on a small number of observations, gathered from disparate sources, under different conditions. There is a need to explore patterns of language acquisition through alternative modes systematically and in more depth, and from a wider range of cultures. The present study compares the use of language structure in speaking children and children using communication aids, both with cerebral palsy and from Hindi-speaking families. It examines the development of language structures over time and accompanying changes in interaction patterns between children and their teachers and caregivers. A brief account of the structure of Hindi and its acquisition is provided here as a context.

Early acquisition of Hindi in typically developing children

Hindi is an inflected language spoken within a fixed word order (although with some exceptions to the rule). The inflections are marked by 'matras' that are often bound forms. There appears to be a semantically distinct relationship between the inflected forms of verbs, nouns, pronouns and adjectives (Abbi, 1980; Kachru, 1980). Some of these patterns are similar to other languages, particularly inflected languages like Hebrew, Serbo-Croatian, Russian and Turkish. Kaul (1993) studied the emergence of syntax and morphology in 49 Hindi-speaking typically developing children between the ages of 18 and 48 months, using Brown's stages of mean length utterance (1973). Two-word utterances emerged between the ages of 18 months and two years, three- and four-word utterances between the ages of two and three years, and five-word utterances from the age of three. In Hindi, and some other inflected languages, aspectual participles appear at the two-word stage, marking initially the verbs, and then postpositions inflect the nouns and pronouns for person, number and gender. These are referred to as 'PNG markers' (Kachru, 1980). Case markers are important in Hindi. Nouns, pronouns and adjectives are modified by postpositions to denote pragmatic and semantic functions: locative, possessive, agentive, instrumental and nominative. As in English, Hindi employs a relatively fixed word order of Subject–Object–Verb (SOV). Children learn the rules of the word order pattern very early. The exceptions seen are in the interrogative and negative sentences where the pattern appears to change for pragmatic reasons, either to emphasize a point or to make communicative intention more clear. By the end of the two-word stage Hindi speaking children, like their counterparts around the world, have acquired much of the basic grammatical machinery they need.

The study

A group comparison was used to explore differences in language and communication development between speaking children and young aided communicators. The three-tiered model of data analysis presented by Light (1993) was used to structure the analysis. In addition to the group comparison, a detailed analysis of one child is presented.

The children

Ten children from Hindi-speaking homes participated in the study. They were selected from the Centre for Special Education, a school for children with cerebral palsy. Their ages at the outset of the study ranged from 6;1 to 9;11 years. The children all had diagnoses of cerebral palsy, including spastic diplegia (six children), athetoid quadriplegia (two children), spastic quadriplegia (one child), and mixed athetoid-spastic (one child). The Picture Test of Receptive Language (Hindi) (Kaul, 1999) was used to assess the children's language comprehension. This test assesses the number of 'information carrying words' that a child can understand (from one-word level to five-word level) based on the Derbyshire Language Scheme (Knowles and Masidlover, 1982). The test scores indicate the percentage of correct responses on the whole test, and the level of understanding of information-carrying words. Non-verbal cognitive abilities were assessed using the Raven Coloured Progressive Matrices (Raven, 1956) and the Boehm Test of Basic Concepts-Revised (1986) was used to assess the children's understanding of verbal concepts. The scores from the Raven test have to be treated with caution. Though the test items are meant to be culture-free, they have not been standardized for a Hindi-speaking Indian population. The Raven Test was scored to assess concrete and abstract concepts whereas the Boehm test scores measured the child's understanding of positional concepts. Table 14.1 provides details of the individual children in the study.

A comparison of the aided communicators and the speaking children indicates that the speaking children had less severe motoric involvement (all had diagnoses of spastic diplegia). As is evident, the children within each group presented heterogeneous profiles with diverse physical, cognitive and communicative abilities. However, the groups were comparable in their receptive language skills as tested on the Picture Test of Receptive Language, with one child in each group functioning at the three-word level, with the rest functioning at the four-word level. In terms of expression, the speaking children all used speech and made no use of either manual signs or aided communication, although they did produce some conventional gestures. The non-speaking children had no functional speech and relied on their communication boards, although they did vocalize and used conventional gestures.

Table 14.1. Description of the children (see text for assessment measures)

Child	Gender	Age	Diagnosis	Assessment	Communication system
Aided communicators					
Sameer	M	10;7	Cerebral palsy, athetoid quadriplegic	4+ word level PTRL 96% Boehms 84% Raven Grade IV	Word board, gestures
Mez	F	9;0	Cerebral palsy, spastic quadriplegic	3+ word level PTRL 74% Boehms 53% Raven Grade IV	Pictographic representations, gestures
Sajid	M	8;4	Cerebral palsy, spastic diplegic	4+ word level PTRL 89% Boehms 85% Raven Grade IV	Pictographic representations, a few spoken words
Tarun	M	8;0	Cerebral palsy, athetoid quadriplegic	4+ word level PTRL 96% Boehms 87% Raven Grade IV	Pictographic representations, gestures
Abhishek	M	7;4	Cerebral palsy, spastic athetoid	4+ word level PTRL 94% Boehms 94% Raven Grade III+	Word board, gestures

(contd)

Table 14.1. (contd).

Child	Gender	Age	Diagnosis	Assessment	Communication system
Speaking children					
Nita	F	8;0	Cerebral palsy, spastic athetoid	4+ word level PTRL 96% Boehms 79% Raven Grade V	Speech
Mukul	M	6;10	Cerebral palsy, spastic diplegic	4+ word level PTRL 81% Boehms 61% Raven Grade IV	Speech
Kirti	F	7;10	Cerebral palsy, spastic diplegic	3+ word level PTRL 76% Boehms 66% Raven Grade IV	Speech
Abdul	M	9;11	Cerebral palsy, spastic diplegic	4+ word level PTRL 66% Boehms 84% Raven Grade IV	Speech
Raju	M	6;1	Cerebral palsy, spastic diplegic	4+ word level PTRL 86% Boehms 84% Raven Grade III	Speech

Procedures

The study was conducted over a period of 19 months. Video recordings of individual interactions in the school with a familiar communication partner were obtained at four different times, with an interval of eight months between the first and second recording, six months between the second and third recording and four months between the third and fourth recordings. Fifty utterances were collected for each child at each recording, yielding a total of 200 utterances per child. On average, it took 2.4 sessions for the aided communicators and 1.4 sessions for the speaking children to produce 50 utterances. In the final session the pattern was more similar in both groups with the aided communicators taking an average of 1.2 sessions and the speaking children 1.0 session to produce 50 utterances.

Since the aim of the study was to observe the language use of speaking children's and children using communication aids and not to elicit responses, each session comprised a spontaneous conversation between the child and a familiar communication partner (the class teacher). The video recording was done in a classroom. The communication partners typically used speech to communicate with the children, with occasional modelling on their boards, verbal prompting and asking for clarifications (checking utterances).

Two interventions were implemented for the aided communicators. After the first recording, the children's boards were redesigned to add more vocabulary and improve access to the communication board. After the second recording, a workshop for communication partners was organized, focusing on strategies to enhance the ability of the aided communicators to participate more effectively in conversations.

Analysis

The procedures outlined by Crystal, Fletcher and Garman (1976) (LARSP) were followed for the grammatical analysis. The children's communication was transcribed and analysed for linguistic structure (clause, phrase, word levels and morphological markers); utterance length (number of single and multi-word utterances, and mean length utterance); communicative functions, discourse strategies and conversation patterns. These last included the number of turns taken to establish a message. Adult communication was analysed for discourse strategies, conversation patterns and communication partner strategies. Appendix 14-A provides details of the coding protocol.

Reliability measures

Ten per cent of each child's entire interaction sample (200 utterances) at each of the four data collection points were randomly selected, transcribed and coded for each level of analysis by an independent rater who had also carried out the rating for the pilot study. The inter-rater reliability was calculated according to the Sackett formula (1978). The results showed 100% agreement for mode of responses and utterance length for all ten children at each of the four phases. For codings of communicative categories and facilitator strategies, 10% of the utterances were randomly selected and coded for each child at each phase. Kappa values (Cohen and Manion, 1960) were calculated for each of the coded categories, with an average value of 0.83 for the aided group and 0.92 for the speaking group.

Lexical access: the children's communication boards

The children had examples of all lexical categories on their boards (nouns, verbs, adjectives, adverbs, prepositions and pronouns). A few morphological markers (PNG markers) were available to all the children on their communication displays from the outset of the study. However, it was at Phase 2 that all the morphological markers within each child's individual receptive language (based on the results of the Picture Test of Receptive Language in Hindi) were added. For three of the children, the markers (matras) were represented in pictographic representations whereas for the word board users the matras were indicated by their intra-syllabic form (as in normal written Hindi text). Table 14.2 tabulates the total vocabularies on the boards used by the aided communicators in the study at the four different time periods, categorized by lexical type and morphosyntactic status.

Results

Across all four video recordings over a 19-month-period utterance patterns of the children in both groups showed developmental trends similar to those observed by Kaul (1993) in her study of typically developing Hindi speaking children at the same receptive language level. Both utterance length and use of grammatical markers increased steadily over time. Kaul (1993) found in her study of Hindi speaking children that, within the receptive language level of three to four words, the adverb phrase and complex sentences emerged last. Similar findings were observed in the speaking children in this study.

As shown in Table 14.3, clauses were most frequently used, followed by noun phrases. Following clauses were usually single words or S-V, O-V or S-C structures (S = subject; V = verb; A = Adverb; C = Complement). Similarities were observed between the speaking children and the aided communicators in the study. The percentage of occurrence of clause and noun phrases was similar. Both groups tended to use more nouns than verbs, to make requests and simple responses and to ask questions. Adjectives and pronouns, which are used most frequently in typically developing children, appeared infrequently in both the speaking children and the aided communicators in this

Table 14.2. Distribution of vocabulary on the children's communication board

Child	Phase	Special block with markers	Phrases	Question words	People	Descriptives	Objects/ places	Position words	Action words
Abhihsek	1	3	10	6	88	40	154	0	20
	2	6	26	8	21	20	51	8	23
	3	4	42	9	100	32	246	14	60
	4	4	42	9	100	32	246	14	60
Sameer	1	13	30	7	50	21	130	14	38
	2	6	20	6	60	29	170	11	35
	3	10	65	9	70	28	313	14	38
	4	10	53	9	70	34	300	14	65
Mez	1	0	1	0	17	12	63	5	22
	2	19	15	7	13	23	87	8	52
	3	19	17	7	23	23	108	8	56
	4	19	17	7	26	34	158	8	59
Tarum	1	0	4	0	9	7	56	3	20
	2	11	17	7	16	30	67	7	40
	3	11	19	7	30	46	109	8	49
	4	11	21	7	32	46	111	8	50
Saajid	1	3	0	4	14	17	34	4	26
	2	24	19	7	10	18	40	8	40
	3	21	24	8	18	18	65	10	47
	4	24	20	8	15	19	59	10	47

Table 14.3. Utterances, lexical categories and markers used by the aided communicators and the natural speakers

	Aided communicators		Natural speakers	
Utterance type	Frq	%	Frq	%
Clause	702	69.2	521	53.6
Noun phrase	239	23.6	232	23.9
Verb phrase	73	7.2	118	12.1
Adverb phrase	0	0.0	30	3.1
Complex	0	0.0	71	7.3
Total	1014		972	
Lexical category	Frq	%	Frq	%
Noun	1091	62.1	663	31.2
Adjective	120	6.8	144	6.8
Pronoun	80	4.6	187	8.8
Verb	304	17.3	703	33.1
Adverb	21	1.2	78	3.7
Question	11	0.6	18	0.9
Affirmative	86	4.9	141	6.6
Negative	45	2.6	189	8.9
Total	1758		2123	
Markers				
Png markers	115	35.8	664	47.1
Auxiliaries	68	21.2	232	16.5
Tense markers	92	28.7	303	21.5
Case markers	46	14.3	210	14.9
Total	321		1409	

study, and questions and negatives were also less frequent. The aided communicators used twice as many nouns overall, and half as many verbs, as the speaking children. The pattern of use of grammatical markers was also similar in both groups.

As a rule, the aided group used fewer markers and relied mostly on noun phrases. Both groups marked nouns and verbs for gender and number and person. Verbs were marked by auxiliaries and tense markers in both the groups but the variations among the aided communicators were greater than for the speaking children. A major difference between the groups was in their use of multi-word utterances. Multi-word utterances were coded when a child used more than one word (vocal or board) to communicate a message. A one-word board utterance and a gesture was not coded as multi-word. Multi-word utterances could take several turns to complete.

Table 14.4 shows the average MLU of the children in each group for each phase, based on Brown's (1973) rules for calculating morpheme count with a few additions and departures keeping in view the specific nature of the Hindi language. In the aided group, MLU increased from 1.54 at Phase 1 to 2.50 at Phase 4, while in the speaking group, MLU increased from 2.72 to MLU 3.23.

Clause and phrase structure in language is closely related to lexical category. In other words, children need to have a range of lexical types in their vocabulary in order to realize different types of clauses and phrases. Words related to action, state, tense and aspect were used by both groups but the frequency and the spread of these words was found to be greater in the speaking group. The children in the speaking group used more verbs than those in the aided group, to express or comment on what they were either doing themselves, or to comment on what they saw other people doing. By contrast, the aided communicators made less use of verbs, even though there were some verbs available on their boards. Although these differences were not statistically significant, qualitative differences in the language used by the children were noted. For example, some children initially expressed request for action through non-linguistic modes, typically using gesture to communicate actions.

A major difference between the groups was in the use of adverb phrases and complex sentences. These did not appear at all in the utterances of the non-speaking children (see Table 14.3). Another difference between the aided and speaking groups was in their use of negatives and affirmatives. The aided communicators used negatives and affirmatives to acknowledge and confirm their messages. Negatives were used infrequently, and more as denial than as control words to refuse or protest. By contrast, the speaking children used *yes* and *no* not only to acknowledge (that is, to indicate that the speaker's message had been understood) but to clarify, confirm and deny, and answer questions or add to information.

Table 14.4. Mean length of utterance (MLU) for the aided communicators and the natural speakers in the four phases

Groups	Phase 1	Phase 2	Phase 3	Phase 4
Aided communicators	1.54	1.64	2.01	2.50
Natural speakers	2.72	2.72	3.26	3.23

Word order

Most of the aided communicators used two- to three-word utterances, with the exception of two children who used three- to four-word utterances. Only one child in the present study used a word order that differed from the spoken input (SVO instead of SOV). This was at Phase 1 and changed towards SOV over time. If the children used two-word subject–verb combinations like *BAALI DO* ('earrings give'), or multi-words, subject–object–verb combinations, *PAPA BIRYANI KHAYA* ('Papa biryani ate') the word order remained consistent with the spoken input, with the verb always coming at the end. Some of the children used multi-modal ways of communicating their messages. For example, one child pointed to a graphic sign on the board and then produced a gesture: *BAALI* ('earrings') DO ('give').

The results from the first set of recordings were consistent with previous research indicating that children who use communication boards tend to apply a more limited range of linguistic structures than typically developing children at a similar stage of language development (Bedrosian, 1997; Smith, 1994; Soto, 1999; Udwin and Yule, 1990); and also a more limited range than peers with cerebral palsy who can speak. However, there was considerable heterogeneity within the groups and it was not clear from the initial record-ings what factors were influencing their use of language. For example, it has been suggested that the use of action words by children with cerebral palsy may be related to the degree of motor impairment (McDonald, 1987; Mirenda and Mathy-Laikko, 1989). The aided communicators in this study all had greater motor difficulties than the speaking children. It is also not clear whether lack of language structure was in fact due to the unavailability of the relevant vocabulary on the children's boards. Soto (1999) noted omissions of verbs and articles by users of aided communication even when instances of these word classes were available.

Changes over time

At the first recording, the children in the aided group used grammatical struc-tures that were different from those of typically developing children, even when the linguistic forms were within their receptive repertoire. Table 14.5 summarizes the features of the children's communication patterns which changed, and which stayed the same over the 19 months of the study. Over the phases, significant effects were noted for child turns, MLU and multi-words.

Several features of the children's language developed over time. Table 14.6 shows how the utterance patterns in the two groups changed over the phases. In the aided group, the use of noun and verb phrase increased.

Initially, the children were relying primarily on single word utterances. Over time, there was a significant increase in their use of noun and verb phrases ('noun + noun', 'adjective + noun' and 'verb + auxiliaries', with nouns and verbs inflected for gender and number). With the exception of

Table 14.5. Two way (mixed) anova results of conversation patterns used by the aided communicators and the natural speakers

Category	Variables	F	df	p
Child turns	Group	18.36	8,1	0.003
	Phase	3.42	24,3	0.033
	Group x Phase	5.89	24,3	0.004
Child conversation space	Group	19.68	8,1	0.002
	Phase	1.91	24,3	ns
	Group x Phase	4.36	24,3	ns
Multi-turns	Group	7.99	8,1	0.022
	Phase	2.03	24,3	ns
	Group x Phase	2.49	24,3	ns
MLU	Group	2.21	8,1	ns
	Phase	5.47	24,3	0.005
	Group x Phase	0.56	24,3	ns
Multi-word	Group	2.65	8,1	ns
	Phase	5.09	24,3	0.007
	Group x Phase	0.49	24,3	ns
Gestures	Group	14.91	8,1	0.005
	Phase	1.32	24,3	ns
	Group x Phase	3.29	24,3	0.038

one child who used multi-modal utterances ('graphic sign + gesture'), the multi-word utterances of the four aided communicators were graphic sign or word board utterances, clearly indicating that once given the restructured boards, the children were using language in a more diverse way. Table 14.7 shows the changes in vocabulary use in both groups across the phases.

Table 14.8 shows the use of grammatical markers over time. Within the aided group variations were noted. Two children significantly increased their use of grammatical markers, whereas the remaining three did not. Analysis of variance shows a phase effect for clause and PNG markers confirming changes over the phases (see Table 14.9).

There were developmental trends in the use of nearly all vocabulary types for both the groups. This was evident from the increase in the frequency of words used by the aided communicators from the first to the fourth recordings. The aided group used a total of 376 words in the recording in Phase 1 and 525 words in Phase 4 (see Table 14.7). By the second recording, two

Table 14.6. Frequency and percentage of the different utterances across the four phases for the aided communicators and the natural speakers

Utterance	Phase 1		Phase 2		Phase 3		Phase 4	
	Frq	%	Frq	%	Frq	%	Frq	%
Aided communicators								
Clause	193	81.1	186	72.9	181	66.5	142	57.0
Noun phrase	36	15.1	53	20.8	68	25.0	82	32.9
Verb phrase	9	3.8	16	6.3	23	8.5	25	10.0
Adverb phrase	0	0.0	0	0.0	0	0.0	0	0.0
Complex	0	0.0	0	0.0	0	0.0	0	0.0
Total	238		255		272		249	
Natural speakers								
Clause	141	55.7	131	53.5	126	54.3	123	50.8
Noun phrase	58	22.9	54	22.0	58	25.0	62	17.2
Verb phrase	33	13.0	39	15.9	18	7.7	28	11.6
Adverb phrase	6	2.4	5	2.0	7	3.0	12	5.0
Complex	15	5.9	16	6.5	23	9.9	17	7.0
Total	253		245		232		242	

children had begun to use adverbs and by the third recording, four children had started to use questions. These findings support Sutton's contention (1997) that a small vocabulary may make grammatical development difficult and that an expansion in vocabulary may facilitate grammatical development. The use of simple clauses decreased from 193 in Phase 1 to 142 in Phase 4 (Table 14.6), while the use of verb phrases increased from nine in Phase 1 to 25 in Phase 4, and noun phrases from 36 in Phase 1 to 82 in Phase 4.

Changes in the use of linguistic structures also appeared to have an effect on the communicative interaction patterns. Over time, the aided communicators began to use different discourse skills and their conversation patterns changed. Of key interest was the use of grammatical structures (particularly the grammatical markers, tenses, PNG markers and case markers). Linguistic markers function to support pragmatic development in the use of discourse. By marking the correct tense or gender of a person or an action, a message can be conveyed more efficiently. For example when the child points to the auxiliary 'thi' as opposed to 'tha' (indicating that the utterance is about a girl), the communication partner is able to understand the message more clearly. If the child points to the adjective 'mota' instead of 'moti', it is understood the utterance is about a fat man. The use of such markers may influence interactive partners, who may find it easier to understand and follow the topics of the conversation and allow the aided communicator to assume more control.

Table 14.7. Frequency and percentage of vocabulary across the four phases for aided and naturally speaking children

Utterance	Phase 1		Phase 2		Phase 3		Phase 4	
	Frq	%	Frq	%	Frq	%	Frq	%
Aided communicators								
Nouns	258	68.6	248	59.9	255	57.7	330	62.9
Adjectives	19	5.1	30	7.3	36	8.1	35	6.7
Pronouns	17	4.5	24	5.8	22	5.0	17	3.2
Verbs	59	15.7	67	16.2	84	19.0	94	17.9
Adverbs	0	0.0	13	3.1	5	1.1	3	0.6
Questions	0	0.0	0	0.0	6	1.4	5	1.0
Affirmatives	16	4.3	20	4.8	24	5.4	26	5.0
Negatives	7	1.9	12	2.9	10	2.3	15	2.9
Total	376		414		442		525	
Natural speakers								
Nouns	163	35.5	139	27.4	186	31.1	175	28.8
Adjectives	25	5.4	29	5.7	48	8.0	42	6.9
Pronouns	32	7.0	34	6.7	71	11.9	50	8.2
Verbs	140	30.5	182	35.8	183	30.6	198	32.6
Adverbs	13	2.8	14	2.8	16	2.7	35	5.8
Questions	4	0.9	4	0.8	5	0.8	5	0.8
Affirmatives	39	8.5	55	10.8	46	7.7	51	8.4
Negatives	43	10.0	51	10.0	43	7.2	52	8.6
Total	459		508		598		608	

Table 14.8. Frequency and percentage of markers at each phase

Marker	Phase 1		Phase 2		Phase 3		Phase 4	
	Frq	%	Frq	%	Frq	%	Frq	%
Aided communicators								
Tense	8	30.8	14	25.9	35	28.0	35	30.2
Auxiliary	4	15.4	7	13.0	21	16.8	36	31.0
PNG	13	50.5	21	38.9	47	37.6	34	29.3
Case marker	1	3.9	12	22.2	22	17.6	11	9.5
Total	26		54		125		116	
Natural speakers								
Tense	63	21.9	81	23.4	75	20.3	84	20.7
Auxiliary	48	16.7	59	17.1	61	16.5	64	15.7
PNG	131	45.5	156	45.1	178	48.2	199	49.0
Case marker	46	16.0	50	14.5	55	14.9	59	14.5
Total	288		346		369		406	

Table 14.9. Two way (mixed) anova results of language patterns used by the aided communicators and the natural speakers

Category	Variables	F	df	p
Clause	Group	3.61	8,1	ns
	Phase	4.08	24,3	0.018
	Group x Phase	1.46	24,3	ns
Adverb	Group	8.54	8,1	0.019
phrase	Phase	1.90	24,3	ns
	Group x Phase	1.02	24,3	ns
Verbs	Group	5.31	8,1	0.050
	Phase	2.75	24,3	ns
	Group x Phase	0.36	24,3	ns
Nouns	Group	6.64	8,1	0.033
	Phase	2.20	24,3	ns
	Group x Phase	1.16	24,3	ns
PNG	Group	6.81	8,1	0.031
markers	Phase	3.18	24,3	0.042
	Group x Phase	0.72	24,3	ns
Tense	Group	5.31	8,1	0.050
markers	Phase	2.13	24,3	ns
	Group x Phase	1.15	24,3	0.038
Auxiliary	Group	5.60	8,1	0.045
	Phase	1.47	24,3	ns
	Group x Phase	0.24	24,3	ns

Table 14.10 shows the development of communicative functions in the two groups. Phase 2 and 3 are of particular interest since they followed the two interventions, the board change before Phase 2 and the communication partner workshop before Phase 3. Variations in the frequency of occurrence of most communicative functions were seen in both groups. The communicative functions which increased for the aided communicators included acknowledgement which increased from 105 at Phase 1 to 429 at Phase 4, and clarification which increased from 46 at Phase 1 to 78 at Phase 4. Differences in the frequency of discourse strategies used across the phases were more evident for the aided communicators than the speaking children (Table 14.11). The aided communicators used a total of 732 discourse strategies at Phase 1 and 994 at Phase 4.

Table 14.10. Frequency and percentage of communicative functions at each phase

Utterance	Phase 1		Phase 2		Phase 3		Phase 4	
	Frq	%	Frq	%	Frq	%	Frq	%
Aided communicators								
Acknowledge	105	14.1	179	25.9	269	35.4	429	40.9
Clarification	46	6.2	53	7.7	50	6.6	78	7.4
Reformulation	12	1.6	16	2.3	17	2.2	11	1.1
Answers	226	30.4	195	28.3	199	26.2	192	18.3
Spontaneous information	8	1.1	11	1.6	9	1.2	27	2.6
Requests	13	1.8	10	1.5	9	1.2	5	0.5
Confirmations	246	33.1	180	26.1	166	21.8	231	22.0
Denials	85	11.4	41	5.9	38	5.0	72	6.9
Expressions of opinion	3	0.4	5	0.7	3	0.4	5	0.5
Total	744		690		760		1050	
Natural speakers								
Acknowledge	12	3.7	24	7.6	39	11.6	0	0.0
Clarification	36	11.2	31	9.8	31	9.2	14	5.4
Reformulation	6	1.9	0	0.0	4	1.2	1	0.4
Answers	149	46.3	146	45.9	142	42.1	156	59.8
Spontaneous information	11	3.4	6	1.9	14	4.1	14	5.4
Requests	4	1.2	7	2.2	7	2.1	5	1.9
Confirmations	70	21.7	63	19.8	61	18.1	47	18.0
Denials	30	9.3	36	11.3	34	10.1	19	7.3
Expressions of opinion	4	1.2	5	1.6	5	1.5	5	1.9
Total	322		318		337		261	

Overall, the results suggest that both changes to the children's displays and training of communication partners helped to develop particular aspects of communication, and that gains were particularly marked for the aided communicators in the study. The interaction between linguistic development and patterns of communication can be illustrated by detailed analysis of one of the children who made the greatest linguistic gains – Sameer.

Sameer

Sameer was a young boy diagnosed with athetoid quadriplegia. At the start of the study, he was aged 11;7 years, and had been using a communication board for over two years. He came from a middle-class Hindi-speaking family, with an older sister and a younger brother, who also had cerebral palsy. His family were very sociable, with many friends who often visited. The parents were very supportive and the mother was a regular participant in the school's parent programme.

Table 14.11. Frequency and percentage of discourse strategies at each phase (CRM strategies are child utterances that maintain the conversation; CRD strategies are child utterances that develop the conversation)

Utterance	Phase 1		Phase 2		Phase 3		Phase 4	
	Frq	%	Frq	%	Frq	%	Frq	%
Aided communicators								
Greet	1	0.1	2	0.3	1	0.1	0	0.0
Initiate	1	0.1	0	0.0	2	0.3	1	0.1
Answer yes or no	192	26.2	262	38.2	320	43.4	493	49.6
Repeat	12	1.6	16	2.3	14	1.9	19	1.9
Reconfirm	158	21.6	90	13.1	94	12.7	119	12.0
Reformulate	8	1.1	11	1.6	11	1.5	9	0.9
Choose topic	1	0.1	1	0.2	2	0.3	1	0.1
Provide more information	349	47.7	299	43.6	288	39.0	345	34.7
Ask for more information	8	1.1	3	0.4	5	0.7	11	1.1
Joke	1	0.1	0	0.0	0	0.0	6	0.6
Shift topic	1	0.1	2	0.3	1	0.1	1	0.1
Close	0	0.0	0	0.0	0	0.0	0	0.0
Total discourse strategies	732		686		738		994	
Total CRM strategies	370		379		439		640	
Total CRD strategies	360		305		296		364	
Natural speakers								
Greet	0	0.0	0	0.0	0	0.0	0	0.0
Initiate	1	0.3	0	0.0	3	0.9	0	0.0
Answer yes or no	20	6.1	28	9.0	40	13.4	6	2.3
Repeat	0	0.0	2	0.6	0	0.0	1	0.4
Reconfirm	60	18.2	49	15.8	41	12.0	31	12.0
Reformulate	1	0.3	1	0.3	1	0.3	1	0.4
Choose topic	1	0.3	0	0.0	2	0.6	1	0.4
Provide more information	243	73.6	223	71.7	237	69.1	209	80.7
Ask for more information	1	0.3	6	1.9	12	3.5	7	2.7
Joke	3	0.9	0	0.0	0	0.0	1	0.4
Shift topic	0	0.0	2	0.6	1	0.3	2	0.8
Close	0	0.0	0	0.0	0	0.0	0	0.0
Total discourse strategies	330		311		343		259	
Total CRM strategies	81		80		88		39	
Total CRD strategies	248		231		252		220	

Assessment showed that Sameer scored between the 10th and 25th percentile for his age on the Raven Progressive Matrices. His teacher reported that he had the ability to perform at the level of peers in his class but, due to his communication problems, Sameer did not participate as actively as she thought he could. On the Boehms Test of Basic Concepts (Form A) he gave correct answers to 41 of the 50 items, indicating that he had a clear understanding of location, direction, dimension and orientation. On the Picture Test for Receptive Language (Hindi) Sameer scored 96%, placing him at 4+ word level of receptive language. He comprehended all the grammatical markers of the Hindi language although he sometimes made errors with the tense forms. Expressively, however, he generally used two-to-three-word phrases but seldom marked them for gender, possessive or tense.

Language and communication profile

Sameer was non-speaking and communicated multi-modally, using gestures and body posture to express 'yes' and 'no'. He also used facial expressions that were understood by a familiar partner. He was initially introduced to a Blissymbol board but had progressed to using a word board. Due to his physical disability, Sameer had problems in accessing his communication board, particularly when excited and anxious to pass on a message. Although he could point to the squares with his right index finger, he often took time to do so because of uncontrolled movements. His speed of communication was slow and, because he was sensitive to not being able to make utterances quickly, his teacher reported that there were many occasions of communication breakdowns or non-responses during class activities. He seemed eager to share ideas and to chat, but seldom initiated in class, mainly because of the time he took to convey a message. This meant that he often kept quiet or let the communication partner guess his messages. He seldom reformulated his messages.

Sameer at Phase 1

Sameer had a 16 inch × 12 inch multi-page display with a total vocabulary of 304 words which included pictures and graphic representations, written within a matrix of 2.5 × 2.5 cm squares. This included 30 phrases, seven question words, 180 nouns, 38 verbs, 20 pronouns, 21 adjectives, six possessives, five tenses and 14 prepositions. Some markers were also available on the board: tha (masculine), thi (feminine), thay (plural) and the auxiliaries hua (has) and hai (is) were represented with written words, and three tense markers were represented by graphic signs:) *PAST,*)(*PRESENT* and (*FUTURE.* One possessive marker was represented by a graphic sign. There were 30 pictograms and 100 Blissymbols. Under each graphic representation, the word was written in either Hindi or English. English words (alphabets) and numerals 1 to 10 were written in English. Words were arranged according to Hindi syntax (SOV order). The vocabulary was arranged over six pages, with an index on each page. Figure 14.1 shows the lay-out of one page in Sameer's communication book. Sameer only expressed 'yes' and 'no' with gestures and body posture, but used several idiosyncratic behaviours to

Sameer	YES	POSSES-SIVE +	hua (Aux.)	hai (is)	Tha thi thay (was)	NO	PAST)	PRESENT)(	FUTURE (
Hello	I/my	You	BIG	SMALL	FOOD	HOUSE	CAR	BIRTH-DAY	EAT
Thanks	Mother	Father	HAPPY	SAD	WATER	SCHOOL	BUS	HOLIDAY	DRINK
Sorry	Father	Abhishek	NEW	OLD	ROTI	TOILET	TRAIN	FEVER	PLAY
Please	Gudiya	Boy	DIRTY	CLEAN	MILK	COM-PUTER	AUTO	MONEY*	FIGHT
WHAT?	Girl	Aunty	GOOD	BAD	TEA	OUTING	WHEEL-CHAIR	MEDI-CINE*	GIVE
WHO?	FRIEND	WE	SICK	ANGRY	BISCUIT	MUSIC	ANIMAL	PRE SENT*	Cry
WHEN?	HE/SHE	Welcome	AFRAID	LOTS	RICE	CLASS	BIRD	FILM*	See
WHERE?	I DO / NOT / KNOW	HUNGRY			VEGE-TABLE	SHOP	WORK	HOME-WORK*	Come
WHY?	I WANT	THIRSTY	WET	DRY	FRUIT	OFFICE	LETTER	PUJA*	
HOW?	BEST / OF / LUCK							PARTY*	

Figure 14.1. One page in Sameer's communication book. English words have been written for the reader. The actual board consists of written Hindi and English words (underlined), Blissymbols (italics), and pictures and line-drawings (italics and *).

convey a variety of meanings. These were only understood by people who knew him well.

Sameer (S) was recorded at Phase 1 conversing with his communication partner (F) about his holidays, taking three sessions to produce 50 utterances. Analysis showed that at this point he communicated mainly responsively. There was only one example of a spontaneous initiation. Communication was multimodal: he used as many gestures (101) as points to his board (93). The total number of turns in the three conversation sessions was 483, with Sameer taking 201 turns and his partner 282, a ratio of 42:58. MLU was 2.08. He produced 29 one-word utterances (58%) and 21 multi-word utterances (42%). These were produced over 45 multi-turns (that is, a sequence of turns dedicated to the production of a single utterance). He was mostly using simple clauses (32) with very little phrase expansion (18). The multi-word utterances used by Sameer were generally noun expansions (12) used to describe and give more information about the subject:

Scooter kharab (scooter spoilt).
Daant bada (teeth big).
Abhishek purana (Abhishek old: 'his brother's school bag is old').

Sameer used generic verbs, like eat, sleep, read and go throughout the conversation. He used six verb phrases with the teacher helping him to expand the words each time to give the linguistically correct word, like in these examples:

S: Papa so (papa sleep)
F: {Papa so Papa so ya ya soya} (Papa slept).
S: Papa so ya (Papa slept).

S: Abhishek Guidiya chal (Abhishek Gudiya go).
F: {Abhishek Guidya chale thay Abhishek Guidya chale thay} (Abhishek Gudiaya went).
S: Abhishek Guidya chale thay (Abhishek Gudiaya went).

Most of the missing markers were the bound markers -ya and -aa; that marked perfect aspect denoting a past action. Sameer did in fact use a few of the markers available, as will be observed later, and these were correct and appropriate. Five were markers of person, number and gender, and three were tense markers and three were auxiliaries. He generally used the present and past auxiliaries correctly:

Dinosaur dekha tha (dinosaur saw: 'saw a dinosaur').
Mera papa nehlata hai (My papa bath-es is: 'my papa bathes me').

This suggests that any limitations in his use of Hindi were due to lack of availability of items rather than deficits in his underlying knowledge.

Changes to the board

Following the analysis of Sameer's interactions at Phase 1, changes were made to his board that increased the size and diversity of vocabulary and the availability of grammatical markers. The size of the board was slightly enlarged and the vocabulary was changed from a mixture of words, graphic signs and pictures to Hindi words only. The board was organized by themes: people, nature talk, home talk, school talk, project work, going out talk, numbers and letters (in English and Hindi). At the bottom of each page was an index with a number code. Each page also included phrases related to the theme, which were selected through discussion with Sameer. The placing of words was consistent from one page to another, and the markers were categorized according to the relevant argument. For example, tense, auxiliary and PNG markers were placed above verbs, and adverbs and case markers were placed above pronouns, nouns and adjectives.

Sameer at Phase 2

In the second recording, 50 utterances were produced in one session. The total number of turns was 589 with Sameer taking 262 turns and the communication partner 327, a ratio of 44:56. Although the communication partner continued to choose the topics in the conversation, Sameer appeared to have more to say about each topic and communicated in somewhat longer sentences, reflected in an increased MLU of 2.62. Twenty-two of the 50 utterances were single and 28 were multi-word utterances, completed over a total of 56 multi-turns. Sameer used this reformatted board with greater ease. He could access the markers because they were placed on each page, above the vocabulary items that were marked for gender, number and person. Often his board pointing was not clear and the communication partner had to check what he had pointed at. If her guess was incorrect, Sameer reformulated the message, using the vocabulary and markers available on the board. In the following extract, the topic is the Holi festival.

> F: *Aaj to bade rang kapade pehan ke aayee ho/school dress pehan ke nahin aayee ho?* (Today you are wearing coloured clothes, you are not wearing your school dress?)
> S: (Smiling) <u>Hum</u> (I).
> F: *Hum* (I).
> S: <u>Humme</u> (we).
> F: *Humme, accha, humme, humme* (we, okay, we, we).
> S: <u>school</u> (school).

F: *school* (school).
S: <u>holi</u> (holi).
F: *mein holi* (in holi). *Hain? Kya holi?* (Yes? What holi?) *School mein holi* (holi (in) school).
S: <u>Khel</u> (play).
F: *Okay, khel* (okay, play).
S: <u>Gen</u> (will play).
F: *Isliye rangeen kapade pehanke ayee ho tum!* (That's why you have worn coloured clothes today!)
S: (Smiles.)

Sameer took six turns to complete this conversation. The communication partner started the conversation with an indirect question to elicit an answer. She also prompted him verbally or by pointing to the word on the board in order to help him expand his message. She repeated each board utterance, filling in the missing marker *mein* (verbal), but when Sameer completed his message using the correct tense marker -<u>gen</u>, the communication partner responded naturally and did not repeat Sameer's entire message. Sameer marked the verbs correctly for both future tense and number as in the following example, completed over eight turns:

<u>Hum hum Holi gila rang khelegen</u> (We, we will play [with] wet colour.)

Here there is an agreement between the subject <u>hum</u> (we) and the verb <u>khelegen</u> (we will play), thereby indicating that he was talking about what he and his friends and family would do at Holi. Sameer also used the PNG markers correctly using plural marking -<u>gen</u> for the subjects (Mummy and Papa), in the following example, completed over six turns:

<u>Mummy Papa nahin khelegen</u> (Mummy, Papa will not play).

Sameer used the bound form -<u>te</u> to denote actions taking place in the past. He used a very adult-like phrase (<u>khilate khate</u>) to describe what he did during Holi at home:

<u>Pakori khilate khate</u> (We feed others pakori [and] eat pakori).

In the following example, despite missing the word mein (in), like in <u>balti mein</u> (in bucket), Sameer was able to convey his message in three multi-turns because he used the inverted auxiliary <u>hoon</u> (would):

<u>Balti gila (rang) chahata hoon</u> ([I] would like wet colour [in the] bucket).
<u>Babuji death ho gaya tha</u> (Babuji had died).

Sameer used the inverted auxiliary with the past markers -ya and the auxiliary tha to give information about his grandfather's death. Again, the possessive -ka (-s) was missing – Babuji ka (Babuji's). Yet by using the verb phrase and markers expressively, he was able to convey his message efficiently in four multi-turns. With regard to the use of the English word death, using English words within a Hindi conversation is typical of Indian children living in a multi-lingual urban environment (Kaul, 1993). Sameer's communication partner added words in English that Sameer frequently used. An indication of his linguistic competence was that he used the correct auxiliary tha to mark the agreement between the subject grandfather and death.

Sameer at Phase 3

The 50 utterances were collected over two sessions. The total number of turns were 804, with Sameer taking 360 turns and the communication partner 444. The ratio thus remains consistent at 45:55. MLU was 3.82. Thirty-four of the 50 utterances were multi-word utterances, produced over 167 multi-turns.

The conversation patterns also changed. The communication partner was now suggesting rather than controlling the topics and the boy would select what he wanted to talk about. The weather and car ride seemed to be his preferred topics. He was now expressing himself quite eloquently, as in the following example, talking about what he would do during his holiday:

Papa (ka) rupaiya paisa rupaiya leke main mauj mast karoonga! ([I] will take Papa's money and have a good time!)

Sameer was also beginning to use a wider range of linguistic markers (32 for person, number and gender, as against five at Phase 1), as shown in the following example describing a monsoon day in Calcutta, taking 24 multi-turns:

Mujhe barsaat mausam accha lag hai (I like the monsoon season).
Bijli chamakti hai (Lightning flashes).
Aakash hava paani andhera chaaya hai (saky, wind, water (are) covered with darkness).

He sometimes missed out the bound marker -ta, which, for example, should have marked lag in the example above. However, when he did use the aspectual marker, he marked the gender correctly: Bijli chamakti (lightning flashes). Bijli (lightning) is marked correctly by the verb ending chamakti (flashes).

When using multi-word utterances, Sameer always used the correct Hindi word order, Subject Object Complement Verb (SOCV), as in the following example, describing what he saw from his car on his way to school on a rainy day:

Kamra gaadi chakka naala darvaaza khidki khidki doobe thay (room(s), wheel(s) of cars, drains, door(s), window(s) were all drowned).

Another change in his communication at this time is that he began to ask for more information using question words, like in Aunty kab? (When is aunty?: 'When is aunty coming?')

Sameer at Phase 4

The 50 utterances were collected over two sessions. Although the number of turns increased as compared to Phase 1, the ratio of child to adult utterances remained constant at 45:55. Sameer produced 324 turns and the adult 390, a total of 714. As at Phase 3, a clear majority of the utterances (36) were multi-word, produced over 104 multiturns. MLU was 4.88, bringing him within the MLU range of typically developing Hindi speakers at the same receptive language level (Kaul, 1993).

Sameer still used multi-modal communication at the end of the study, including vocalization for confirmation. However, his points to the board had increased steadily from 93 at Phase 1 (46% of turns) to 194 at Time 4 (60% of turns). He used 84 gestures to confirm, acknowledge or deny. Whereas at Phase 1, the use of board points and gestures was more or less equal, by Phase 4, the board was being used almost twice as much as gestures. Linguistically, Sameer had consistently increased his use of grammatical markers. At Phase 4 he used 24, the majority (23) being tense markers including the past auxiliary tha (masculine), thi (feminine) and thay (plural), correctly indicating gender and number. By this time, Sameer was actively choosing topics himself and appeared to be more in control of the conversation. He seemed to have more to talk about, and this is perhaps reflected in an increase of his checking behaviours (turns designed to ensure that the partner has got the message), which virtually doubled from 98 at Phase 1 to 182 at Phase 4. The following extracts illustrate the conversation at Phase 4.

Sameer chose a topic in the conversation and the communication partner responded with enthusiasm and genuine interest:

S: 6 (index number to 'home' page).
F: (Turning to page 6) *Page six mein jaana hai?* (You want to go to page 6?)
S: 'Yes' (nods). (Starts to give information about his family) Holi nahin khelengi (will not play holi).

F: *Mummy kyon nahin khelengi?* (Why won't Mummy play?)
S: <u>Papa</u> (Papa).
F: *Papa, theek hai* (Papa, right).
S: <u>-ka</u> (-s).
F: *Papa ke, Papake* (Papa's, Papa's, never mind). *Koi baat nahi, Papake* (carry on then, Papa's). *chalo . . . phir* (????)
S: Papa (papa).
F: *Hain? Papa ka Papa* (What? What do you call Papa's papa?) *ko kya kaheten ho?* (????)
S: (Turns to new page) <u>Papa ke Papa</u> (Papa's papa).
F: *Kaun hein?* (Who is?)
S: <u>Babuji</u> (grandfather).
F: <u>Babuji bolte thay aap, hain</u> (you called him Babuji, right?)
S: (Searching for word on board) <u>Dead</u> (dead).
F: *Death, death, accha* (Death, death, okay).

Sameer conveyed the message about his grandfather's death quite clearly (Papa's Papa), but the communication partner encouraged him to use the word <u>Babuji</u> (grandfather).

At this phase, although the communication partner was asking questions, Sameer appeared more in control. As seen in the examples given above, he chose the information he wanted to give, selected the words he wanted to use and often decided not to pick up the suggestions made by the communication partner (as in <u>Babuji</u>). As he was using more extensive vocabulary, he seemed to be gaining more control of his conversation. If he made an error, he corrected himself. If the communication partner did not understand, he repeated or reformed his message.

In the following example, Sameer described a winter's day in response to the communication partner asking for information about Solan (a hill station):

S: <u>Olley</u> (hail).
F: *Kya girti hai vahan pe?* (What falls in there?)
S: <u>Olley</u> (hail).
F: *Olley* (hail).
S: <u>Baraf</u> (snow).
F: *Olley aur baraf* (hail and snow).
S: (Searching on board.)
F: *Olley aur baraf* (hail and snow).
S: <u>Gir</u> (fall).
F: Very good (patting Sameer's head). *Gir, uske baad?* (very good, and then?)
S: <u>Ti</u> (falling).
F: *Ti . . . girti* (points) (falling).
S: <u>Thi</u> (did fall).
F: *Thi* (did fall: 'fell').

Sameer was now using some case markers spontaneously. By using the marker -se, Sameer was able to get his message across more quickly, as when describing bathing in winter, over three turns:

Garam paani se (with hot water).

He also now spontaneously formulated questions in complete sentences:

Kahan gayee thay? (Where did you all go?)

Here he correctly marked the verb -ee and the auxiliary thay (plural). He was also using the inverted auxiliary:

Main CSE school padta hoon (I study in CSE school).

Sameer's utterances show how linguistic competence appears to be directly related to the availability and organization of vocabulary and grammatical markers on the communication board. The communication partner always waited for Sameer to formulate the message, and prompted only if he appeared to be stuck or the message was unclear. She would then point to the marker or word that Sameer needed to complete his message. However, it was not only the redesigning of the board that helped Sameer to develop his communication. His communication partner also changed her own patterns of interaction in response to his increased skills.

Communication partner at Phase 1

The communication partner chose all the topics in the conversation. She was very familiar with Sameer's home routine and his interests, so she chose topics that he generally liked to talk about, particularly his family, friends and outings. She changed the topic whenever she felt the conversation was flagging. Sometimes Sameer was observed to take time in responding to the partner's message. The communication partner responded to these communication breakdowns by often over-prompting verbally. She appeared anxious to make Sameer use linguistically correct sentences, therefore appearing too talkative. At this time, the most frequently used communicative function by the communication partner was asking for information (40%). Almost 28% of the questions were close ended and only 13% (37 questions) were open ended. She tended to follow an open-ended question immediately by a closed without waiting for an answer. The communication partner checked Sameer's utterances 98 times during the conversation. She repeated each word after Sameer had pointed on the board. Sometimes he did not get a chance to expand on his message and was interrupted by the communication partner, who was in total control of the conversation in all the three sessions. Sameer readily answered questions and gave information and much of the conversation space was occupied by Sameer using gestures (101) to either acknowledge or clarify his message. Sameer appeared to be totally dependent on the communication partner leading the conversation but he obviously enjoyed chatting with her.

F: *Gudiya, Abhishek?* (Gudiya, Abhishek?) *Mama nahin gayii thi?* (Didn't Mama go?)
S: 'No' (shakes head).
F: *Mama ko chod diya ghar mein?* (Left Mama at home?)
S: (Smiles).
F: *Saachi?* (really?)
S: 'Yes' (nods).

Sameer responded to yes/no questions by gestures. This was the general pattern seen in his answers to closed questions at this phase.

Communication partner at Phase 2

At Phase 2, the most frequently used communicative function by the communication partner continued to be asking for information (33%). However, the marked change was the increase of open-ended questions from 11% at Phase 1 to 19% at Phase 2. Open-ended questions increased to 82, a marked change from Phase 1 where the communication partner asked only 37 open-ended questions. Prompts were used more frequently (159), most of them being board prompts (modelling):

F: *Kya kiya chuttiyon mein?* (What did you do in the holidays?)
S: <u>Sameer.</u>
F: *Sameer, hain?* (Sameer, yes?)
S: <u>Pad</u> (read).
F: {*Ta hai* <u>ta hai</u>}(has read).
S: <u>Padta hai</u> (read).
F: *Padta hai* (read + aspect marker *-ta* = reads) *Baap re!! Padta hai!* (Goodness me! Reads!)

The communication partner provided the correct marker *-ta* to help Sameer complete his message in a syntactically appropriate manner.

Communication partner at Phase 3

At Phase 3 there was a change in the use of pauses by the communication partner. Sameer seemed more ready to initiate and to join in the conversation.

Therefore there was no need for the communication partner to pause to give him opportunities to participate. She paused 28 times, compared with Phases 1 and 2 where she paused 44 and 51 times, respectively, in order to give Sameer a chance to make a response and to expand his message. As Sameer gave more information, the communication partner changed her strategies as well. She modelled more and her prompts clearly helped Sameer to communicate more effectively. Sameer now took more responsibility in the communicative interactions. He chose the topics for conversation, began to reform his messages, provided spontaneous information and expressed opinion. The communication partner asked more open-ended questions, often teasing Sameer in order to elicit a response. In the following conversation about his new present of a school bag, she uses a mixture of open and closed questions, and Sameer provides new information, correcting her at one point.

F: *Kaun laya bag? Kaun kharid ke laya bag aapke liye?* (Who bought the bag? Who bought you the bag?)
S: Mummy (Mummy).
F: *Accha mummy, hoon?* (OK Mummy, yes?)
S: Papa (Papa).
F: *Papa, hain Papa* (Papa, yes Papa).
F: *Kiska bag hai? Ye?* (Whose bag? This one?) *Kallu vala hai kya? Ke ration vala hai* (Kallu [pointing to school bag] ration bag?)
S: Naya (new).
F: *Naya . . . theek hai Mummy papa naya kya layee hein, battao, battao, shabash* (new, OK, Mummy Papa brought what? Tell me. Good.)
S: Bag (bag).
F: *Bag, bag laya* (bag/ [he] brought bag).
S: La ye ([they] brought).
F: *Hain naya bag layee hain!* (Right, they brought [you] a new bag!)
S: 'Yes' (nods).

Communication partner at Phase 4

The communication partner continued to play a major role by asking for information. She continued to repeat Sameer's utterances as she had done at Phase 1, but now more for confirmation than clarification. There appeared to be a shift in the responses of the two communication partners, with Sameer taking on a more active and a more balanced role in the conversation, so that the communication partner's input was now to maintain the conversation, more than – as before – taking responsibility for its development.

The most effective strategy that the communication partner appeared to be using at Phase 4 was asking open-ended questions (16%), compared to Phase 1 when the communication partner used more close-ended questions

(24%) and fewer open-ended questions (11%). In phase 4 the prompts (26%) were given to help Sameer expand his message by providing a linguistically correct utterance or sometimes expanding on a linguistic structure used by Sameer. The communication partner prompted with care, starting by verbal prompting, then board prompting (area prompting going on to column and then direct pointing at the word) thereby giving ample opportunity for Sameer to participate in the conversation with some degree or measure of control. When the communication partner asked an open-ended question, Sameer often used multi-words to give more information. The following extract illustrates the prompting strategies used by the communication partner:

F: *Kya kya kiya chuttiyon mein battao?* (What else did you do in the holidays? Tell me).
S: Pita (father).
F: *Accha, pita* (OK father).
S: Abhishek (Abhishek).
F: *Abhishek* (Abhishek).
S: Gudiya (Gudiya).
F: *Hain, Gudiya, hein?* (Yes, Gudiya, yes?)
S: Chal (go).
F: (Interrupts) *chale thay* (go + aux thay: [they] went).
S: Chale thay ([they] went).

Here the communication partner prompted the correct linguistic structure in order to help Sameer clarify his message. These examples illustrate that over the phases, the communication partner used different strategies to augment Sameer's language development and his communication. The evidence from Phase 4 suggests that Sameer appeared to be consolidating his linguistic skills, and that the communication partner's interaction style changes in response to this.

Discussion

This study exemplifies Brown and Yule's (1983) definition of discourse as 'language in use'. The findings indicate that linguistic competence does impact on communicative interaction patterns and thereby on communicative competence. Light (1989) proposes that linguistic and operational competencies refer to knowledge and skills in the use of the tools of communication, whereas social and strategic competencies reflect functional knowledge and judgement in interaction. Warrick (1989) suggests that often aided communicators are more 'challenged' by social relational inadequacies than by cognitive or physical limitations. The five aided communicators and their communication partners clearly showed differences in these four competencies, but the change in discourse strategies in all of them indicates that social competencies had clearly changed. The balance in the use of utterances that develop a conversation and utterances maintaining a conversation by all the children demonstrates a change in functional knowledge and judgement. A point to keep in mind is that the children showed different views of conversation control. Some appeared to happily 'let go' of control to ensure their communication partners' participation in the conversation, while others tried to gain control by actively 'holding' a conversation. In the case of Sameer, the increase in the use of linguistic markers appeared to lead to more reciprocal symmetry within the conversation. This is reflected in the changes in conversation space occupied by both partners over the phases. The increase in the extent to which the children's utterances maintained the conversation indicates an increased level of participation.

The development of linguistic competence

The study raises questions about how linguistic competence can best be scaffolded for children using aided communication. Two key factors here are the modality of expression, and the role of the communication partner. It is important to note that access to morphological and syntactic markers was provided through orthographic representations, rather than pictorial signs. For fluent readers, orthography maps directly on to spoken language, thus restoring symmetry in the modalities of input and output. However, in the process of developing literacy, children go through a stage of treating written words as holistic gestalts (Frith, 1985). It is not clear from the study whether the children were using phonological representations to access the markers (thereby demonstrating phoneme–grapheme correspondence) or whether they were acquiring them as gestalts. There are different implications for teaching and learning in each case. If mastery of the orthographic code is required for children to start to use linguistic markers effectively, then their use may be inaccessible to children who cannot read fluently. However, the fact that some of the children were able to use a mixture of pictorial and orthographic representations suggests that it may be possible to accommodate a range of codes, and access linguistic segments through a holistic, rather than a segmental, strategy. Buckley (1993) suggests that many children have been directed to graphic representations who may in fact be capable of mastering orthography. We clearly need more research into ways of developing literacy in children using aided communication.

The present results demonstrate that word-order problems are not a necessary concomitant of the use of aided communication. It seems likely that the clear structure available on the boards, arranged according to Hindi word order, combined with different facilitation strategies, such as modelling or verbal prompting, and opportunity for expanding their linguistic structures, helped the children to translate word order from the auditory input to the visual output. Translation is one of two options for the realization of constituent order – the alternative is to generate a structure within the non-speech mode and independent of the input. It has been suggested that there is an inherent logic to the visuo-spatial modality, such that objects are positioned then acted upon, resulting in patient–action structures (Nakanishi, 1994; Sutton and Morford, 1998). Provided that communication partners are sensitive enough to recognize the child's system, this may be a viable alternative route, but there are obvious advantages to the development of a system that is compatible with that of the linguistic environment.

The second issue is how best to scaffold linguistic competence. In this study, where the children had clearly indicated that they knew the meaning of the particular linguistic or grammatical feature (as tested receptively), the communication partner modelled and prompted the children to use the grammatical markers in order to provide opportunity to use language for better communication. This was not a prescriptive teaching approach: the aim was not to teach grammar, but to provide opportunities for more efficient communication that could be understood by many communication partners. Naturally occurring opportunities were taken to use modelling and expansion within the child's expressive mode of communication. This is similar to the strategies employed by parents in child-directed speech (Snow, 1995). Utterances that do not match the adult input are frequently expanded into syntactically more correct forms in adult–child discourse (Hirsh-Pasek, Treiman and Schneiderman, 1984). Expansions appear to be perceived as cues to imitation (Scherer and Olswang, 1984), as indeed occurred in this study. The communication partners provided structured guidance using certain linguistic structures that were known to be within each child's receptive repertoire so that ultimately the children gained autonomous control of their use of language.

These findings suggest that both guidance from communicative partners and the provision of appropriately designed systems are critical to the acquisition of native language structures for children using aided communication. A possible tension exists between communicative and linguistic competence. Pragmatically, the effort involved in constructing a full sentence may be too great for the communicative payload (see Sperber and Wilson, 1986). Pragmatic considerations may mean that, at times, individuals choose to limit linguistic structure in order to communicate the maximum information with the least effort. In this chapter, it is argued that communicative efficiency is increased through the provision of structure, because this means a reduction in ambiguity. Research using experimental paradigms, such as referential communication tasks, are needed to clarify how and when it is useful for children to use particular linguistic features (see, for example, Richardson and Klecan-Aker, 2000). The selection is likely to be motivated by discourse function.

The observations reveal both transactional and interactional use of language. When the children wished to convey information, they used linguistic codes, particularly at Phase 4. But when they wished to maintain the conversation to keep the 'social closeness' within the conversation going, they often used gestures or body language to confirm, deny, clarify or acknowledge messages.

Communication partners

Communication is a dynamic process in which all parties influence each other in mutual co-regulation. Here, the communication partners exerted critical influence on the conversations with the aided communicators. The conversations were of a particular type – occurring within the school setting, but relating to the children's interests and concerns, rather than involving explicitly pedagogical topics. The children seemed happy to engage in conversations that were of a personal nature in the school setting. The communication partners showed examples of scaffolding, providing 'structured guidance' by expanding and reforming their partners' messages, and they increased their range of strategies as the children's communicative competence developed.

Appendix 14-A: Coding protocol

Turn

One or more utterances exchanged within interaction.

Utterance

One word or more exchanges by child or adult to convey a message.

Utterance unit

A complete message conveyed through multi-modal means (speech, gesture or board). With the aided communicators these exchanges may require turns by both partners to complete a single utterance because of direct repetition of words (equates to MLU of a speaking child). The utterances of aided communicators are often not complete until he or she has confirmed (verbally or non-verbally) that the utterance has been understood correctly. Confirmation of the message (usually in the form of gesturing or indicating 'yes') is not included in the child's utterance unit. If the child itself conveys elaboration, then the expanded message becomes part of the utterance.

Utterance boundaries

An utterance begins when the aided communicator either answers a question or gives a spontaneous message. The utterance may continue over many turns until the message is completed.

Single word

When a child uses single words in one turn or a string of single words over many turns.

Multi-word

When a child uses more than one word (vocal or board) it is termed multi-word. A one-word board indication and a gesture are not coded as multi-word.

Child's conversation space

This is calculated using the following formula:

child utterances/total utterances × 100 = per cent of conversation space

Proportion of child turns

This is calculated using the following formula:

(adult turns – child turns)/total turns (child and adult) × 100 = per cent of child turns

CHAPTER 15

A developmental approach towards teacher training: a contradiction in terms?

ERNA ALANT

The importance of teacher–child interaction is widely acknowledged as professionals and parents realize the impact of the relationship on young school-going children's communication and emotional development. The relationship is characterized not only by the facilitation of knowledge and skills, but also in terms of the personal and social development of children. Barnes (1975) states that 'If teachers understand the patterns of communication in their lessons they can take more responsibility for what their pupils learn' (p. 20). The teacher's understanding of the nature of interaction in the class as well as individual children's ways of expression and participation thus forms an essential part of teaching practice. To place a communicative challenge within a child's zone of proximal development, the teacher must understand the nature of this zone, and thus what the child can do and how the child is able to do it. This means that the teacher needs to be able to learn from observing problem-solving behaviour of the child in order to extend the child's development. The role of augmentative and alternative communication strategies in enhancing teacher–child interaction by facilitating problem-solving behaviour as an integral part of the communication process is thus pivotal to understanding issues surrounding the sustainability of augmentative and alternative communication in the classroom.

Anecdotal accounts and research studies have often reported difficulties in sustaining the use of augmentative and alternative communication in the classroom. Practitioners and researchers (Allen, Moore, Dunn and Anderson, 1986; Rivarola, Schiaffino, Veruggio, Oldrini, Scarioni and Chiari, 2000) have commented on the dwindling use of augmentative and alternative communication in classrooms and how communication aids are either collecting dust or are locked up in cupboards without being used. Clearly, there are a variety of reasons for the reduced use of such aids in the classroom, ranging from reduced interest in using manual signs or communication devices (the new gadget becomes old), teachers' lack of expertise and imagination, lack of support from professionals outside school to a lack of time to focus on an alternative form of communication. Non-use of communication devices is, however, seldom attributed to the constraints that the alternative modes of communication impose on human interactions. Relatively little reflection is evident on the use of different communication systems in enhancing problem-solving behaviour as part of the communication process. Communication involves the development of meaning, which is a negotiated process. For alternative communication forms to be effective, it thus has to enable participants to engage in a process of shared meaning in an effort to develop common ground that can provide a basis for further understanding and extension.

Training in classrooms with children who have no speech or unintelligible speech, and interactions with teachers during the past 10 years, has highlighted some of the difficulties experienced by teachers in this process. It seemed as if teachers have generally accepted this group of children in the classroom, but experience difficulties in integrating children who use augmentative and alternative communication within the broader setting of classroom interaction. As teachers are involved in the interaction process it is difficult for them to objectify the process to facilitate understanding of the systemic nature of interactions in the classroom. Even though teachers would try to relate to children using augmentative and alternative communication according to their cognitive and linguistic abilities, this remains a challenging process as teachers also need to communicate with the rest of the class. Teachers thus often express a feeling of powerlessness because of the difficulties involved in balancing individual attention to children and attending to the group. In my experience, this has been particularly prevalent in situations where teachers had larger numbers of children in the class and used a whole-group teaching approach.

These observations raise questions concerning the relevance of the training approaches used to assist teachers to use augmentative and alternative communication as a tool for understanding the individual child. Formal training invariably focuses on competency areas (see, for example, Light, 1989) to assist teachers in understanding the use of augmentative and alternative communication. Training is also often conducted during an intensive period (Deegan, 1992) with some follow-up visits in the classroom focusing on curriculum instruction (Beliveau et al., 2000; Bornman and Alant, 1999; Burkhart, West and Garber, 1992; Loeding, Zangari and Lloyd, 1990). Relatively little attention is paid to the task of assisting teachers in developing skills to engage in dialogue with children using augmentative and alternative communication. Similarly, the challenges in balancing individual and group classroom needs often remain pervasive in teacher training. Augmentative and alternative communication intervention consequently often manifests as the process of implementation of specific strategies rather than the use of specific augmentative and alternative communication to facilitate the development of meaning in interaction, that is, scaffolding.

In the introduction to this book, von Tetzchner and Grove describe the process of scaffolding by emphasizing the role of adults in guiding children in negotiating meaning. They point out that following as well as directing children's attention are important parts of the scaffolding process as children need to learn to adapt to societal rules and norms for participation whilst developing their own individual ways of expression and interaction. George Herbert Mead (1955) made the differentiation between the 'I' (individualistic) and 'Me' (social-oriented) component of the self and emphasized that the integration between these two components is essential in forming an integrated personality. The over-accentuation of either of these components is not only negative in the short term, but could also have a long-term effect on the development of the individual. From this it is logical that non-use of manual sign systems and communication aids could also be attributed to the way in which these systems are used in the process of scaffolding – that is, the process of developing meaning in interaction. If a system is not flexible enough to allow communication partners to create new meaning, information transfer will remain the primary goal of interaction, thus limiting the use of the alternative communication system to specific controlled situations and functions. This could be described as a non-scaffolding process characterized by a conventionalized exchange of messages. In this kind of situation, it is reasonable to suppose that the need for the use of the augmentative and alternative communication system might dwindle.

For the use of augmentative and alternative communication to be sustainable teachers therefore need to understand why this form of communication is essential for the development of children with no speech or unintelligible speech and how it can add to their own understanding and interaction with these children. Teachers need to relate to the alternative communication system as a way to facilitate engagement with the child rather than as a process of getting the child to use predetermined messages. In the second instance, they need to acquire the skill to include the use of augmentative and alternative communication within the broader framework of classroom interaction. This accommodation of the use of alternative communication systems within traditional classroom interaction needs to be explored to allow professionals specializing in the augmentative and alternative communication to support teachers more meaningfully during this process.

Classroom interaction as dialogue

Classroom discourse differs markedly from interaction in other settings, in that its purpose is to instruct and inform, and this is reflected in the discourse structure and functions (Hammersley, 1981). Generally, in conversations, topic changes are unpredictable and often only loosely defined, whereas in the classroom the teacher typically chooses the topic, decides how to subdivide the topic and how to cope with clarifications and digressions. Traditional classroom interactions tend to be teacher directed and non-scaffolding in nature. Children are expected to listen and to participate when appropriate. The focus on child-centred approaches in teaching, however, emphasize the need for a stronger developmental approach towards classroom interaction. The nature of this asymmetric communication situation requires specific sensitivity to enhance language and communication development in school-going children.

Communication is a dialogical process whereby both adults and children engage in a process of creating meaning. The intersubjective nature of this relationship implies that both children and adults have the sensitivity to develop 'new meaning' in their interaction. Apart from joint meanings, the sensitivity towards subjective interpretation is pivotal in enhancing communication development. This implies that the teacher needs to understand the motives and interest of the child to engage in meaningful interaction. In line with the 'co-operative principle' suggested by Grice (1989), speakers try to be informative, relevant and clear while listeners interpret what they say to try to live up to these expectations.

This principle of dialogue and co-operation clearly presents the teacher with challenges, particularly in classrooms where children are of diverse abilities and from varied linguistic and cultural contexts. To relate to the developmental achievements of children and hence to develop useful strategies for facilitating this development requires sufficient understanding not only of the individual child but also of the other students in the class to enable class dialogue to be meaningful group interaction: 'Ultimately, understanding what another person means is always a matter of understanding both what is said and what to do with what is said' (Bridges, Sinha and Walkerdine, 1981, p. 122). Strategies therefore need to be effective not only for understanding children with disabilities but also for using this knowledge to facilitate general participation in the classroom. Although the emphasis in this chapter is on the interaction between a teacher and a communication aid user, the role of the teacher in facilitating peer interaction between the aided communicator and other children is equally important. Reality is that for children with no or unintelligible speech, the school – but, in particular, the classroom – probably constitutes a most important supplement to the communication at home. For a large number of children there may not be many communication and interaction opportunities outside of these two settings.

The challenge that this interactional situation poses for the implementation of augmentative and alternative communication in the classroom is extensive. Not only does the teacher need to learn how to interact with a child using manual or graphic signs to facilitate the child's communication development but the teacher also needs to explore ways in which to integrate these communication forms with all the communication going on in the class to ensure harmonious group interaction. For class interaction to be meaningful it must involve a great sensitivity towards principles of scaffolding in group interaction, and must ensure that children with varying abilities participate in the process. Skills acquired in scaffolding in interacting with one student can thus have an important impact on the teacher's interactional style with the rest of the class if adequate training support is provided for this extension of skills.

Implementation of augmentative and alternative communication in the classroom

Attitudes and expectations of teachers have been identified as important contributing factors in determining how they engage in interaction with children with no or unintelligible speech. Perceptions of special school teachers indicated a positive relationship between teachers' own competence in providing communication training and their perceptions of students' abilities (Soto, 1997b). Teachers' perceptions of their own skills in interacting with children with limited speech are thus closely associated with their perception of the students' abilities to perform. From this one could deduce that teachers who are able to engage in scaffolding processes with their students tend to be better at recognizing these children's potential for learning. Similarly, Locke and Mirenda (1992) report that teachers' level of participation in intervention with augmentative and alternative communication seems to increase as they become more knowledgeable and confident in the field.

The pivotal role of the teacher in facilitating the use and development of the communication system of young children is reflected in a variety of in-service and other training programmes for teachers. The findings of, for example, Bornman and Alant (1999) and Rowland and Schweigert (1993) emphasize the importance of teachers' skills in creating communication opportunities in the classroom. These studies confirm that, whilst focusing on one child with limited speech, the teacher can be assisted successfully in creating more communication opportunities for all the children in the classroom. The term 'communication opportunities' can, in this case, be contrasted with the term 'communication challenges'. Communication opportunities in practice refer to the provision of specific conditions for interactions. These interactions do not, however, necessarily imply the use of a word or a manual or graphic sign to enhance its use in new or different settings or situations. 'Communication challenges' on the other hand, focuses more on the creative process of language use, thus the process of scaffolding.

Most approaches towards language and communication intervention would acknowledge the importance of focusing on meaning rather than form. The challenges in making this approach a reality in the classroom, particularly in interaction with a child using augmentative and alternative communication, are considerable. There may, for example, be graphic signs on communication boards or pre-recorded utterances on communication aids to enable children to participate in classroom interactions. Active participation is therefore encouraged on an action-based level to facilitate social interaction in the classroom activities. Externally identified goals for communication are identified to facilitate participation, but pre-recorded messages may become non-scaffolding repetition. However, externally identified goals or opportunities for communication can be used to facilitate the student's awareness and participation in communication as an important first step. As mentioned earlier, directing children's attention to specific opportunities and providing them with communication opportunities is a recognized component of scaffolding. The challenge is to prevent this interaction from remaining a technical 'exchange of messages on demand' and to use this communication to observe children's behaviour to adapt the communication process in order to allow for problem-solving and the provision of creative challenges.

Due to the nature of augmentative and alternative communication strategies, the communication action remains individual oriented. When communication aids with speech output are used, focus is often on individual children's use of pre-recorded utterances. Although individual children thus have access to some communal language and communication items, interaction between the aided communicator and peers in the class remains challenging as teachers or parents go through the process of message recording and selection. Development of meaning between the individual child, teacher and peers therefore tends to be static and stultifying unless great sensitivity towards the aided communicator's motives and interests is maintained. Gerber and Kraat (1992) emphasize the difficulties involved in using pre-programming in augmentative and alternative communication by pointing out that the linguistic productions are usually shorter, the medium tends to dictate form, productions do not necessarily reflect the linguistic competence of children, children using augmentative and alternative communication rely heavily on multiple modes of communication and their partners assume atypical roles in their conversations with the children.

A focus on external motivation, rather than intrinsic motivation, of children in the process of communication is relatively common. The difficulties that people experience in understanding the comprehension and use of children using augmentative and alternative communication, misinterpretations of the communication efforts and difficulties in coping with them within the class setting all contribute to the challenges of augmentative and alternative communication, and in particular to classroom-based interactions using it. It is well documented that teachers, like other adults, tend to compensate for children who have limited speech by taking more turns due to the reciprocal nature of interaction, initiating interactions more frequently, using more direct questions as well as using more attention directing utterances and requests (Basil, 1992; Cicognani and Zani, 1992; Light, 1989). As it was argued that the use of a voice-output device can provide children with easy access to communication and improve the quality of interactions, a study was conducted to determine whether providing a child with a voice-output device can reverse the negative trends in a teacher's interactions with the child and to describe the nature of the changes observed (Popich and Alant, 1997, 1999). Changes were also described in relation to the teacher's interaction with the other students in the class to provide a broader developmental background for the impact of the intervention. The study was conducted in a special school for children with physical disabilities and mild learning problems and was primarily concerned with the teacher's verbalizations in an attempt to sensitize the teacher towards her own verbalizations in interaction with a child using a communication aid.

The study presented here (Popich and Alant, 1999) describes the overall proportion of interaction directed at a child with limited speech and the speaking children in the same class and the changes that occurred in the teacher's communicative interactions during the four phases of the study. It also investigates the comparative role of teacher training in the process of improving quality of interaction between teachers and aided communicators.

Method

There were nine children in the classroom, varying between 3;0 and 4;8 years of age. One 4;8-year-old child was provided with a communication aid with speech output where the messages were changed according to the topic of the class. There were two additional children with unintelligible speech who had no access to alternative communication. The teacher was a 35-year-old woman with 10 years' teaching experience.

The observations were conducted in four phases:

- Pre-implementation. During this phase, the child had no communication device.
- Post-implementation. During this phase, the child was familiar with the device. The teacher had been shown how to record and delete messages but had no training in using the device in communicative interaction.

- Post-training phase. During this phase the teacher received training in using the communication aid in interaction, by focusing on communication functions and different types of questions that can be used to enhance the expressive communication of the communicator.
- Withdrawal phase. This phase was conducted eight weeks after training was ended.

After a phase of two weeks, covering the pre-implementation and post-implementation phases, the teacher and the aided communicator received training in using a digital speaker. Training was intensive and focused on this dyad for one week. It included five training sessions of one hour each on five consecutive days. The content of the individual training sessions included operational skills and making the teacher aware of different utterance types (functions) and how to use different kinds of questions (according to Bloom's taxonomy) in interacting with the aided communicator.

Observations were obtained by recording and analysing classroom storytime interactions. The number of interactions directed at each child, types of questions used, as well as messages recorded on the communication aid were determined for each phase. Interactions between the teacher and the aided communicator, as well as between the teacher and the whole class, were investigated within each phase.

Forty-eight recordings were made, 12 recordings during each of the four phases of the research. Twenty-four of the recordings were of interaction in the classroom and 24 of interaction between the teacher and the aided communicator. An independent observer transcribed all tapes and final decisions were based on 100% agreement between two raters.

Quantitative changes in the teacher's communication

Figures 15.1 to 15.4 present an overview of the overall proportion of interaction directed at each child during group sessions in pre-implementation and post-training phases. The verbalizations of the teacher directed at the whole class decreased from 72% (pre-implementation), 65% (post-implementation), 56% (post-training) to 53% (withdrawal). The teacher's individual interactions with the children increased, and in particular with the child using a communication aid (A). More of the verbalizations were directed at the aided communicator than at any of the other children.

Although this could be regarded as a positive indicator for the child using the communication device, it is pertinent to view this change against the background of the aided communicator's experience as well as that of the group. An increase in communication efforts directed at the child using a communication aid by the teacher does not necessarily reflect an increased comprehension of the child's understanding and developmental achievements. The teacher clearly understood how to programme the device and was able to pre-record messages to facilitate exchanges with the child. The decrease in interaction with the other children in the class does, however, reflect her focus on the communication aid user and the use of the digital speaker in the classroom.

Figure 15.5 demonstrates the decreasing interaction pattern between the teacher and the other children in the class. There seems to be a small albeit noteworthy increase in the teacher's verbal interactions with the two other children with limited speech in the class (F and I). This might indicate some increase in awareness of potential abilities from the teacher in interacting with these two children who had no access to communication systems and communicated by ordinary gestures. This might be indicative of a general change in perception of the teacher as she becomes aware of the importance of investing effort into communication with these children. Training might therefore have created a positive situation for her to explore the process of scaffolding in with the other children with limited speech.

As the teacher became more aware of interaction with the aided communicator, she proportionally reduced interaction with the speaking children in the class (B, D, E, H). One could argue that this could represent a Hawthorn effect as the teacher was conscious of the recordings in the class. Recordings were made over a couple of weeks (12 recordings during each phase) in an attempt to diminish the impact of recordings. This still remains a difficult issue, however, as recordings were made during one timetable period during the day, such as story time.

Another explanation for the increase in interaction could revolve around the teacher and her increased commitment and orientation towards communicating with the aided communicator. The communication pattern in the class was changing and at the end of training it had not yet reached a point of stabilization. An extension of the recording period would clearly have been most useful to identify changes in the interaction pattern and observing stabilization of interaction patterns over time. Similarly, using some other timetable periods in addition to story time might have confirmed or refuted observations made during the story-time period.

Observations show that the communication aid user more closely resembled the speaking children than the other children with limited speech in terms of the frequency of teacher-directed verbalizations, even before the implementation (Figure 15.1). This could reflect a perceived advantage on her part in interacting with him as a basis for her enthusiasm for child A to receive a communication aid. Hammersley (1974) raises the importance of understanding the conditions or implicit attitudes contributing to whether

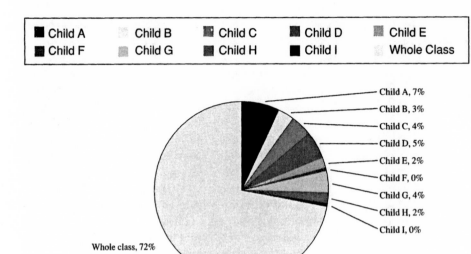

Figure 15.1

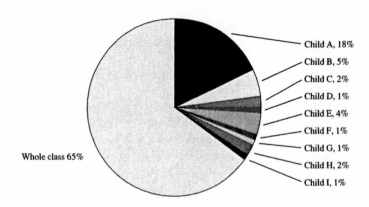

Figure 15.2

Figures 15.1 to 15.4. The proportion of teacher verbalizations directed at each child during the four phases: Pre-implementation, post-implementation, post-training, post-withdrawal.

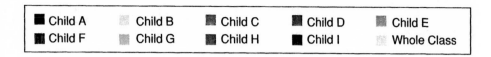

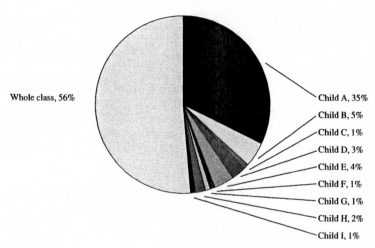

Whole class, 56%

Child A, 35%
Child B, 5%
Child C, 1%
Child D, 3%
Child E, 4%
Child F, 1%
Child G, 1%
Child H, 2%
Child I, 1%

Figures 15.3

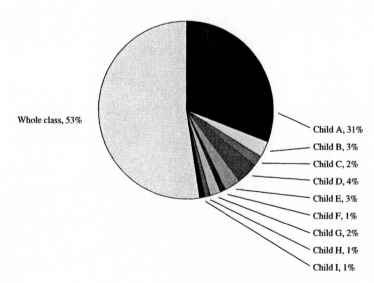

Whole class, 53%

Child A, 31%
Child B, 3%
Child C, 2%
Child D, 4%
Child E, 3%
Child F, 1%
Child G, 2%
Child H, 1%
Child I, 1%

Figure 15.4

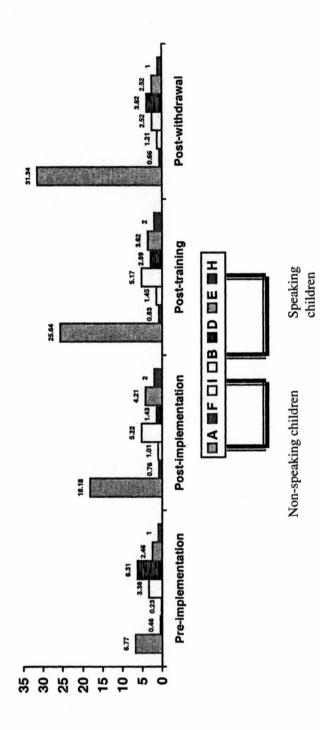

Figure 15.5. The proportion of teacher verbalizations during group sessions directed at the speaking children and the children with limited speech.

children are included or excluded in class interaction and similarly how they are being evaluated by the teachers. 'My focus . . . is the way in which the teachers in a particular school work to organize pupil participation in classrooms and the relevance of that organization for the "intelligence" pupils are required to show' (Hammersley, 1974, p. 355).

Qualitative changes in the teacher's communication

The observations show that three types of verbal interactions were most frequently directed at all the children over a five-week period (Figure 15.6). The teacher used requesting (for example, *show me*) and attention directing (for example, *look there*) more frequently with all three children with limited speech, whilst she used affirming (for example, *that's right*) and answering questions (for example, *because if he doesn't put on a jersey he will get cold*) most frequently with the six speaking children. Although the teacher used affirming quite frequently with the communication-aid user, the same did not apply to the two other children with limited speech. This might indicate that the aided communicator was exposed to more creative challenges than the other children with limited speech, who had fewer challenges that might have elicited affirmation.

The different kind of feedback received by the speaking children and the children with limited speech reflects a tendency of the teacher to be relatively more responsive (answering questions, being affirming) to the children who were speaking, hence the quality of feedback given in the classroom is different. This is particularly important when considering the creation of an engaging environment in the classroom (Hendrickson and Frank, 1993). It is noteworthy that there were no significant differences between the types of verbalizations used by the teacher during each of the intervention phases even though her interaction with the communication aid user increased. This suggests that changes occurred in the frequency of the teachers' interaction but that the quality of the interaction remained the same. This supports the observation of Saville-Troike (1982) that communication in the majority of classrooms can be described as 'rigid'. There are rigid turn-taking rules, implicit control precepts and a great deal of teacher directions.

The teacher-training programme addressed different ways of using language in the classroom in an attempt to increase the variation of language functions used in interaction with the children. The present observations seem to point to a couple of issues: firstly, that the training programme did not allow enough time for the teacher to practise the different language functions and thus to feel at ease in using them. On the other hand, the training was not explicitly oriented towards using the different language functions to facilitate the development of meaning between teacher and

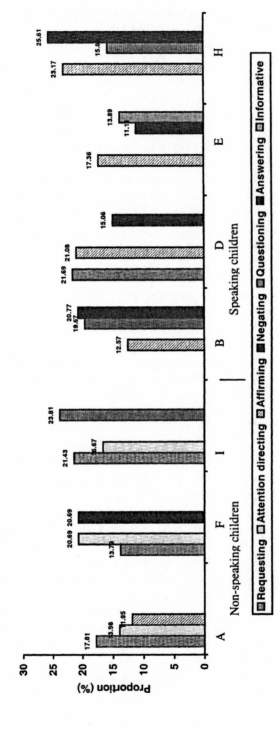

Figure 15.6. Three most frequent types of verbalizations used with each of the children.

child. Little focus was placed on observing the children's behaviour and exploring ways to extend current communication efforts with them. The introduction of language teaching without a developmental approach thus could have oriented the teacher towards a more clinical approach to the use of different language functions. The focus was more on the structure or different formulations of functions than on attempting to use these to facilitate understanding of and interaction with the child.

Apart from a critical view of the teaching methodology, this also suggests some of the difficulties involved in changing a communication interaction pattern within a classroom setting. Not only is an interaction style habit forming, but it is also closely associated with the kind of activities that take place in the classroom. One may not expect the teacher to use different language functions in the classroom (or to extend her repertoire) without allowing enough time to familiarize herself with their use in different classroom activities. However, changing interaction patterns are difficult, particularly in a classroom where the teacher is concerned with one communication aid user as well as other children with varying abilities. A developmental approach towards intervention requires a focus on the individual child, and an orientation towards individual understanding. The challenge is to integrate this approach within the classroom to ensure meaningful (not stultifying) group interaction.

Figure 15.7 describes the teacher's use of different types of verbalizations with the aided communicator as part of the group during the four different phases. Figure 15.8 describes the teacher's use of different types of verbalizations with the aided communicator during individual sessions. The figure shows that the teacher gradually more often answered the child's questions (answering) and repeated the child's utterances (imitation) over the four phases. This suggests that the aided communicator did start to ask more questions and verbalize in individual interaction with the teacher. It also reflects an increase in the teacher's sensitivity towards the utterances of the child. During the process of training, it thus seems as if the teacher did become more focused on the child's communication efforts during individual interactions.

Figure 15.7 and 15.8 both show a consistent pattern during the four phases of the study. There is, however, a marked increase in information being supplied by the teacher during individual interactions, suggesting that the teacher tended to provide more information directed at the child when they were alone together. This could be the teacher's way of compensating for the child's limited speech by providing more information, thus also maintaining an asymmetrical interactional situation (Garcia, 1992). However, it could also reflect a change in perception as she realized that the child was able to cope with more input. Once again, however, the caution is focusing

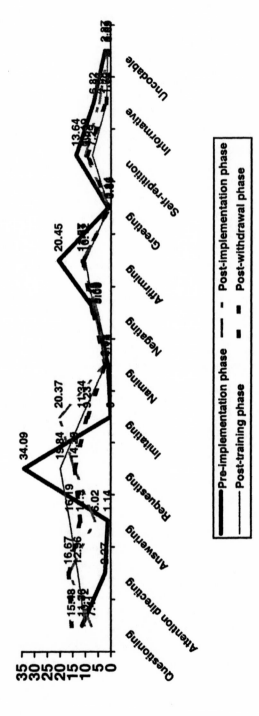

Figure 15.7. Different types of verbalizations used with aided communicator during group sessions in the four phases.

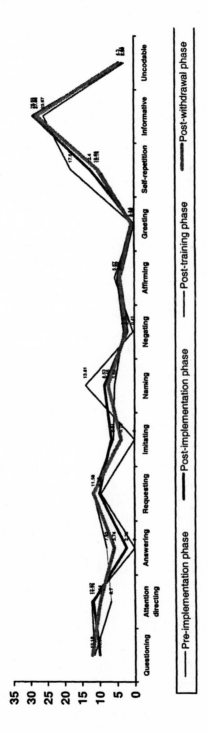

Figure 15.8. Different types of verbalizations used with the aided communicator in individual sessions in the four phases.

on the content or structure of interaction rather than the development of meaning. Facilitating the development of communication necessitates a consistent sensitivity towards comprehension as a collaborative process. Using scaffolding to facilitate development of meaning around specific information would thus be important.

What does become clear from these observations is that intervention changed in relation to the frequency of interaction between the aided communicator and the teacher, but relatively few qualitative changes were observed in the teacher's general interaction pattern in the classroom. One could argue that the change in frequency of use of different functions might facilitate a change in the quality of interaction over time. However, as intervention with the teacher was terminated at that time, this is doubtful.

Questions

Questions play an important role in communication with children who have a large gap between what they understand and what they can express, and who have limited means to express themselves. This was addressed during training and included making the teacher aware of the different levels of questioning (Bloom's taxonomy) to facilitate the use of a broader range of questions in the classroom. Hendrickson and Frank (1993) report that teachers can use questions for a variety of purposes and that more effective teachers tend to use questions to gauge the understanding of children. They maintain that question strategies are, however, often limited due to teachers' limited understanding of the range of communication purposes that questioning can fulfil.

Figure 15.9 shows the types of questions used by the teacher during each phase of the study. Initially, the teacher asked only questions oriented at testing understanding and knowledge and a few application questions. Gradually, however, the use of other categories of questions systematically increased – for example, evaluation, synthesis and analysis. The teacher changed her questioning behaviour over the study period and seemed to become more aware of the variety of functions for which questions can be used. Hendrickson and Frank (1993) refer to the different types of questions in relation to the basic question–answer sequence and to lead questions and response-dependent questions, and emphasize that teachers need to be able to use these for different interactional purposes during teaching. They emphasize that these types of questions are not nearly as critical as the manner in which the questions are applied to enhance learning.

The teacher seemed to extend her use of questioning whilst the same was not observed with the other functions focused on during training. The focus on one specific function (requesting or questioning) as a means of facilitating

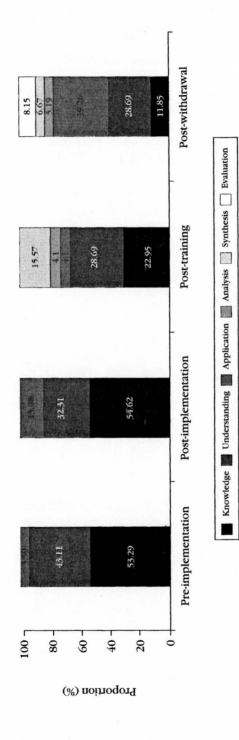

Figure 15.9. Different kinds of questions used by teacher over the four phases in the classroom.

the development of meaning was well understood by the teacher. She was also able to extend the use of different kinds of questions to other students in the class (Figure 15.10).

A similar trend was identified in the utterances recorded by the teacher on the communication aid during individual and group interactions. The communication aid user's access to different kinds of messages increased as the teacher became more skilful in pre-recording utterances of different types to encourage his participation in the class. This trend was evident in both individual and group interactions. The question is, however, whether an increase in the teacher's behaviour was a reflection of her own sensitivity towards interaction with the child or whether it merely reflected her becoming skilled in using questions and a speech-output communication aid with a young child. Although the use of more answering and imitation of the child's utterances by the teacher suggest that the child was starting to initiate, it remains a central issue in the implementation of augmentative and alternative communication. Planning communication for any user of augmentative and alternative communication remains a delicate process that requires caution to ensure that the system used facilitates and does not stultify human interaction.

Implications for teacher training

The present study of the training of teachers to interact with a child using a communication aid emphasizes some of the most demanding issues in relation to teacher training. It not only highlights the need for professionals specializing in augmentative and alternative communication to reflect on the underlying assumptions of their training but it alludes to the challenges in using a developmental approach in classroom intervention.

The use of scaffolding as part of this process needs to be well understood and focused on during training. The process may start with pre-recorded messages by the teacher in interaction with the aided communicator, but this needs to be placed within the framework of creative problem solving in interaction. To achieve this, teachers have to be guided as to how to move beyond just requesting the production of predetermined utterances to use available communication items in more creative ways and for more challenging purposes.

The observations in the present study show that changes occurred in the teacher's behaviour towards the children. However, it is important to note that the focus of the study was on the teacher and did not include an analysis of the children's utterances. The slight increase in answering of questions from the aided communicator by the teacher indicates some change in the child's behaviour, but does not provide any information about the child's

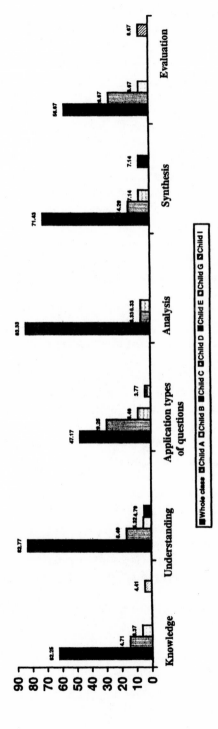

Figure 15.10. The total proportion of each type of question the teacher directed at each child.

reaction to the increased verbalizations. This is important as one needs to sensitize the teacher to the communication skills and initiations of the children to prevent one-way teacher-directed verbal interaction.

Bricker (1992), Warren and Rogers-Warren (1985) and Stokes and Bear (1977) discuss the importance of learner-oriented approaches in intervention by emphasizing the use of naturalistic training strategies that depend heavily on following the learner's cues. This implies a de-emphasis of the traditional teacher interaction model whereby the interaction is adult focused or directed and relies on small-group didactic instruction. Classroom interaction, however, demands that the teacher is able to maintain harmonious interaction with all the children in the class. Individual attention to children therefore has to be accommodated within the broader framework of class interactions.

The increase in the quantity rather than quality of interaction over this period could be part of an evolutionary process whereby the interaction between teacher and children increases as part of the process leading towards more qualitative interactional changes. This raises the question of whether it is possible to increase the quality of the interaction without increasing the quantity. As relatively few qualitative changes were observed in the teacher's interaction, however, it is unclear how long training would need to be followed up to ensure that this process of changing an interaction pattern would be facilitated.

Sustainability of augmentative and alternative communication implies consistent and recurrent use of the alternative communication form to ensure long-term impact. The most logical point of departure for sustainability is the intrinsic motivation to want to communicate, thus to engage in the process of developing meaning with another individual. Facilitating this process between a teacher and a user of augmentative and alternative communication in the classroom implies involvement from specialists in augmentative and alternative communication not only in the alternative communication used, but also in assisting the teacher in integrating newly learned strategies into group interactions. The nature of classroom interaction requires that the teacher is able to shift from an individual to a group interaction style. Training in the classroom should therefore move beyond the implementation of an individual child's augmentative and alternative communication system to assist teachers to use the principles of scaffolding interaction in the broader interactional setting.

CHAPTER 16

Blissymbol learners, their language and their learning partners: development through three decades

SHIRLEY MCNAUGHTON

I like to consider the development of alternative communication users as they acquire their language and communication competencies as resting upon a three-legged stool. The first leg is alternative communication users' abilities and their image of themselves as learners and communicators. The second leg is the alternative communication medium that is introduced, and the third leg consists of the abilities and attitudes of those who are the users' partners in learning. In the same manner in which the strength and stability of any stool's underpinning determines its effectiveness as a platform to reach new heights, the support provided by the three language and communication legs determines the strength and stability of alternative communication users' language and communication competencies and future achievements.

To assist me in examining the legs that have supported language and communication development for Blissymbol users over the past 30 years, Kari Harrington has given her permission to share a retrospective description of her language and communication experiences throughout her formative years. I have known Kari since she was a student in my first Blissymbol class in 1971. Along with about half of her cohort group, she made the transition from communicating, reading and writing with Blissymbols to communicating, reading and writing with orthographic script.

The professional team that initiated Blissymbol instruction in 1971, of which I was a member, did so to enhance communicative opportunities for children who lacked functional speech. We learned throughout the following years how many areas of children's development were affected by speech limitations, especially when such impairments were coupled with physical limitations. Our development as learning partners began with our explorations into alternate ways of communicating, but quickly took us to the domains of language, literacy, cognition, visual processing and social adjustment. As the children developed, so did we.

I asked Kari if I might describe her developmental pathway from infancy to adulthood as a route for examining Blissymbol acquisition, not because of exceptional abilities: her abilities have been assessed throughout the years as average or slightly below average. It is Kari's language and communication achievements, given her non-exceptional abilities, and the records that exist of these achievements that make her story so valuable. Blissymbolics was Kari's first expressive language form, a core component within her multi-modal alternative communication, and a support to literacy development. Throughout Kari's development and that of her peer cohort, it has been evident that in addition to the first leg – her abilities as an alternative communication user – the other two legs of the language and communication stool have been critical in their contribution to development and mature adult competence. Language acquisition is not a one-way influence, but the result of a transactional process (see Sameroff and Chandler, 1975). For a person whose development to a large extent depends on the planned adaptations provided by professionals (von Tetzchner, 1988), both the professionals' theoretical insights and their ability to gain knowledge from the disabled person are decisive. In the early years of Blissymbol use, professionals' learning came primarily from the children as they began to use Blissymbols. My colleagues and I were truly the children's learning partners. Through the years, our professional knowledge evolved as the children grew to adults, as the domain of augmentative and alternative communication expanded, and as research into language development and reading acquisition progressed. The developmental story of professional knowledge within this field thus interacts with the story of Kari's development of communication and language competence.

Theoretical overview

In the gestation days of augmentative and alternative communication, the literature available to professionals was limited. Virtually all of the learning had to be based on personal experience and informal contacts with other pioneers within the field. Awareness had to be nurtured, even within the professional community, of what constituted communication and the importance of communication competence for children's language, cognitive and literacy development.

There were, however, theoretical influences right from the beginning that guided the direction our programme would take. The work of Piaget (1959) led to the provision of opportunities for children to experiment and make discoveries within a learning environment adapted to their developmental abilities. The insights of Vygotsky (1962) heightened the awareness of the need for children to engage in dialogue with adults within activities that provided problem-solving opportunities along with assistance, consistent with the children's zone of proximal development in different domains.

The view of language development that most influenced me and the team I worked with during the early days of the Blissymbol project was an adaptation of the model suggested by Myklebust (1967), in which receptive language was viewed as receiving input from the speech of others and from the environment, and providing a framework for perception, environmental observation, awareness and evaluation. Expressive language was viewed as contributing to the development of communication, thinking, language development, self-concept, concepts, personal behaviour regulation, expression of emotion, and body and spatial awareness, as well as stimulating motivation through greater interaction with the environment. The role of both receptive and expressive language was depicted as the foundation upon which understanding, reading and writing were based. The team positioned Blissymbols with expressive language, and considered them as contributing to the children's total development in much the same way as speech does for speaking children. This model continued to guide the thinking of professionals working with Blissymbols throughout the years, during which increased attention was given to the contribution to be made by Blissymbols to the acquisition of reading and writing skills.

In the 1970s, three seminal publications were welcomed by professionals working with Blissymbolics: the paper by McDonald and Schultz (1973) regarding the use of communication boards with written words; Vickers' (1974) report of a nine-year project using pictures to supplement speech; and the manual on non-vocal communication techniques and aids produced by Vanderheiden and Grilley (1976).

As the atypical development and experiences of children with physical limitations became more apparent, the writing of Jerome Bruner and Margaret Donaldson proved helpful in observing and interpreting the children's behaviour. Bruner (1968) provided a valuable way to describe levels of representation – enactive (demonstrated by actions), iconic (summary images like a diagram or picture) and symbolic (set of symbolic propositions governed by rules) – that could be related to the development of abilities pertaining to graphics. Donaldson (1978) identified the need for balancing the responsibility of the teacher and learner within the teaching and learning process. Her exploration of the relationship between cognitive development and language development provided a framework for the asking of questions regarding the Blissymbol communication dyads that were part of the daily classroom activities.

For individuals who depend on graphic communication, the highest level of competence may be achieved through the acquisition of reading and writing skills for everyday communication. The theoretical paradigm relating to reading acquisition that strongly affected the early teachers and team was that of the whole language approach (Goodman, 1976; Smith, 1971, 1973, 1979). Our instructional philosophy would expand to consider language development, and phonological and graphic processing as well, as we were influenced by the new research findings of the 1980s and 1990s. In the beginning years, however, the major emphasis was upon the functional dimensions of text, on providing reading experiences that were highly motivating, and on giving children the confidence to 'hypothesize' or make an informed guess using context cues when encountering an unknown word. The first model integrating Blissymbolics and literacy development appeared 20 years later. The Language and Literacy Pathway (McNaughton and Lindsay, 1995) shown in Figure 16.1 is based upon the models of Snow (1991) and Keating (1990) and depicts literacy within the language continuum. To Snow's social, auditory, motor and symbolic strands, the visual strand is added as an essential component for children acquiring alternative communication systems.

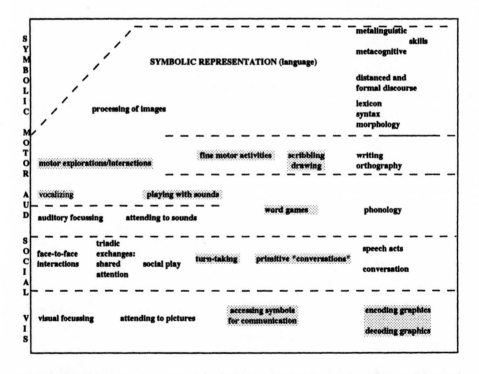

Figure 16.1. The Language and Literacy Pathway with visual, social, audiotory, motor and symbolic strands.

Figure 16.2 shows the second theoretical model specific to augmentative and alternative communication to result from the 30 years of children acquiring Blissymbols. It depicts reading development as beginning with the holistic processing of pictures and progressing through the analytical processing of Blissymbols and then of orthographic writing. The analogy of a ramp was chosen to emphasize the need for a supported and adapted road to literacy for children who are unable to acquire all the language competencies acquired through speech or to use all the phonological contributors to reading acquisition (McNaughton, in press). This depiction of literacy development draws attention to the various stages of graphic representation that can contribute to children's literacy development and rests firmly upon the support provided to the ramp through its five-stranded language foundation.

The Augmentative and Alternative Communication Literacy Ramp, resting as it does upon a strong language base, offers an additional metaphor to that of the three-legged stool. Both metaphors are applied in the account of alternative language and communication development that follows.

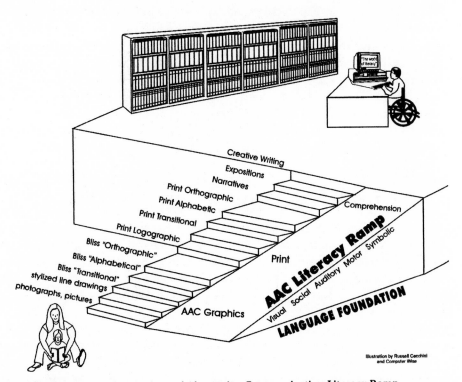

Figure 16.2. The Augmentative and Alternative Communication Literacy Ramp.

Method

The sources for the review of Kari's development include anecdotal information, school records, research information and examples of Kari's writing, selected from a large collection of Kari's creative output through the years. Details relating to Kari's childhood experiences have been derived from Harrington and Harrington (1988) and Harrington and Harrington (personal communication, July, 1992). The anecdotal information has been selected to include significant events that best characterize Kari's developmental pathway. The determination of an event as 'significant' was influenced:

- by Light's (1989) model of communication competence with its four areas of competence – linguistic, operational, social and strategic;
- by the depiction of a language and literacy pathway (McNaughton, 1992a, 1992b; McNaughton and Lindsay, 1995); and
- by a recognition of the importance of environmental factors in literacy acquisition (Koppenhaver, Evans and Yoder, 1991; Koppenhaver and Yoder, 1993; McNaughton, 1998).

The 'selection team' that initially assessed the significance of the occurrences comprised Kari, her mother, Kari's first Blissymbolics teacher (this author) and Kari's first teacher in her community public school. Excerpts from the paper by Harrington and Harrington (1988) along with excerpts from Kari's school reports and examples of Kari's stories and poems may be found on http://home.istar.ca/~bci. Formal documentation of Kari's communication and reading capabilities is derived from Silverman, McNaughton and Kates (1978) and McNaughton (1998). In examining Kari's writing between the ages of 10 and 25, an evaluation structure developed by Salvia and Hughes (1990) is used.

Kari's early development: birth to age six years

Kari was born on 6 January 1965, at a time when the field of augmentative and alternative communication did not exist, when little distinction was made in North America between cerebral palsy and intellectual impairment, and when the existence of Blissymbols was known by only those few scholars who responded to Charles Bliss upon receiving a description of his international language.

During the first months of Kari's life, her parents treated her in the same manner as their first child, although it was evident to them that there were delays in her development. At that time, their family doctor assured them that 'all children develop at their own rate and Kari's rate was a slow one'. It was not until she was 11 months old, that Kari was diagnosed as having cerebral palsy. At the time, many children and adults with cerebral palsy were institutionalized on the advice of their family physicians. Of those children with cerebral palsy who remained in their own homes, few were admitted to the public schools and even fewer (only the lucky ones with parents who advocated strongly for them) had home tutors. Some were able to attend activity programmes established by parents for a few hours a day.

When Kari was 18 months old, she and her parents began attending a newly established parent information service at Ontario Crippled Children's Centre, where parents and children met one morning a week with therapists and a social worker. They were assisted in dealing with Kari's physical limitations, but no attention was given to communication. The Centre doctor told them that intellectual impairment accompanied Kari's cerebral palsy and it was recommended that she attend a nursery for 'trainable mentally retarded children' for social stimulation. At three years of age, Kari began attending this nursery two mornings a week, and when she was four this was extended to three mornings a week. Both the staff and her parents noticed that Kari seemed more alert than many of the other children. Kari's parents were encouraged to continue their efforts at home to stimulate her and provide her with learning opportunities. Still the focus was primarily on activities that could improve Kari's physical dexterity and fine motor skills, like sorting beads by colour and shape, wooden puzzles and stacking toys.

Although Kari's mother does not remember that any special attention was given to Kari's language and pre-literacy development, Kari's early years were rich, nonetheless, in learning opportunities and in emerging literacy events. Her family read stories to her every day and ensured that Kari shared in all their activities. The arrival of her sister, Linda, when Kari was three and her brother, Rob, was five, implied that Kari would be surrounded by children's play during all of her pre-school years. Kari's first (non-electric) wheelchair when she was three years old gave her independent seating and allowed her to view the activities of the busy household. Kari's parents noticed her motivation to be an active participant in group activities.

As Kari became involved in the songs and play activities of the nursery for 'trainable mentally retarded children', her parents observed that she was doing the gestures to the songs on her own and in proper sequence. There was also consistency in the vocalizations that accompanied the gestures. This indicated to them that she had an accurate representation of the words and phrases in the songs. Their recollections of her communication within the family and in her nursery and pre-school programmes, however, relate only to her comprehension of spoken language. Her reactions to people who were speaking to her and the interest and attention she gave to conversations, story books and the activities of her brother and sister and other children indicated to the parents that she was similar to her brother and sister in her understanding of the events in her world (Harrington and Harrington, 1988). Kari's expressive communication at this time was limited to pointing directly at objects she wanted. She would often become upset and cry when she was not understood or when her needs and wishes were not anticipated by her family.

At the age of five, Kari was given an intellectual assessment at a centre for children with intellectual disability. Her parents were told that Kari's disability was more physical than intellectual. Following this, Kari started to attend the out-patient programme of the Ontario Crippled Children's Centre, which provided her with regular physiotherapy and speech therapy. She attended a nursery programme, half days, five days a week. By the end of the year, Kari was participating motorically as much in nursery activities as her physical abilities allowed. During this year, a brief attempt was made to introduce a picture board for choosing at snack time, but it was soon discontinued. Since Kari was used to pointing to the objects she wanted (at snack time and on other occasions), the pictures did not appear to offer her any advantage. Kari would indicate to her teacher what she wanted by rolling to a specific toy or activity. She also liked to scribble small notes with pencil and paper. While this enabled her to produce 'work' like some of the other children, it served no communicative purpose.

Middle childhood: age six to 10

In the fall of 1971, when Kari was six years old, she was placed in a special education primary class in which a traditional beginning reading programme of the early 1970s was practised, using primer readers. Kari was encouraged to use her left hand to practice copy typing of words, phrases and sentences on a typewriter. After seven months, her teacher reported that Kari knew 23 words and had reached page 32 in the primer. She could write the lower case letters of the typewriter when they were named and knew 'many of the capital letters as well'. By June, she had read to page 57 in the primer and had completed the accompanying workbook pages. Her knowledge of orthographic writing, however, was insufficient for her to initiate communication or to express her thoughts in this medium. Her means of communication were limited to pointing with hand and eye and responding to yes/no questions.

The pilot symbol programme

An experimental programme called the Symbol Communication Project was established at the Ontario Crippled Children's Centre in the fall of 1971. The project team's mandate was to explore possible communication techniques with six children selected as being the most responsive to their school programme among those who lacked functional speech. A primary criterion was a wide discrepancy between receptive and expressive language. The project's goal of developing a method of communication other than speech was looked upon with scepticism, and in some instances with resistance, by a number of the professionals at the Centre. The early 1970s was a time when communication was equated with speech and the focus of language intervention was upon producing recognizable sounds. This intervention met the needs of some of the children but there were many children for whom speech production was unrealistic.

Kari was chosen as one of six students aged five to eight years to participate in the pilot programme and in October 1971 her school time became divided between the Blissymbol class and the special education primary class. In addition to a gap between functional speech and receptive language ability, the main criteria were good form discrimination and ability to derive meaning from symbols. At first, the project team attempted to develop its own symbols, but when this author found a chapter describing Blissymbolics in *Signs and Symbols around the World* (Helfman, 1967), this was adopted as the project's graphic system. The team first designed an introductory set of 30 Blissymbols, then a board with 100 Blissymbols, which was expanded to boards with 200, 340 and 400 Blissymbols.

Kari received each board as it became available. Her progress in learning Blissymbols was typical of those children who were physically able to point directly to their communication boards and thus could communicate quite quickly. Other students in Kari's class required adapted technology or coding systems in order to reduce the motor demands or the number of locations that must be accessed. For this group, the progress proved to be slower. Prototype technology began to be developed and tested, but this was not functional for daily use. In most instances the children still had to rely solely upon manual boards. Some children began to use directed scanning in order to enhance the size of the vocabulary that could be accessed. However, in these pioneering days, the emphasis was on the children's development of motor independence in order to try to achieve independent language production, and every attempt was made for each child to select Blissymbols without help.

Early learning by partners

When the Blissymbolics programme began, the only references that could be found regarding the communication by those who lacked functional speech were a few newspaper clippings relating to the use of the Possum, an adapted typewriter used in the UK. The inference in much of the professional literature was that the impairments associated with cerebral palsy would preclude literacy and academic achievement even if individual examples contradicted this claim.

An acquisition topic that received considerable attention by the team was the selection and organization of vocabulary. The rationale for selecting vocabulary was based on the grammatical distinction between content or lexical words and function or grammatical words. Content words include nouns, verbs and adjectives; function words include the definite and indefinite articles, prepositions, conjunctions, verbal auxiliaries, and so forth. Blissymbols were readily available in both categories and this was viewed as a strong advantage. The Blissymbols were ordered according to the Fitzgerald key, with the grammatical ordering of words in a typical sentence appearing from left to right on the board. An important addition to the early vocabulary was the Blissymbol *COMBINE* that allowed the children to compose their own Blissymbols and indicate to their partners that a new compound Blissymbol was intended rather than a sentence. Also *OPPOSITE-MEANING* and *SIMILAR-TO* significantly increased the meanings that could be expressed (see Figure 16.3). The children were taught to use 'extended meanings' and the instructors to look for such meanings when interpreting the children's utterances.

Within a month of receiving the new display, Kari and three other children were applying the combining strategy effectively. They used the strategies to expand the number of meanings they could derive from a limited set of Blissymbols. They also used letters of the alphabet to denote specific persons, places and things (see Figure 16.3).

Blissymbols as the main means of communication in the class

In the first year, Blissymbols were taught in the mornings only by withdrawing the children from their regular classes. The following year, Kari and her peers were placed in classes where Blissymbols were used throughout the day. The children were divided into two groups according to their ability to access the Blissymbols. The children who could point independently were able to expand their vocabularies more quickly than those children who required assistance to indicate the Blissymbols they wanted. For those who were skilful in pointing, greater attention could be given to literacy along with their Blissymbol activities. When Kari entered this class in September 1972, she was 'conversant with the 340 Blissymbol display, except for the prepositions, some of the adverbs, and the conjunctions. Kari used Blissymbols spontaneously and with English order' (McNaughton, 1973, p. 25).

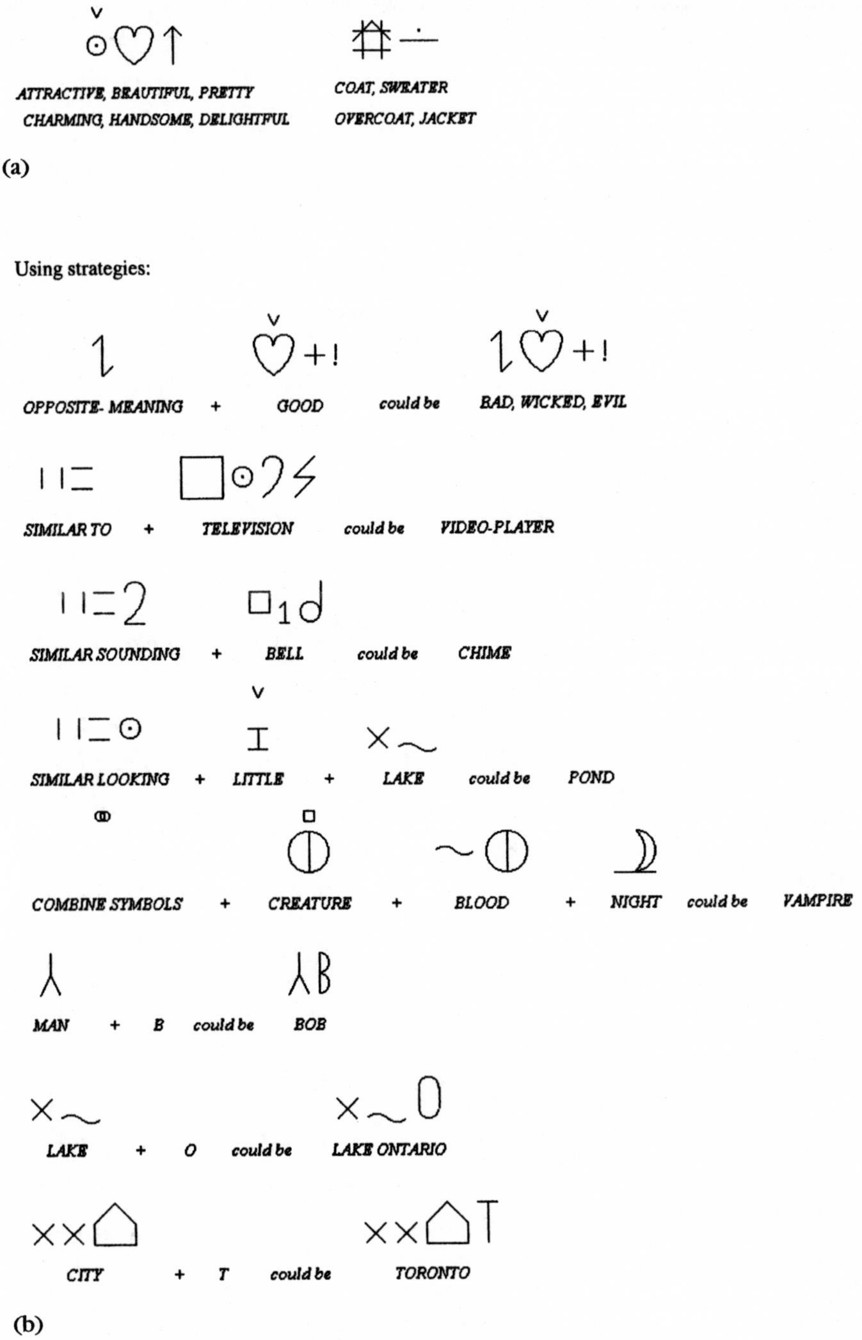

ATTRACTIVE, BEAUTIFUL, PRETTY
CHARMING, HANDSOME, DELIGHTFUL

COAT, SWEATER
OVERCOAT, JACKET

(a)

Using strategies:

OPPOSITE- MEANING + GOOD could be BAD, WICKED, EVIL

SIMILAR TO + TELEVISION could be VIDEO-PLAYER

SIMILAR SOUNDING + BELL could be CHIME

SIMILAR LOOKING + LITTLE + LAKE could be POND

COMBINE SYMBOLS + CREATURE + BLOOD + NIGHT could be VAMPIRE

MAN + B could be BOB

LAKE + O could be LAKE ONTARIO

CITY + T could be TORONTO

(b)

Figure 16.3. Extended meanings with Blissymbols.

However, the set of 340 Blissymbols still made many meanings difficult to express. This is demonstrated by the lexical additions that were made during the autumn of 1972:

1. Particles, such as *PERSON-WHO* and *PLACE-WHERE*
2. *TO-BE*
3. *PAST-TENSE* and *FUTURE-TENSE*
4. Blissymbols for seasons
5. Blissymbols for days of the week
6. Blissymbols for family members
7. *SIMILAR-TO,* for example combined with senses, to produce meanings like 'smells like' and 'feels like'
8. Blissymbols for special themes and seasonal activities created by children and teachers
9. Blissymbols for exclamations, like *WOW* and *YUCK*
10. Ten Blissymbols required as key words in Stott reading games
11. An alphabet as arranged on typewriters

The additions above illustrate well the manner in which the early Blissymbol programme evolved, and how the children's development and learning interacted with that of their teachers and other team members. By the end of the year, Kari's communication board consisted of 380 Blissymbols. Her use of Blissymbols was described as being 'imaginative and innovative and displaying independent and well-organized thinking ability'. For example, she spontaneously combined *THINK* and *SLEEP* to say 'dream' and expressed a 'problem' as *DIFFICULT-THINK.*

The reason for introducing Blissymbols was to make it possible for the children to get their meanings across through adding to, rather than attempting to replace, the communication methods they already used, mainly gestures, vocalizing and responding to yes/no questions. Besides the lessons where new Blissymbols were presented and explained, the main method of 'instruction' was that of Blissymbols being used throughout the day for communication. Blissymbols were written on the blackboard to record the date, the weather, mystery messages, daily activities and class-room projects. They were written on experience charts and overhead projector transparencies during group activities so that the children's stories, answers to questions and contributions to group conversation could be shared by all. The children were encouraged to use Blissymbols in any writing activities at home. Figure 16.4 shows a letter in Blissymbols written by Kari to her teacher when on holidays at her summer cottage.

After one year with Blissymbols as the main means of communication in the class, a consistent heavy use of single Blissymbols and telegraphic sentences were noted during group discussions at circle time. There were

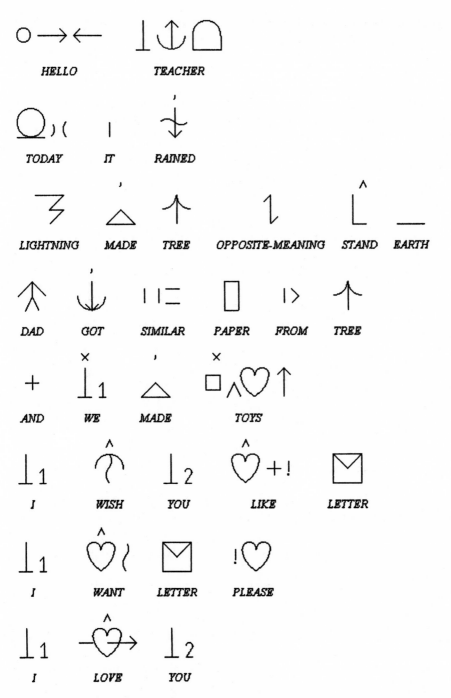

Figure 16.4. Letter written by Kari to her teacher.

few questions and requests, as well as utterances produced with *OPPOSITE-MEANING* and *SIMILAR-TO*. Spelling and the first consonant were infrequently used by the group as a whole at this stage. However, this documentation was accompanied by the comment that the results obtained from the group discussion records did not coincide with the impressions gained from conversations with individual children outside circle time, where questions and requests played a more prominent role, and the use of the Blissymbols *OPPOSITE-MEANING* and *SIMILAR-TO* and spelling seemed to be more regular (McNaughton, 1973).

The children communicated differently in different social settings. These observations demonstrate the different dynamics involved in group discussions where for the first time, these children were having the opportunity to 'talk' with their peers, and one-on-one conversation with an encouraging adult. With adults, the children seemed more comfortable and demonstrated a higher level of output. With their peers, their limited experience in interacting directly with each other seemed to be affecting their output.

This view was supported by reports from a parent meeting in the school that Kari was not very involved in activities with her peers. The children worked in parallel rather than together. In an attempt to increase peer communication, more peer conversations and role playing (of another classmate) was introduced in the classroom. The latter proved to be very challenging for the children. Role playing the teacher seemed to be an easier first step. Following this initiative, Kari began to interact more readily with others. This emphasizes the dependence on planning, even for participation in ordinary peer conversations (see also Tavares and Peixoto, this volume).

Outside school, too, Kari began to request information, solve problems, express concern and request explanations – 'How do you know?' became a common query. At last Kari had a way to say things without having to rely on endless questions asked by others and the frustration of not being understood. One day Linda, Kari's younger sister, was confronted with an empty ketchup bottle and a plate of chips at the dinner table. Kari tugged at Linda's arm and told her with Blissymbols to put water in the bottle. At the age of seven years, Kari was for the first time able to contribute a suggestion to the family, although Linda found that water added to ketchup makes for awful, soggy chips (Harrington and Harrington, 1988).

In 1973, Kari's mother reported that Kari had developed a strategy for using the book *Semantography* (Bliss, 1965) as a resource book to help her understand the meaning of new words. During activities at home, she would search for the Blissymbol to provide her with the information that users of spoken and written English would find in a dictionary – what the component parts meant, and how this information contributed to a composite meaning. This was a strategy that Kari used well into adulthood. As a result of Kari's initiative, a personal Blissymbol dictionary was made for each child. A published edition of all the Blissymbols in the standard vocabulary of the 1970s was not available until 1980 (Hehner, 1980). It was at this time when the provision of standard displays of 100, 200 and 400 Blissymbols was replaced by Blissymbol stamps and blank grids in North America. This enabled each child's communication display or book to be customized.

The increasing expressive abilities demonstrated by Kari and the other children changed their environment in significant ways, both in school and at home. During their first school year, Kari and the other children were often regarded as dull or intellectually impaired when moving about within the Centre without a Blissymbol tray. In the following year, however, as the children began participating in Centre activities with their Blissymbol board attached to their wheelchair, people seemed to consider the children as being 'bright'. When Kari expressed concern that an orange seed she had swallowed might grow into a baby inside of her, her parents realized that she was taking in much of what was going on around her and began to explain things to her in a way they never had before. Kari's ability to combine Blissymbols for a single meaning both surprised and amazed them. They had prepared themselves for serious limitations in her mind as well as her body. Kari's ability to learn and use Blissymbols effectively proved to everyone that she had significant capabilities.

Kari's full communicative use of Blissymbols was demonstrated when she fell out of bed one night and awoke crying. She was inconsolable, and with the light from a flashlight in order not to disturb Kari's sleeping sister, her mother watched Kari explain that she had dreamed that she was able to walk and had tried to get out of bed, only to crumple to the floor. It was important for both Kari and her mother that Kari could share her dream and that her mother could comfort her with the knowledge of the reason for her distress. Blissymbols were indeed not only a tool for education, but had become an everyday expressive language form that Kari shared with her family. It was the realization of the developmental goal of the programme to enable children to express their thoughts, emotions, concerns and ideas.

In December 1974, when Kari was 9;11 years old, her language skills were regarded as sufficient for her to take both the verbal and the performance parts of the Wechsler Intelligence Scale for Children (Wechsler, 1949). Her overall age score was estimated to be between seven and eight years. The test results showed a scattering of functioning with strengths in verbal reasoning and attention to visual detail, and weaknesses in arithmetic skills and general information.

During this school year, information was also collected on the use of Blissymbols by the children in Kari's class (Silverman et al., 1978). Kari was rated as excellent in 'spontaneously offering an alternative Blissymbol message when her first message was not understood', in using *OPPOSITE-MEANING* and *COMBINE* to expand her vocabulary, and in her use of verb tenses. She was rated as good in her use of the indicators of 'part of speech'. In an analysis of 108 examples of 'best Blissymbol utterances' submitted to the study of Silverman and associates, 21 sentence types were identified, ranging from 'Agent plus Action' and 'Agent plus Object' to 'Agent plus Action plus Object plus Dative', 'Agent plus Action plus Clause' and 'Object plus intransitive Action plus Object or Modifier'. The number of Blissymbols in best utterances ranged from two to 17 with a mean of nine, and the number of Blissymbols in typical utterances ranged from one to 15 with mean of five (Silverman et al., 1978, p. 59). This demonstrated to the team the children's extensive and creative use of the language capabilities of Blissymbolics.

Two important discoveries relating to speech and hearing during the 1973–4 school year alerted the team to the importance of considering all aspects of communication within any programme relating to alternative communication. All of the children were vocalizing more and this resulted in five of them becoming eligible for speech therapy for the first time. It appeared that the need and pressure for speech production had been decreased within the classroom, and they were able to verbalize more readily. Being able to use the Blissymbols seemed to make the children more relaxed in producing their messages. In future years some of the children did indeed progress to a reliance upon speech and a gradual reduction in the use of Blissymbols. As a result of a hearing assessment, it was found that Kari had a severe hearing loss in one ear that had been undetected during her first two years in the communication programme. Both discoveries were important warnings that the programme must maintain a broad view that included all the abilities related to communication. They could have been overlooked given the intense focus upon the alternative communication form.

Reading and writing

To participate fully in the broad literate world requires the ability to read and write. For non-speaking persons the mastery of orthographic writing, reading and spelling brings with it the liberation of producing an endless number of words and sentences through manipulating in countless ways a small set of sound-based characters – the letters of the orthographic alphabet. Blissymbolics also allows the manipulation of units, this time semantically based characters, to express countless meanings, but the set of characters that is required is extensive (over 800) and the receptive audience is small. Orthographic writing was therefore always a developmental goal for Kari and the other children. When they, in their different ways, used Blissymbols, they gained experience with expressive language, an essential reading ingredient, and the interpretation of Blissymbols presented by others implied practice in a form of reading. Thus, by using the ideographic and pictorial Blissymbols and the language structure of Blissymbolics, the children not only developed their expressive language – they were learning to read. That these first experiences with reading did not require knowledge of letter–sound correspondences greatly simplified the task (McNaughton, 1973).

Kari had started to follow traditional reading classes when she began school. However, when she began the Blissymbol programme, after one year in the primary educational programme, letters and words were mainly used to complement Blissymbol communication. In the second year of the Blissymbol programme, the orthographic reading programme was integrated with instruction based on Blissymbols, first in the form of the 'initial consonant strategy' – that is, to indicate the first letter of a word to make the meaning of a Blissymbol more specific. Blissymbols were used to teach phonic skills by relating the sounds corresponding to letters of the vocabulary that appeared as Blissymbols on the communication boards. Blissymbols were also substituted for spoken words in student games and assignments relating to initial letter and rhyme word recognition. The composing and reading of Blissymbol stories and letters was a regular component of the school day.

In the spring of 1973, when Kari was 7;8 years, her recognition of words that appeared on her Blissymbol board was assessed. With the Blissymbol removed, she correctly pointed out 23 of 25 written words when the words were spoken (word recognition), and indicated the Blissymbols (without the glosses) corresponding to 17 of 20 written words that were presented on cards (word retrieval). She was one of the best readers of orthographic writing in her class of Blissymbol users but she was still dependent on Blissymbols because her spelling was far from sufficiently developed for her to use it as her major communication form in ordinary conversations.

In the following school year, a heavier emphasis began to be placed on literacy development by building on the children's knowledge of Blissymbols. They were using communication boards with 400 Blissymbols and were using the words that accompanied the Blissymbols within their reading instructional programme. When, at the age of eight years, the use of letters began to accompany Blissymbols as Kari's primary line of communication development (see Renner, this volume), it was with a deeper understanding of the meaning of words and of what reading and writing could do for her.

By the end of this school year, Kari's teacher wrote that Kari's reading comprehension and word attack skills had increased and that she was becoming more independent and receptive to word-oriented challenges. However, compared with typically developing children, her understanding of grapheme–phoneme correspondences was limited. When writing independently, she thought of her utterance in Blissymbols and copied the necessary words from her board. She was unable to rely on decoding skills to identify an unfamiliar written word. When trying to decipher orthographically written words she used contextual clues, but would also often ignore or guess an unfamiliar written word. Kari's early progress in reading was thus in large part due to her learning to guess better when she attempted to identify unknown words. For this she relied on her general language abilities to better understand the meaning of running text. This behaviour was consistent with one of our teaching objectives at the time, as influenced by the writings of Frank Smith (1971), who emphasizes the importance of a learner's willingness to make mistakes and of the teacher's tolerance of them.

An analogy strategy was applied in linking Blissymbol reading and orthographic reading: the explaining of the component parts of Blissymbols was extended to explaining the component parts of orthographically written words, and attention was drawn to the different roles of the different characters: providing the meaning of characters in Blissymbols and providing the sounds of letters in print. These semantic derivations made it easier for the children to remember the Blissymbols and in many instances they provided the children with explanations for concepts that were unfamiliar to them. This strategy of explication predated the shift that came about in reading acquisition theory during the 1980s, when an extensive research literature provided support to the need for explicit instruction in phonological decoding in beginning reading (Gough and Hillinger, 1980; Rayner and Pollatsek, 1989; Stanovich, 1984, 1986).

During the fall of 1973, when Kari was 8;8 years old, as orthographic writing was receiving more attention academically, Kari still demonstrated a strong reliance on Blissymbols to express her intent within conversations. According to her teacher's report, Kari also continued to use a combination of vocalizations and gestures to supplement and clarify her Blissymbol utterances, but to a much lesser degree. As her communication with Blissymbols became clearer, her gestures and body posture appeared to be an extension of emotional expression rather than a clarification of her meaning (for a discussion on the relationship between language and gesture, see Launonen and Grove, this volume).

A significant event in Kari's development at this time was the phasing out of the daily communication notes that had passed between home and nursery and between home and school. Kari could now independently relay any information that was needed. At school, her teachers were reporting that she was spending time with orthographically written materials of all kinds, becoming increasingly confident about her reading skill and demonstrating a greater willingness to try words that were unfamiliar to her. She showed an interest in the spelling of words, and was anxious to work independently. By the end of this third school year in the Blissymbol program, Kari had worked through eight levels of the Holt Basic Reading system - the entire Grade One material – since January. She was attempting to use complete sentences in her typing, and showed interest in the different verb tenses as they appeared in orthographically written words. Her Blissymbol usage was described as exhibiting a variety of styles, with full sentences being her usual output pattern. She was enjoying typing from Blissymbol copy to English. Kari's growing interest in writing became more evident this year as she spent more of her hours of spare time at home writing stories, colouring pictures to accompany them and making books of her stories.

The other children in Kari's class developed in a similar way. The team could observe the unique unfolding of each child's range of abilities, and their educational programming could be planned in a much more responsive and individualized manner. By the 1974–5 school year, all were demonstrating a unique developmental path within the Blissymbolic strand described in the Language and Literacy Pathway (see Figure 16.1).

Late childhood: age 10–12 years

In the autumn of 1975, when Kari was 10;8 years old, her language environment was changed significantly. Her expressive communication was considered sufficiently developed for her to function in a less restricted environment, even if she was still dependent on Blissymbols and an adapted curriculum. From a language acquisition point of view, her ability to communicate with persons who were familiar to her and the independent use of an electric typewriter, was emphasized. Only one of the other children in Kari's class was also considered to have the necessary communicative skills for functioning in a less restricted educational environment.

She moved to the same public school that her brother and sister attended. It was a half block from her home, and she could go to school on her own. She was partially segregated: the core educational programme was in a classroom with other disabled children and part of the time she was within an ordinary class where she could socialize and participate in activities with speaking children. The primary special class contained 12 children with mixed exceptionalities. Kari received individualized instruction, with an emphasis on Blissymbol communication, but the teacher saw the potential Blissymbols held for promoting language skills in the other children. Kari became the class expert in Blissymbols and the spelling resource person for the other children because the glosses appearing with each Blissymbol could be pointed to by Kari upon request. This tutor role represented communicative challenges that were an important basis for her further development of language competence.

Her written work was in full sentences, including Blissymbols for words she could not yet spell. By the end of the school year Kari was reading at a grade two level, but was still to a great extent dependent on non-spelling strategies when reading or working on language exercises. By the end of the second year in her community school, Kari was reading at a grade three level and, according to the teacher, 'with enjoyment, comprehension and independence'. At age 12, Kari's reading had developed by a grade level for two successive school years.

Adolescence: age 13–16 years

Kari had used a small number of gestures and home signs since early childhood, but manual signing had not been pursued as a communication option in any formal way. At a camp during the summer of 1977, she learned to sign several songs and began to use signing at home and within her class's singing performances. She thus extended by herself her multi-component alternative communication system and increased her communicative repertoire and flexibility.

When at the age of 12;9, Kari moved to the junior special class, her school work included independent research projects, independent work contracts and formal workbooks. She still relied heavily on Blissymbols in her interpersonal communication, but letters were playing an increasing role. Her orthographic written work exhibited longer sentences and more elaboration. She completed the grade four reading level, with high performance on the comprehension tests in her reader.

At the beginning of Kari's second year in the junior special class she had a new teacher who tended only to lecture and did not give individualized teaching. Because of her hearing impairment, Kari did not hear everything the teacher said during group lessons, and the teaching pace was too fast without enough time for the provision of background knowledge. The teacher felt badly about the situation but there were many demands for her attention. She did not give the time required for Kari's Blissymbol communication. This meant that Kari became a less active participant and communicator in the class, and hence learned less. This school year was an unfortunate demonstration that teaching is not a one-way provision of 'information', but that teaching and learning is a collaborative activity where sufficient time for communication is a prerequisite. Young aided communicators need extended time devoted to dialogue in order to gain the same advantage from education as speaking children.

Late adolescence and early adulthood

Although Kari's spelling was gradually improving, Blissymbols continued to be used for much of her interpersonal communication through adolescence and into adulthood. Now Kari was using a variety of communication techniques, according to the communication partner and her own physical state. Her computer with speech output was used at school and at home when she was at a distance from the family member to whom she was conversing. She used manual signing with her mother at the end of the day when they both were tired. She used her Blissymbol board when she wanted a private conversation with a friend and an alphabet board when she needed a simple way to communicate during meals in restaurants.

One teacher noticed that Kari had developed problem-solving strategies that were demonstrated in her continual upgrading of her vocabulary. Kari felt it necessary to develop a logical communication board that was efficient for her and meaningful to others. In 1986, Kari designed a new and for her more efficient Blissymbol display, relying on her experience in acquiring and using aided communication. She had few difficulties with spelling and language arts at level 6, and continued to use the word-processing powers of the computer both in orthographic text and Blissymbols (see below).

Communication is not only dialogues and conversations in small groups. It extends for many of us to giving presentations to large groups. This became a goal for Kari and three other communication aid users and they entered a training programme for presenters to give community presentations. Kari became much more confident and assertive as she gained experience. She enjoyed giving public presentations, despite frequent breakdowns of the technology.

Kari's increased communicative confidence was evident when in 1988 she had to enter the hospital with thrombosis. She took charge of her interactions with the medical staff and successfully communicated with the doctors and nurses during her hospital stay. Kari considered this a significant event for this time in her life, and to this she added a second event to be noted. Upon returning home from the hospital, she began having friends visit her on Saturday nights. This indication of inclusion by her peers was very important to her. Kari was now 23 years of age.

Adolescence and early adulthood marked an era of prolific writing. Kari wrote many poems and short stories and, in 1987, began writing regularly for the magazine *Communicating Together.* The adolescents in her segregated high school class had much lower cognitive abilities than Kari, and the adolescents in her non-segregated classes showed different social skills and had different interests from Kari. Her writing gave her an outlet for her thoughts and a way to communicate about her feelings.

The language environment

The support Kari received through her language environment in school varied greatly as her teachers displayed a range of attitudes with regard to her communication. In the orthopaedic class, she was given the time that is needed to use Blissymbols, whereas in the English class her teacher claimed that time constraints forced her to rely on yes/no questions in communicating with Kari. Kari's continuing acquisition of new language skills, even when the learning environment lacked the support she needed, can be attributed to her growing confidence from her successful experiences outside the school and to the practice she got with Blissymbols and orthographic writing in some of the classes she attended. As Kari's mother noted:

> Kari did quite well in her subjects within the main stream, but not without our continued help and support on the home front. We read difficult text together – discussed it and related it, if possible, to things within her own experience. We listened to and answered her questions and, in general, did whatever we could to help clarify things for her. Kari has often said that without that input from us, she would never have survived in those classes. (Harrington and Harrington, 1988)

The growing awareness in the augmentative and alternative communication field of the importance of support in all environments could not be more ably demonstrated than in this report of the family help that was so critical to Kari's achievement.

Technology

The year 1981 represented the beginning of the computer age for Kari and other disabled individuals. Kari was 16 years old and had entered an orthopaedic class at Langstaff secondary school. At this time, she began to use the school computer to do her own writing and to correct her written work. The speech synthesizer was a great help when she was editing her work independently. In 1982, she learned to access and print Blissymbols in a research project two evenings per week, but it was not until 1984 that Kari received her first personal computer, an Apple 2E.

In 1986, Kari was able to lease an Epson with Speech PAC voice-output device through the newly established Assistive Devices Programme of the Ontario Ministry of Health. She found people more accepting of her communication when she used this technology than when she used Blissymbols without speech. She assisted in teaching another student how to use the computerized Talking BlissApple system.

The telephone was an everyday tool for most of Kari's speaking peers, but her use of it came later than most and only when she gained proficiency with her voice output device. She compensated, however, by early use of electronic mail. In 1984, Kari began using Confer, a teleconferencing program that enabled her to send and receive written messages from friends (see Harrington, 1984a, 1984b).

Literacy skills in adulthood: age 30

At the age of 30, Kari was a participant in a study that evaluated the literacy acquisition of 31 users of Blissymbols (McNaughton, 1998). In most of the reading-related tasks within the assessment battery, Kari performed within the average range or above the average performance of her cohort group (Table 16.1). On sentence comprehension, she received a grade score of 6.5 on the Peabody Individual Achievement Test (Dunn and Markwardt, 1970), which denotes the median score of grade six classes within public education in the US in 1970. The average grade level for Kari's cohort was 3.3 (standard deviation 1.8). Her reading comprehension quotient was 90 when using the norms for the 16 to 18 year olds.

Discussion

Kari's developmental pathway has been unusual compared with normally speaking children – a pathway that required a form of environmental support from the family and the teachers that was different from other children. Throughout her school years, the content and style of her instructional programme varied, sometimes meeting her special support requirements, sometimes failing to do so. She gained expressive communication skills much later than other children, including the use of orthographic writing, which for her also had an important function in direct communication with other people. The use of orthographic writing was developed on the foundation of another graphic communication form, Blissymbolics. Table 16.2 gives an overview of her progress over the years.

There were several reasons for the delayed onset of an alternative communication system. When Kari first entered the nursery for 'trainable mentally retarded children' in 1968, the focus was on socialization and group activities. Her response to the activities in the programme and the observations of the teachers and her parents indicated a learning potential that had not previ-

Table 16.1. Kari's reading profile compared to the rest of the reading children in her class (McNaughton, 1998)

	Kari	Group mean (sd)	
CVC-NC (non-conventional) word task	65	76.43	(14.64)
Visual analysis retrieval (with Blissymbols)	60	80.00	(16.33)
Recognition decoding pseudoword task	100	85.71	(19.02)
Spelling word pair	100	83.57	(16.99)
Homophone word pair	83	60.29	(19.05)

Table 16.2. Summary of Kari's communication and language development 1967–1995

Year	Age	
1967	2	Gestures and home signs.
1968	3	Assumed to have some understanding.
1970	5	Pointed to objects, rolled across room to gain access and indicate specific item (mother).
1972	7;6	Knowledge of orthographic writing insufficient for her to initiate communication or to express her thoughts.
1972	7:9	Communication board with 340 Blissymbols, but has problems with prepositions, some adverbs and the conjunctions. Used Blissymbols spontaneously and with English order.
1972	7;11	Communication board with 380 Blissymbols. Use was imaginative and innovative. Displayed independent and well-organized reasoning.
1973	8	Requested information, solved problems, expressing concern, requested explanations: How do you know?
1974	9	Thought of her utterance in Blissymbols and copied the necessary words from her display.
1974	9;11	Communicated well enough for being assessed with the verbal part of the WISC. Results showed strength in verbal reasoning and attention to visual detail. Blissymbol usage exhibited a variety of styles with full sentences being her usual ones.
1976	11;6	Reading at grade 2 level.
1977	12	Learned to sign several songs at summer camp. Began using signing at home and with class when singing.
1979	14;6	Beginning grade 4 reading level.
1981	16	Employed all her language skills successfully.
1981	16;6	Beginning grade 6 reading level.
1995	30	Reading at grade 9–10 level.

ously been recognized by the professionals who had assessed her. In her time at the Ontario Crippled Children Centre from 1970 to 1975, the emphasis was first on her physical and experiential development in the nursery programme, and then secondly on communication integrated with language, reading and cognitive development within the Blissymbolics programme. Similar non-communicative early priorities are reported in other countries (Basil and Soro-Camats, 1996; von Tetzchner, 1997).

When Kari entered the primary programme in her community school in 1975, the curriculum was individualized in order to accommodate and support her communication form. In the intermediate and senior years, such adaptations proved to be very difficult for some teachers due to time constraints, the class size, the behaviour of other students and the teachers' strict adherence to their pre-designed course. As Kari studied within the secondary school programme, 1981 to 1988, her ongoing literacy and language development was witness to the outcome that is possible when a strong language foundation has been acquired and there is ongoing support of the learner's communication form. Her development could not be described as the result of a continuous optimal language environment or 'language acquisition support system' (see Bruner, 1983), but it could be considered as benefiting from the strong support she received in her early formative years.

Reading and writing

During her early Blissymbol years, Kari excelled in learning Blissymbols. Her ability to recognize and use Blissymbol components was rated as 'fair' when she was nine years old, and as 'good' when she was 10 years old (Silverman et al., 1978). As an adult, however, her performance was low on tasks requiring visual analysis without the support of known phonological information. On both a non-conventional word task and a task involving visual analysis and retrieval with Blissymbols, both requiring visual analysis of non-conventional characters, Kari's performance was below that of most of her reading peers, although her overall reading performance placed her at the high end of this group. In contrast, her scores on tasks that provided known phonological information were higher than the average for the group of independent readers (McNaughton, 1998).

These overall findings in the McNaughton (1998) study demonstrate that a different type of processing may be required in picture identification and a visual matching than is required in the visual analysis and retrieval of Blissymbols, and that visual analysis and retrieval ability comes later in development than picture recognition and visual matching. The results also indicate that there is a positive relationship between performance on the visual analysis retrieval tasks and the lowest developmental level of a phonological recoding (which involves both phonological and visual decoding) only at an early developmental level within reading acquisition. There is no indication of any relationship at more advanced reading levels. From these results the position can be taken that a relationship between skill in visual analysis and reading achievement may be developmentally limited. Hence, the possibility of support being derived at the earliest stage of phonological recoding from regular exposure to visual decoding, cannot be discounted –

especially if the learning partner captures the child's interest in the analytic processing of both Blissymbols and orthographic script.

The results of the McNaughton (1998) study support the transactional model of development (see Sameroff, 1987), in that the impact of severe congenital and physical impairments upon family and educational support, language and literacy learning opportunities, and the expectations of the individual, family and school regarding literacy acquisition may be seen as initiating a series of restricting external events rather than as directly causing reading difficulties. The attitudes engendered by severe congenital speech and physical impairment may well be a primary factor that influences expectations for reading acquisition and sets in motion a complex of inter-related behaviours and beliefs, resulting in limited reading experiences and eventually in reduced levels of reading proficiency. Limited reading performance, which in the past has been attributed to physical impairment and anarthria, may in fact be found to be related to environmental conditions and experiences that in turn restrict an understanding of the potential of persons with this diagnosis (McNaughton, 1998). In Kari's case, her family's attitudes did not follow the pattern often found for persons with severe congenital speech and physical impairment. Her ecological rating was among the four highest of the 32 subjects in the McNaughton study and Kari's literacy achievement was typical of those subjects with strong ecological support.

The lesson to be learned from Kari's reading progress is that the building of a language foundation must be gradual and according to the individual's position on his or her developmental path. The early reading milestones typically exhibited by speaking children are not replicated by those who base their literacy on a non-speech communication form instead of speech, and who are acquiring expressive communication skills along with ordinary reading and writing skills. If time and attention are given to developing a strong language foundation, however, a child communicating with Blissymbols may progress through new reading levels and may continue to do so beyond the school years. In this endeavour, the two major language environments of children – the home and school – both play decisive roles for the young aided communicators. The language environment provided at school must include additional resources. The school has the responsibility of making appropriate language forms available in all the natural environments of the child and of helping the child apply these forms to the acquisition of new skills. Kari's family enriched her positive school language experiences and compensated when the school environment was ineffective. Her home always provided communication partners who were patient and responsive to Kari's communicative efforts. When comparing Kari's communication and reading skills with those of the other children in the study, it may well be that her higher performance was due in part to her fortunate biological attributes.

However, it is equally likely that the differences were in large measure due to the overall quality of her 'language acquisition support system' (see Bruner, 1983).

Salvia and Hughes (1990) identify four components for the evaluation of writing: grammar, mechanics, diction, and diversity. *Grammar* refers to the sequencing and interrelationships among words that give meaning to written expression and includes parts of speech, sentence construction, pronoun case (different forms of the same word), agreement in number and gender between pronouns and antecedents and consistency in number between subjects and verbs: verb tense, voice and mood. *Mechanics* refer to the conventions used to write English and has as subcomponents punctuation, capitalization, font styles, abbreviations, number usage, referencing and general format. *Diction* refers to word usage and considers the following aspects: using the word that means precisely what the writer intends, wordiness and omission of words. *Diversity* refers to the use of different vocabulary, sentence structures and grammatical transformations. This structure is applied to an examination of Kari's writing in Table 16.3.

Throughout her development, Kari's writing, while creative and extensive, appears to have been about four years behind that of the typical developmental pattern of non-disabled children. However, her writing performance indicates skills in keeping with the grade level in which she was working and her writing as an adult demonstrates a high level of competency.

Blissymbols, language and literacy

The number of non-speaking people in North America who use Blissymbolics has been greatly reduced in the 1990s. Many adults, like Kari, made the transition to orthographic writing. Some were given pictographic systems like PCS and PIC, often without the user being consulted. Others have continued to use Blissymbols because they found it valuable and would not relinquish it. A similar trend may be found in some countries outside North America (von Tetzchner and Jensen, 1996). As literacy for users on non-speech communication systems began to gain attention in North America, the features of Blissymbolics were again examined. The links to literacy that were postulated in the 1970s became more clearly identified in the 1990s, and there has been a re-discovery of the importance of its language capabilities.

The definition of language provided by Lindblom (1990) may be applied to provide a clear distinction between the language features of Blissymbolics and the representational features of pictures and line drawings. His explanation of the duality of language offers a rationale for differentiating between symbol types:

Table 16.3.

Grammar

Age 10   Complete sentences, pronouns, the possessive case, an auxiliary verb and consistency in number between subject and verb.

Age 11   Frequent usage, sometimes incorrectly, of the possessive; confusing possessive with plural; exploring different tense forms of the verb; some inconsistency in number between subject and verb; and misuse of article.

Age 15   Agreement between subject and verb; exploring variety of sentence types; and direct quotation used.

Age 16   Use of descriptives; variety of sentence constructions; and extensive use of direct quotations.

Age 25   Correct use of questions, assertive sentences, direct quotations; and flexibility of verb forms.

Mechanics

Age 10   Punctuation and capitalization.

Age 11   Punctuation and capitalization with longer sentences.

Age 15   Use of exclamation mark and brackets.

Age 16   Use of question marks and exclamation marks.

Age 25   Correct use of punctuation throughout.

Diction

Age 10   Appropriate word usage for grade one reading level.

Age 11   Appropriate word usage for grade two reading level.

Age 15   Appropriate word usage for grade three reading level.

Age 16   Expanded word usage.

Age 25   Appropriate for the story.

Diversity

Age 10   The limited type of sentence structure, vocabulary and grammatical transformations typical of the grade one student.

Age 11   Variety of sentence and word types used.

Age 15   Variety of sentence forms, appropriate style for topic.

Age 16   Increasing variety in style of sentence forms and words used (typical of grades 5-6 student).

Age 25   Continued growth in variety of sentence forms.

Human languages make combinatorial use of discrete units at two levels of structure. At the phonological level they combine vowels and consonants to form words and other forms. And at the level of syntax they use rules for combining words into phrases and sentences. This combinatorial method is so powerful that, for practical purposes, it sets no upper limit on the number of messages that languages can convey. It is the key to their expressive power. Since it operates both on the units of phonology and on the units of syntax, it has dual structure. In the terminology of the linguist, human languages are said to exhibit duality (Lindblom, 1990, p. 227).

For speaking children, the duality of the language of their environment is applied every time they utter or write a new word or produce an original phrase or sentence. The 'combinatorial capability' is mastered through day-to-day interaction. They learn their language through listening to the talk of others, through talking with those in their environment and through early explorations with writing within their drawings. For aided communication users who understand spoken language, the duality of their native language is presented to them receptively as they listen to the speaking of those who interact with them – sometimes also to their own artificial voice if they use speech-output communication devices – and as they observe the orthographically written sentences in books. Users of communication aids can only acquire 'combinatorial capability' expressively, however, if their communication system provides duality and they are able to access and manipulate individual lexical units and sentence elements (see Smith, 1996; Soto, 1999; Sutton, 1999; von Tetzchner et al., 1996). Blissymbolics may serve in this expressive capacity both on manual communication boards and as the representation system through which communication aids with synthetic speech are accessed.

Integration

The qualities of language environments as they contribute to the development of children using alternative communication are closely related to the discussion of segregation and inclusion. During the timespan that covers Kari's education, I and my colleagues have arrived at a position regarding integration that may deserve consideration 30 years after Kari began school. Returning to the three-legged stool analogy, according to this position, alternative communication users require a strong communication, language and literacy foundation – usually facilitated through primary education in a segregated setting – before they can benefit from whatever developmental support they may be provided with in the regular school programme. Only with sturdy legs can the stool be strong.

In looking back upon the 1970s from the year 2002, it seems that the attitudes towards segregation and inclusion are now reversed. Today, with inclusion being the general practice in North America, specialized classrooms and individualized instruction can only be obtained through lengthy assessments and documentation of the child's limitations. In the 1970s, it was necessary to demonstrate the child's strengths in order for them to be considered for placement in an inclusive school setting. From the vantage point of an educator who taught in the 1970s, the earlier approach appears much more constructive. In my view, the ideal for children who acquire aided communication is partial segregation during the pre-school and primary years, receiving individualized language, communication and literacy instruction within a group of children who share the need for and the interest in alternative communication. In addition, as part of a planned language development programme, there must be opportunities to socialize and participate in activities with speaking children. These socialization and language learning opportunities should not be viewed, however, as providing or substituting for a segregated core language development and educational programme. The slower communication speed, the different experiential background, the need to have special opportunities to ensure active participation in the learning programme, the need to share learning with those with common communication challenges and the need for specialized knowledge on the part of the teacher all require provisions that can rarely be met within the regular classroom in North America. Typically these conditions can best be provided in a segregated classroom with a specialized staff. The school placement model that was followed with Kari in 1975 was based on her having a strong language, communication and literacy foundation before she moved from the segregated to the inclusive setting. When the legs of the stool were firmly in place, it was deemed time for her to make the move. The decision proved to be a very good one. During her eight years of secondary education, from the age of 16 to 23 years, Kari earned a total of seven credits. By age 30, she performed at a grade nine to 10 level in reading and continued to take correspondence courses. These outcomes demonstrate a remarkable developmental journey for a young woman originally assessed as 'trainable mental retarded'. They speak as well to the need for extended time for development and the benefit derived from ongoing consistent support from home.

Implications for intervention

The development of Kari and other Blissymbol users has made the primary importance of the language environment – both at home and in the educational setting – very evident. The achievements of those who progressed to orthography is a strong reminder of the importance of including literacy competency as an outcome of language development for non-speaking children. The development of literacy is a result of the mutual transactional influences of external support during the learning-to-read stage and the individual's language and cognitive competencies. A number of studies have demonstrated the importance of communication partners (Kraat, 1985; Light, McNaughton and Parnes, 1994). Kari's development and that of her cohorts who have achieved literacy competence provide strong anecdotal evidence for the role played by the language environment during their formative years.

The greatest value of Blissymbolics in development may well be its two-fold role – (a) as a transition 'language' between pictographic systems and orthographic writing for those like Kari who can achieve literacy, and (b) as a long-term expressive language form for those who do not become fluent in spelling but who independently generate new meanings. It is the language structure and developmental scaffolding that Blissymbolics provides for the user that is one of its important strengths. In intervention, one should be concerned with (a) the children's development of strategies to compensate for having to communicate in a cumbersome way (not having natural speech), and (b) children's development of language in order to gain metalinguistic competency and a mastery of orthographic script in as many forms as possible: spelling, reading and writing. This means that in addition to the attention given to language development and visual analysis, there must be a strong emphasis on cognitive and phonological processing and a recognition that the phonological domain is likely to present difficulty. The answer is innovative teaching and the integration of all aspects of language development within the educational programme (McNaughton, 1995).

Acknowledgement

Kari was indeed fortunate in the assistance she received both from her learning partners at home and school and from Blissymbolics. In return, Kari has taught much to her family, her teachers and to the many friends and colleagues who have interacted directly with her. I thank her for allowing her learning to become ours.

Blissymbols used herein derived from the symbols described in the work, *Semantography*, original copyright© C.K. Bliss. In September, 1982, C.K. Bliss granted an exclusive, non-cancellable and perpetual, world-wide licence to the Blissymbolics Communication Institute, for the application of Blissymbols, for use by handicapped persons and persons having communication difficulties.

References and Citation Index

Abbi, A. (1980). *Semantic Grammar of Hindi*. Delhi, India: Bahiri. **303**

Abrahamsen, A.A., Cavallo, M. and McCluer, J. (1985). Is the sign advantage a robust phenomenon? *Merrill-Palmer Quarterly, 31,* 177–209. **118, 119, 149**

Abrahamsen, A.A., Lamb, M., Brown-Williams, J. and McCarthy, S. (1990). Boundary conditions on language emergence; contributions from atypical learners and input. In P. Siple and S. Fischer (Eds), *Theoretical Issues in Sign Language Research* (pp. 231–54). Chicago, Illinois: University of Chicago Press. **3, 4**

Akhtar, N. and Tomasello, M. (1996). Two-year-olds learn words for absent objects and actions. *British Journal of Developmental Psychology, 14,* 79–93. **289**

Allen, D., Moore, E., Dunn, N. and Anderson, V. (1986). Transition from an urban residential setting to a rural public school setting: Do augmentative communication systems work in the real world? *Augmentative and Alternative Communication, 2,* 69. **335**

Alm, N. and Newell, A.F. (1996). Being an interesting conversation partner. In S. von Tetzchner and M.H. Jensen (Eds), *Augmentative and Alternative Communication: European Perspectives* (pp. 171–81). London, UK: Whurr. **256, 274**

Alsaker, F.D. and Flammer, A. (1999). *The Adolescent Experience*. London, UK: Lawrence Erlbaum. **273**

Arvidson, H.H. and Lloyd, L.L. (1997). History of AAC. In L.L. Lloyd, D.R. Fuller and H.H. Arvidson (Eds), *Augmentative and Alternative Communication: A Handbook of Principles and Practices* (pp. 18–26). London, UK: Allyn & Bacon. **2**

Baddeley, A.D. (1986). *Working Memory*. Oxford, UK: Clarendon. **44**

Baddeley, A.D. and Hitch, G.J. (1974). Working memory. In G. Bower (Ed.), *The Psychology of Learning and Motivation: Advances in Research and Theory, Volume 8* (pp. 47–90). New York: Academic Press. **43**

Bakeman, R. and Adamson, L. (1984). Coordinating attention to people and objects in mother-infant and peer-infant interaction. *Child Development, 55,* 1278–89. **29**

Baker-Ward, L., Ornstein, P.A. and Holden, D.J. (1984). The expression of memorization in early childhood. *Journal of Experimental Child Psychology, 37,* 555–75. **41, 54**

Balandin, S. and Iacono, T. (1998). A few well-chosen words. *Augmentative and Alternative Communication, 14,* 147–61. **74**

Baldwin, D.A. (1991). Infants' contribution to the achievement of joint reference. *Child Development, 62,* 875–90. **30, 31**

Bankson, N.W. (1977). *Bankson Language Screening Test*. Baltimore, Maryland: University Park Press. **275**

Bara, B., Bosco, F.M. and Bucciarelli, M. (1999). Developmental pragmatics in normal and abnormal children. *Brain and Language, 68,* 507–28. **86**

Barnes, D. (1975). *From Communication to Curriculum.* New York: Penguin. **335**

Baron-Cohen, S. (1989). Perceptual role-taking and protodeclarative pointing in autism. *British Journal of Developmental Psychology, 7,* 113-27. **35**

Baron-Cohen, S. (1995). *Mindblindness: An essay on autism and Theory of Mind.* Cambridge, Massachusetts: MIT Press. **35, 212**

Barrett, M. (1995). Early lexical development. In P. Fletcher and B. MacWhinney (Eds), *The Handbook of Child Language* (pp. 362-92). Cambridge, Massachusetts: Basil Blackwell. **85, 117**

Barrouillet, P. and Poirier, L. (1997). Comparing and transforming: an application of Piaget's morphisms theory to the development of class inclusion and arithmetic problem solving. *Human Development, 40,* 216-34. **155**

Barton, M. and Tomasello, M. (1994). The rest of the family: the role of fathers and siblings in early language development. In C. Gallaway and B. Richards (Eds), *Input and Interaction in Language Acquisition* (pp. 109-34). London, UK: Cambridge University Press. **158, 159**

Basil, C. (1992). Social interaction and learned helplessness in severely disabled children. *Augmentative and Alternative Communication, 8,* 188-99. **9, 204, 207, 213, 226, 274, 341**

Basil, C. (2001). Comunicación aumentativa y alternativa en la práctica: El reto de identificar intervenciones significativas. In F. Alcantud Marín and M. Lobato Galindo (Eds), *2001 - Odisea de la comunicación: Ponencias y comunicaciones de las II Jornadas sobre Comunicación Aumentativa y Alternativa* (pp. 68-77). Valencia, Spain: Sociedad Española de Comunicación Aumentativa y Alternativa - ISAAC España. **274**

Basil, C. and Soro-Camats, E. (1996). Supporting graphic language acquisition by a girl with multiple impairments. In S. von Tetzchner and M.H. Jensen (Eds), *Augmentative and Alternative Communication: European Perspectives* (pp. 270-91). London, UK: Whurr. **16, 285, 380**

Bates, E. (1976). *Language and Context: The Acquisition of Pragmatics.* New York: Academic Press. **230, 300**

Bates, E. (1979). *The Emergence of Symbols.* London, UK: Academic Press. **77**

Bates, E., Bretherton, I. and Snyder, L. (1988). *From First Words to Grammar: Individual Differences and Dissociable Mechanisms.* Cambridge, UK: Cambridge University Press. **40, 248**

Bates, E., Camaioni, L. and Volterra, V. (1975). The acquisition of performatives prior to speech. *Merrill-Palmer Quarterly, 21,* 205-26. **84**

Bates, E., Dale, P. and Thal, D. (1995). Individual differences and their implications for theories of language development. In P. Fletcher and B. MacWhinney (Eds), *The Handbook of Child Language* (pp. 96-151). Cambridge, Massachusetts: Basil Blackwell. **19, 119, 205**

Bauer, P.J. and Werkera, S.S. (1995). One- to two-year-olds' recall of events: The more expressed, the more impressed. *Journal of Experimental Child Psychology, 59,* 475-96. **248**

Bauer, P.J. and Werkera, S.S. (1997). Saying is revealing: Verbal expression of event memory in the transition from infancy to early childhood. In P.W. van den Broek, P.J. Bauer and T. Bourg (Eds), *Developmental Spans in Event Comprehension and Representation: Bridging Fictional and Actual Events* (pp. 139-68). Hillsdale, New Jersey: Lawrence Erlbaum. **248**

Baumwell, L., Tamis-LeMonda, C.S. and Bornstein, M.H. (1997). Maternal verbal sensitivity and child language comprehension. *Infant Behaviour and Development, 20,* 247-58. **30**

Bedrosian, J.L. (1997). AAC technology and communicative competence: Issues and directions for future research. In J. Brodin and E. Björck-Åkesson (Eds), *Methodological Issues in Research in Augmentative and Alternative Communication* (pp. 62-6). Vällingby, Sweden: Swedish Handicap Institute. **312**

Bedrosian, J. (1999). Efficacy research issues in AAC: Interactive storybook reading. *Augmentative and Alternative Communication, 15,* 45-55. **233**

Beliveau, C., Howery, K., Pon, C., Lycan, S. and Schmidt, J. (2000, August). I CAN Camp: Students and educational support personnel training. Conference Proceedings of the 9th Biennial Conference of the International Society of Augmentative and Alternative Communication, Washington, USA. **336**

Bennett-Kastor, T. (1988). *Analyzing Children's Language.* Oxford, UK: Basil Blackwell. **155**

Berko-Gleason, J. (1975). *Fathers and Other Strangers: Men's Speech to Young Children. Georgetown University Roundtable on Language and Linguistics.* Washington DC: Georgetown University Press. **159**

Besio, S. and Chinato, M.G. (1996). A semiotic analysis of the possibilities and limitations of Blissymbols. In S. von Tetzchner and M.H. Jensen (Eds), *Augmentative and Alternative Communication: European Perspectives* (pp. 182-94). London, UK: Whurr. **58**

Beukelman, D., McGinnis, J. and Morrow, D. (1991). Vocabulary selection in augmentative and alternative communication. *Augmentative and Alternative Communication, 7,* 171-85. **74**

Beukelman, D.R. and Mirenda, P. (1992). *Augmentative and Alternative Communication.* Baltimore, Maryland: Paul H. Brookes. **57**

Beukelman, D.R. and Mirenda, P. (1998). *Augmentative and Alternative Communication,* Second edition. Baltimore, Maryland: Paul H. Brookes. **38, 81, 274, 286**

Bialystok, E. (1999). Cognitive complexity and attentional control in the bilingual mind. *Child Development, 70,* 636-44. **20**

Bialystok, E. and Ryan, E.B. (1985). A metacognitive framework for the development of first and second language skills. In D.L. Forrest-Pressley, G.E. MacKinnon and T.G. Waller (Eds), *Metacognition, Cognition, and Human Performance, Volume 1: Theoretical perspectives* (pp. 207-52). Orlando, Florida: Academic Press. **64**

Bickerton, D. (1981). *Roots of Language.* Ann Arbor, Michigan: Karoma. **207**

Bijou, S.W. (1993). *Behavior Analysis of Child Development.* Reno, North Virginia: Context Press. **7**

Bird, F., Dores, P.A., Moniz, D. and Robinson, J. (1989). Reducing severe aggressive and self-injurious behaviors with functional communication training. *American Journal on Mental Retardation, 94,* 37-48. **181**

Bishop, D.V.M. (1982). *Test of Reception of Grammar.* Manchester, UK: Department of Psychology, University of Manchester. **161**

Bishop, D.V.M. (1997). *Uncommon Understanding: Development and Disorders of Language Understanding in Children.* Hove, UK: Psychology Press. **3**

Bishop, D.V.M. and Edmondson, A. (1987). Language-impaired 4-year-olds: Distinguishing transient from persistent impairment. *Journal of Speech and Hearing Disorders, 52,* 156-73. **229**

Bjorklund, D.F. (2000). *Children's thinking: Developmental function and individual differences.* Third edition. Belmont, California: Wadsworth. **44, 45**

Bjorklund, D.F. and Coyle, T.R. (1995). Utilization deficiencies in the development of memory strategies. In F.E. Weinert and W. Schneider (Eds), *Memory Performance and Competencies: Issues in Growth and Development* (pp. 283-300). Mahwah, New Jersey: Lawrence Erlbaum. **49**

Bjorklund, D.F., Muir-Broaddus, J.E. and Schneider, W. (1990). The role of knowledge in the development of strategies. In D.F. Bjorklund (Ed.), *Children's Strategies: Contemporary Views of Cognitive Development* (pp. 93-128). Hillsdale, New Jersey: Lawrence Erlbaum. **41, 47**

Blischak, D.M. and Lloyd, L.L. (1996). Multimodal augmentative and alternative communication. *Augmentative and Alternative Communication, 12,* 37-46. **177**

Blischak, D.M. and McDaniels, M.A. (1995). Effects of picture size and placement on memory for written words. *Journal of Speech and Hearing Research, 38,* 1356-62. **205**

Bliss, C.K. (1965). *Semantography (Blissymbolics).* Sydney: Semantography Publications. **176, 370**

Bloom, L. (1973). *One Word at a Time.* The Hague, The Netherlands: Mouton. **3**

Bloom, L. (1993). *The Transition from Infancy to Language: Acquiring the Power of Expression.* Cambridge, UK: Cambridge University Press. **211, 212, 234, 289**

Bloom, P. (2000). *How Children Learn the Meanings of Words.* Cambridge, Massachusetts: MIT Press. **30, 31, 36**

Boehm, A.E. (1986). *Boehm's Test of Basic Concepts - Revised manual.* New York: The Psychological Corporation. **304, 319**

Bol, G. and Kuiken, F. (1990). Grammatical analysis of developmental language disorders: a study of the morphosyntax of children with specific language disorders, with hearing impairment and with Down's syndrome. *Clinical Linguistics and Phonetics, 4,* 77-86. **150**

Bonvillian, J.D. and Blackburn, D.W. (1991). Manual communication and autism: Factors relating to sign language acquisition. In P. Siple and S.D. Fischer (Eds), *Theoretical issues in sign language research, Volume 2: Psychology* (pp. 255-77). Chicago, Illinois: Chicago University Press. **2, 4, 19, 21**

Bonvillian, J.D. and Nelson, K.E. (1978) Development of sign language in language-handicapped individuals. In P. Siple (Ed.), *Understanding language through sign language research* (pp. 187-212). New York: Academic Press. **8**

Borkowski, J.G. and Muthukrishna, N. (1995). Learning environments and skill generalization: How contexts facilitate regulatory processes and efficacy beliefs. In F.E. Weinert and W. Schneider (Eds), *Memory Performance and Competencies: Issues in Growth and Development* (pp. 283-300). Mahwah, New Jersey: Lawrence Erlbaum. **50, 51**

Bornman, J. and Alant, E. (1999). Training teachers to facilitate classroom interaction with autistic children using digital voice output devices in the classroom context. *South African Journal of Education, 17* (1), 15-20. **336, 339**

Botvin, G. and Sutton-Smith, B. (1977). The development of structural complexity in children's fantasy narratives. *Developmental Psychology, 13,* 377-88. **231**

Boudreau, D. and Chapman, R. (2000). The relationship between event representation and linguistic skill in narratives of children and adolescents with Down Syndrome. *Journal of Speech, Language and Hearing Research, 43,* 1146-59. **232**

Braine, M.D.S. (1963). The ontogeny of English phrase structure: The first phase. *Language, 39,* 1-14. **120**

Bray, M. and Woolnough, L. (1988). The language skills of children with Down's syndrome aged 12 to 16 years. *Child Language Teaching and Therapy, 4,* 311-24. **85, 150, 233**

Bray, N. (1990). A cognitive model for Minspeak. In *The Fifth Annual Minspeak Conference Proceedings.* Wooster, Ohio: Prentke Romich. **61**

Brennan, M. (1994). Word order: Introducing the issues. In M. Brennan and G. Turner (Eds), *Word order issues in sign language: Working papers presented at a workshop in Durham, 18-22 September 1991* (pp. 9-46). Durham, UK: International Sign Linguistics Association. **301**

Bricker, D. (1992). The changing nature of communication and language intervention. In S.F. Warren and J. Reichle (Eds), *Causes and Effects in Communication and Language Intervention* (pp. 361-76). Baltimore, Maryland: Paul H. Brookes. **356**

Bridges, A., Sinha, C. and Walkerdine, V. (1981). The development of comprehension. In G. Wells (Ed.), *Learning through Interaction* (pp. 116-56). Cambridge, UK: Cambridge University Press. **338**

Brinton, B., Fujiki, M., Loeb, D. and Winkler, E. (1986). Development of conversational repair strategies in response to requests for clarification. *Journal of Speech and Hearing Research, 29,* 75-81. **52**

Brookner, S.P. and Murphy, N.O. (1975). The use of a total communication approach with a nondeaf child: a case study. *Language, Speech, and Hearing Services in Schools, 6,* 131-9. **177**

Brown, A.L. and Campione, J.C. (1994). Guided discovery in a community of learners. In K. McGilly (Ed.), *Classroom Lessons: Integrating Cognitive Theory and Classroom Practice* (pp. 229-70). Cambridge, Massachusetts: MIT Press. **290**

Brown, A.L. and DeLoache, J.S. (1978). Skills, plans and self-regulation. In R. Siegler (Ed.), *Children's Thinking: What Develops?* (pp. 3-36). Hillsdale, New Jersey: Lawrence Erlbaum. **59**

Brown, G. and Yule, G. (1983). *Discourse Analysis.* Cambridge, UK: Cambridge University Press. **330**

Brown, R. (1973). *A First Language: The Early Stages.* London, UK: Allen & Unwin. **303, 311**

Brown-Sweeney, S.G. and Smith, B.L. (1997). The development of speech production abilities in children with Down syndrome. *Clinical Linguistics and Phonetics, 11,* 345-62. **85, 150**

Bruner, J.S. (1964). The course of cognitive growth. *American Psychologist, 19,* 1-15. **65**

Bruner, J.S (1968). *Toward a Theory of Instruction.* New York: Norton. **359**

Bruner, J.S. (1975). The ontogenesis of speech acts. *Journal of Child Language, 2,* 1-19. **11, 29, 31, 123**

Bruner, J.S. (1983). *Child's Talk.* Oxford, UK: Oxford University Press. **11, 29, 76, 177, 200, 211, 225, 226, 287, 381, 383**

Bruno, J. (1988). *Interaction, Education and Play: A Minspeak Application Program.* Wooster, Ohio: Prentke Romich. **55, 65**

Bruno, J. (1991). Comparison of picture and word association performance in adults and preliterate children. *Augmentative and Alternative Communication, 7,* 70-9. **45, 46, 57**

Bruno, J. (2001). Designing communication displays to facilitate interactive communication. In W. Loebl, J. Szwiec and P.A. Szczawinski (Eds), *Proceedings of the Third Regional Eastern and Central European Conference on Augmentative and Alternative communication* (pp. 197-202). Warsaw, Poland: Stowarzyzzenie 'Mówic bes slow'. **177**

Bruno, J. and Dribben, M. (1998). Outcomes in AAC: Evaluating the effectiveness of a parent training program. *Augmentative and Alternative Communication, 14,* 59-70. **42**

Buckley, S. (1993). *The Development of Language and Reading in Children with Down Syndrome.* Portsmouth, UK: Sarah Duffen Centre. **331**

Bühler, K. (1930). *Die geistige Entwicklung des Kindes (The mental Development of the Child).* Jena, Germany: Fischer. **70**

Bukowski, W.M., Newcomb, A.F. and Hartup, W.W. (Eds) (1996). *The Company they Keep: Friendship in Childhood and Adolescence.* Cambridge, UK: Cambridge University Press. **286**

Burford, B. and Trevarthen, C. (1997). Evoking communication in Rett syndrome: Comparisons with conversations and games in mother infant interaction. *European Child and Adolescent Psychiatry, 6* (Supplement 1), 26-30. **212**

Burkhart, L. (1994, October). Organizing vocabulary on dynamic display devices: Practical ideas and strategies. Presented at the Sixth Biennial Conference of the International Society for Augmentative and Alternative Communication, Maastricht, the Netherlands. **66**

Burkhart, L.J., West, S. and Garber, S. (1992). Empowering local teams: Training augmentative and alternative communication strategies through direct service. *Augmentative and Alternative Communication, 8,* 121. **336**

Calculator, S.N. (1988). Evaluating the effectiveness of AAC programmes for persons with severe handicaps. *Augmentative and Alternative Communication, 4,* 177-9. **207**

Calculator, S.N. (1997). Fostering early language acquisition and AAC use: Exploring reciprocal influences between children and their environments. *Augmentative and Alternative Communication, 13,* 149-57. **16, 35, 201**

Capps, I., Losh, M. and Thurber, C. (2000). The frog ate the boy and made his mouth sad: Narrative competence in children with autism. *Journal of Abnormal Child Psychology, 28,* 193-204. **232**

Carey, S. (1978). The child as a word learner. In M. Halle, J. Bresnan and G.A. Mutter (Eds), *Linguistic Theory and Psychological Reality* (pp. 264-93). Cambridge, Massachusetts. MIT Press. **40**

Carlson, F. (1981). A format for selecting vocabulary for the nonspeaking child. *Language, Speech, and Hearing Services in Schools, 12,* 140-5. **204**

Carpenter, M., Nagell, K. and Tomasello, M. (1998). Social cognition, joint attention, and communicative competence from 9 to 15 months of age. *Monographs of the Society for Research in Child Development, 63* (4). **79**

Carr, E.G., Kologinsky, E. and Leff-Simon, S. (1987). Acquisition of sign language by autistic children. III: Generalized descriptive phrases. *Journal of Autism and Developmental Disorders, 17,* 217-29. **2**

Case, R. (1995). Capacity-based explanations of working memory growth: a brief history and reevaluation. In F.E. Weinert and W. Schneider (Eds), *Memory Performance and Competencies: Issues in Growth and Development* (pp. 283-300). Mahwah, New Jersey: Lawrence Erlbaum. **43**

Casey, L.O. (1978). Development of communicative behavior in autistic children: A parent program using manual signs. *Journal of Autism and Childhood Schizophrenia, 8,* 45-59. **118**

Casto, G. (1987). Plasticity and the handicapped child: A review of efficacy research. In J.J. Gallagher and C.T. Ramey (Eds), *The Malleability of Children* (pp. 103-13). Baltimore, Maryland: Paul H. Brookes. **86**

Chapman, R.S. (1995). Language development in children and adolescents with Down syndrome. In P. Fletcher and B. MacWhinney (Eds), *The Handbook of Child Language* (pp. 641-63). Cambridge, Massachusetts: Basil Blackwell. **85**

Chapman, R.S., Seung, H.-K., Schwartz, S.E. and Bird, E.K.-R. (1998). Language skills of children and adolescents with Down syndrome: II. Production deficits. *Journal of Speech and Hearing Research, 41*, 861-73. **151**

Cheepen, C. (1988). *The Predictability of Informal Conversation.* Oxford, UK: Pinter. **257, 266**

Chiat, S. and Hunt, J. (1993). Connections between phonology and semantics: an exploration of lexical processing in a language impaired child. *Child Language Teaching and Therapy, 9*, 201-13. **151**

Chomsky, N. (1959). Review of Skinner's 'Verbal behavior'. *Language, 35*, 26-58. **10**

Chomsky, N. (1968). *Language and Mind.* New York: Harcourt Brace Jovanovich. **10**

Chomsky, N. (1972). *Language and Mind.* Enlarged edition. New York: Harcourt Brace Jovanovich. **155**

Chomsky, N. (1988). *Language and Problems of Knowledge.* Cambridge, Massachusetts: MIT Press. **10**

Cicognani, E. and Zani, B. (1992). Teacher-children interactions in a nursery school: an exploratory study. *Language and Education, 6*, 1-12. **341**

Cirlot-New, J., Civils, C.A. and Oxley, J.D. (2001). Increasing turn taking to improve social interaction. In *The 22nd Annual Southeast Augmentative Communication Conference Proceedings.* Birmingham, Alabama: Southeast Augmentative Communication Publications Clinician Series. **42**

Clark, E.V. (1995). Later lexical development and word formation. In P. Fletcher and B. MacWhinney (Eds), *The Handbook of Child Language* (pp. 393-412). Cambridge, Massachusetts: Basil Blackwell. **115, 117**

Clark, R. (1982). Theory and method in child-language research: Are we assuming too much? In S. Kuczaj, II (Ed.), *Language Development, Volume 1: Syntax and semantics* (pp. 1-36). Hillsdale, New Jersey: Lawrence Erlbaum. **208**

Clibbens, J. (2001). Signing and lexical development in children with Down syndrome. *Down Syndrome Research and Practice, 7*, 101-5. **29, 33, 34**

Clibbens, J., Powell, G.G. and Atkinson, E. (2002). Strategies for achieving joint attention when signing to children with Down syndrome. *International Journal of Language and Communication Disorders 37*, 309-23. **34, 36**

Clibbens, J., Powell, G.G. and Grove, N. (1997). Manual signing and AAC: Issues for research and practice. *Communication Matters, 11* (2), 17-18. **29, 34**

Cohen, L. and Manion, L. (1990). *Research methods in education,* Fourth edition. London, UK: Routledge. **308**

Collins, S. (1996). Referring expressions in conversations between aided and natural speakers. In S. von Tetzchner and M.H. Jensen (Eds), *Augmentative and Alternative Communication: European Perspectives* (pp. 89-100). London, UK: Whurr. **206, 225**

Conti-Ramsden, G. (1994). Language interaction with atypical language learners. In C. Gallaway and B. Richards (Eds), *Input and Interaction in Language Acquisition* (pp. 183-195). London, UK: Cambridge University Press. **32, 160**

Conti-Ramsden, G., Hutcheson, G. and Grove, J. (1995). Contingency and breakdown: Children with SLI and their conversations with mothers and fathers. *Journal of Speech and Hearing Research, 38*, 1290-302. **160**

Crais, E. and Chapman, R. (1987). Story recall and inferencing skills in language/learning-disabled and nondisabled children. *Journal of Speech and Hearing Disorders, 52*, 50-5. **230, 231**

Creedon, M.P. (1973). Language development in nonverbal autistic children using a simultaneous communication system. Presented at the Annual Meeting of the Society for Research in Child Development, Philadelphia, Pennsylvania, USA. **118, 150, 152**

Crystal, D., Fletcher, P. and Garman, M. (1976). *The Grammatical Analysis of Language Disability: A procedure for assessment and remediation*. London, UK: Edward Arnold. **307**

Damon, W. and Phelps, E. (1989). Strategic uses of peer learning in children's education. In T.J. Berndt and G-W. Ladd (Eds), *Peer Relationships in Child Development* (pp. 135-57). New York: John Wiley. **295**

Darwin, C. (1877). A biographical sketch of an infant. *Mind, 2*, 285-94. **3**

Deegan, S. (1992). Augmentative and alternative communication training for professionals in Zimbabwe. *Augmentative and Alternative Communication, 8*, 127. **336**

DeLoache, J.S. (1987). Rapid change in symbolic functioning of very young children. *Science, 238*, 1556-7. **57**

DeLoache, J.S. (2000). Dual representation and young children's use of scale models. *Child Development, 71*, 329-38. **57**

DeLoache, J.S. and Burns, N.M. (1994). Early understanding of the representational function of pictures. *Cognition, 52*, 83-110. **57**

DeLoache, J.S. and Marzolf, D.P. (1992). When a picture is not worth a thousand words: Young children's understanding of pictures and models. *Child Development, 62*, 111-26. **57**

DeLoache, J.S., Miller, K.F. and Rosengren, K.S. (1997). The credible shrinking room: very young children's performance with symbolic and nonsymbolic relations. *Psychological Science, 8*, 308-13. **57**

DeLoache, J.S., Uttal, D.H. and Pierroutsakos, S.L. (1998). The development of early symbolization: educational implications. *Learning and Instruction, 8*, 325-39. **57**

Dempster, F.N. (1981). Memory span: sources of individual developmental differences. *Psychological Bulletin, 89*, 63-100. **43**

Denney, N. (1974). Evidence for developmental changes in categorization criteria for children and adults. *Human Development, 17*, 41-53. **62**

Derlega, V.J. and Grzelak, J. (1979). Appropriateness of self-disclosure. In G.J. Chelune (Ed.), *Self-disclosure: Origins, Patterns, and Implications of Openness in Interpersonal Relationships* (pp. 151-76). San Francisco, California: Jossey-Bass. **273**

de Saussure, F. (1974). *Course in General Linguistics*. Glasgow, UK: Collins. **74, 209**

Devenny, D.A. and Silverman, W.P. (1990). Speech dysfluency and manual specialization in Down's syndrome. *Journal of Mental Deficiency Research, 34*, 253-60. **85, 150**

Devenny, D.A., Silverman, W., Balgley, H., Wall, M.J. and Sidtis, J.J. (1990). Specific motor abilities associated with speech dysfluency in Down's syndrome. *Journal of Mental Deficiency Research, 34*, 437-43. **150**

Dockrell, J., Messer, D., George, R. and Wilson, G. (1998). Children with word-finding difficulties – prevalence, presentation and naming problems. *International Journal of Language and Communication Disorders, 33*, 445-54. **151**

Dodd, B., McCormack, P. and Woodyatt, G. (1994). Evaluation of an intervention program: relation between children's phonology and parents' communicative behavior. *American Journal on Mental Retardation, 98*, 632-45. **85, 150**

Dollaghan, C. (1985). Child meets word: 'Fast mapping' in preschool children. *Journal of Speech and Hearing Research, 28,* 449-54. **40**

Donaldson, M. (1978). *Children's Minds.* Glasgow, UK: Fontana. **359**

Dore, J. (1986). The development of conversational competence. In R.L. Schiefelbusch (Ed.), *Language Competence: Assessment and Intervention* (pp. 3-60). London, UK: Taylor & Francis. **203**

Dunn, J. (1988). *The Beginnings of Social Understanding.* Oxford, UK: Basil Blackwell. **112, 252**

Dunn, J. (1999). Siblings, friends and the development of social understanding. In W.A. Collins and B. Laursen (Eds), *Relationships as Developmental Contexts* (pp. 263-79). Mahwah, New Jersey: Lawrence Erlbaum. **112, 207, 286**

Dunn, L.M., Dunn, L., Whetton, C. and Pintillie, D. (1982). *British Picture Vocabulary Scales.* London, UK: NFER-Nelson. **161**

Dunn, L.M. and Markwardt, F.C. (1970). *Peabody Individual Achievement Test.* Circle Pines, Minnesota: American Guidance Service. **379**

Dunst, C.J. (1978). A cognitive-social approach to assessment of early nonverbal communicative behaviour. *Journal of Childhood Communication Disorders, 2,* 10-123. **300**

Dunst, C.J. (1985). Rethinking early intervention. *Analysis and Intervention in Developmental Disabilities, 5,* 165-201. **112**

Dunst, C.J., Trivette, C. and Deal, A. (1988). *Enabling and Empowering Families: Principles and Guidelines for Practice.* Cambridge, Massachusetts: Brookline Books. **113**

Dykens, E.M., Hodapp, R.M. and Evans, D.W. (1994). Profiles and development of adaptive behavior in children with Down syndrome. *American Journal on Mental Retardation, 98,* 580-7. **85**

Eaton, J., Collis, G. and Lewis, V. (1999). Evaluative explanations in children's narratives of a video sequence without dialogue. *Journal of Child Language, 26,* 699-720. **231, 257**

Eimas, P.D. (1985). The perception of speech in early infancy. *Scientific American, 252,* 46-52. **17**

Eisenberg, A.R. (1985). Learning to describe past experiences in conversation. *Discourse Processes, 8,* 177-204. **257**

Ekman, P. (Ed.) (1982). *Emotion in the Human Face: Studies in Emotion and Social Interaction.* Cambridge, UK: Cambridge University Press. **234**

Elder, P., Goossens', C. and Bray, N. (1990). *Semantic Compaction Competency Profile.* Wooster, Ohio: Prentke Romich. **46**

Elkonin, D.B. (1988). *Legens Psykologi (The Psychology of Play).* Moscow, Russia: Progres. **290**

Ellenberger, R. and Steyaert, M. (1978). A child's representation of action in American sign language. In P. Siple (Ed.), *Understanding Language through Sign Language Research* (pp. 261-9). London, UK: Academic Press. **3**

Elliot, C., Murray, D. and Pearson, L. (1983). *British Abilities Scale.* Revised edition. Windsor, UK: NFER-Nelson. **233**

Ellis, S. (1997). Strategy choice in sociocultural context. *Developmental Review, 17,* 490-524. **51**

Elman, J.L., Bates, E.A., Johnson, M.H., Karmiloff-Smith, A., Parisi, D. and Plunkett, K. (1996). *Rethinking Innateness: A Connectionist Perspective on Development.* London, UK: MIT Press. **11**

Engel, S. (1995). *The Stories Children Tell: Making Sense of the Narratives in Childhood.* New York: Freeman. **229**

Fabbretti, D., Pizzuto, E., Vicari, S. and Volterra, V. (1997). A story description task in children with Down's syndrome: Lexical and morphosyntactic abilities. *Journal of Intellectual Disability Research, 41,* 165-79. **232**

Fabricius, W.V. and Cavalier, L. (1989). The role of causal theories about memory in young children's memory strategy choice. *Child Development, 60,* 298-308. **50**

Fenn, G. and Rowe, J. (1975). An experiment in manual communication. *British Journal of Disorders of Human Communication, 10,* 3-16. **302**

Fey, M. (1986). *Language Intervention with Young Children.* London, UK: Taylor & Francis. **156**

Fischer, M.A. (1987). Mother-child interaction in preverbal children with Down syndrome. *Journal of Speech and Hearing Disorders, 52,* 179-90. **84, 112**

Fivush, R. (1984). Learning about school: The development of kindergartners' school scripts. *Child Development, 55,* 1697-709. **230**

Fivush, R. (1991). Gender and emotion in mother-child conversations about the past. *Journal of Narrative and Life History, 1,* 325-41. **298**

Fivush, R. (1997). Event memory in early childhood. In N. Cowan (Ed.), *The Development of Memory in Childhood* (pp. 139-61). London, UK: Psychology Press. **230**

Fivush, R. and Hamond, N.R. (1990). Autobiographical memory across the preschool years: Toward reconceptualizing childhood amnesia. In R. Fivush and J.A. Hudson (Eds), *Knowing and Remembering in Young Children* (pp. 223-248). Cambridge: Cambridge University Press. **298**

Flavell, J.H. and Wellman, H.M. (1977). Metamemory. In R.V. Kail and J.W. Hagen (Eds), *Perspectives on the Development of Memory and Cognition* (pp. 3-33). Hillsdale, New Jersey: Lawrence Erlbaum. **65**

Fletcher, K.L. and Bray, N. (1996). External memory strategy use in preschool children. *Merrill-Palmer Quarterly, 42,* 379-96. **50, 65**

Fletcher, P. and MacWhinney, B. (Eds) (1995). *Handbook of Child Language.* Oxford, UK: Basil Blackwell. **3, 272**

Fodor, J. (1983). *Modularity of Mind. An Essay on Faculty Psychology.* Cambridge, Massachusetts: MIT Press. **10, 155**

Forest, M., Pearpoint, J. and O'Brien, J. (1996). MAPs, circles of friends, and PATH: Powerful tools to help build caring communities. In S. Stainback and W. Stainback (Eds), *Inclusion: A Guide for Educators* (pp. 67-86). Baltimore, Maryland: Paul H. Brookes. **296**

Fox, C. (1993). *At the Very Edge of the Forest: The Influence of Literature on Storytelling by Children.* London, UK: Cassell. **251**

Frederiksen, J., Martin, M., Pereira, L.M., Puig de la Bellacasa, R. and von Tetzchner, S. (1991). Impairment, disability and handicap. In S. von Tetzchner (Ed.), *Issues in Telecommunication and Disability* (pp. 39-47). Luxembourg: Office for Official Publications of the European Communities. **285**

Fried-Oken, M. and More, L. (1992). Initial vocabulary for nonspeaking preschool children based on developmental and environmental language samples. *Augmentative and Alternative Communication, 8,* 1-16. **14, 74, 204**

Frith, U. (1985). Beneath the surface of developmental dyslexia. In K. Patterson, J. Marshall and M. Coltheart (Eds), *Surface Dyslexia* (pp. 301-30). London, UK: Lawrence Erlbaum. **331**

Fulwiler, R.L. and Fouts, R.S. (1976). Acquisition of American sign language by a noncommunicating autistic child. *Journal of Autism and Childhood Schizophrenia, 6,* 43–51. **4, 8**

Gangkofer, M. and Tetzchner, S. (1996). Cleaning ladies and broken busses – a case study on the use of Blissymbols and traditional orthography. In S. von Tetzchner and M.H. Jensen (Eds), *Augmentative and Alternative Communication: European Perspectives* (pp. 292–308). London: Whurr. **209**

Garcia, G.E. (1992). Ethnography and classroom conversation: Taking an emic perspective. *Topics in Language Disorders, 12* (3), 45–66. **349**

George, T.P. and Hartmann, D.P. (1996). Friendship networks of unpopular, average, and popular children. *Child Development, 67,* 2301–16. **293**

Gerber, S. and Kraat, A.W. (1992). Use of a developmental model of language acquisition: applications to children using augmentative and alternative communication systems. *Augmentative and Alternative Communication, 8,* 19–31. **5, 65, 177, 225, 340**

German, D.J. (1992). Word-finding intervention for children and adolescents. *Topics in Language Disorders, 13,* 33–50. **152**

German, D.J. (1996). The effect of word-finding difficulties on intellectual assessment. *Journal of Psychoeducational Assessment, 14,* 373–84. **151**

Gibson, J.J. (1979). *The Ecological Approach to Visual Perception.* Boston, Massachusetts: Houghton Mifflin. **5**

Gleitman, L.R. and Wanner, E. (1982). Language acquisition: The state of the art. In E. Wanner and L.R. Gleitman (Eds), *Language Acquisition: The State of the Art* (pp. 3–48). Cambridge, UK: Cambridge University Press. **231**

Goffman, E. (1963). *Stigma: Notes on the Management of Spoiled Identity.* London, UK: Penguin. **299**

Goffman, E. (1981). *Forms of Talk.* Philadelphia, Pennsylvania: University of Pennsylvania Press. **208**

Goldin-Meadow, S. and Feldman, H. (1975). The creation of a communication system: a study of deaf children of hearing parents. *Sign Language Studies, 8,* 225–34. **149, 302**

Golinkoff, R.M., Mervis, C.B. and Hirsh-Pasek, K. (1994). Early object labels: The case for a developmental lexical principles framework. *Journal of Child Language, 21,* 125–55. **30**

Goodman, G.S., Rudy, L., Bottoms, B. and Aman, C. (1990). Children's concerns and memory: Issues of ecological validity in the study of children's eyewitness testimony. In R. Fivus and J. Hudson (Ed.), *Knowing and Remembering in Young Children* (pp. 249–84). Cambridge, UK: Cambridge University Press. **257**

Goodman, K.S. (1976). Reading: A psycholinguistic guessing game. In H. Singer and R. Ruddell (Eds), *Theoretical Models and Processes of Reading* (pp. 479–508). Newark, Delaware: International Reading Association. **360**

Goodnow, J.J. (1990). The socialization of cognition: What's involved? In J.W. Stigler, R.A. Shweder, and G. Herdt (Eds), *Cultural Psychology: Essays of Comparative Human Development* (pp. 259–86). New York, Cambridge University Press. **51**

Goodz, N.S. (1989). Parental language mixing in bilingual families. *Infant Mental Health Journal, 10,* 25–44. **158**

Goossens', C.A. (1989). Aided communication intervention before assessment: A case study of a child with cerebral palsy. *Augmentative and Alternative Communication, 3,* 14–26. **177**

Goossens', C.A., Elder, P.S. and Bray, N.W. (1990). A preliminary validity study of the

Semantic Compaction Competency Profile. *Fifth Annual Minspeak Conference Proceedings*. Wooster, Ohio: Prentke Romich. **46, 62**

Goossens', C.A., Elder, P.S. and Crain, S. (1992). *Engineering the Preschool Environment for Interactive Symbolic Communication*. Birmingham, Alabama: Southeast Augmentative Communication Conference Publications. **66**

Gough, P.B. and Hillinger, M.L. (1980). Learning to read: An unnatural act. *Bulletin of the Orton Society, 30,* 179–96. **374**

Greenhalgh, S. and Hurwitz, B. (1998). *Narrative Based Medicine*. London, UK: BMJ Books. **229**

Grice, P. (1989). *Studies in the Ways of Words*. Cambridge, Massachusetts: Harvard University Press. **338**

Groce, N.E. (1985). *Everyone here Spoke Sign Language. Hereditary Deafness on Martha's Vineyard*. Cambridge, Massachusetts: Harvard University Press. **81**

Grotnes, B. and Urnes, H. (2000). Språktilegnelse i en sosial kontekst (Language acquisition in a social context). Unpublished thesis, Institute of Psychology, University of Oslo, Norway. **23**

Grove, N. (1995). An analysis of the linguistic skills of signers with learning disabilities. Unpublished PhD thesis, Institute of Education, University of London, UK. **12, 22, 150**

Grove, N. (1997). Gesture, language and multimodality: Implications for research and practice. In E. Björck-Åkesson and P. Lindsay (Eds), *Communication Naturally. Theoretical and Methodological Issues in Augmentative and Alternative Communication* (pp. 92–101). Västerås, Sweden: Mälardalen University Press. **74, 153**

Grove, N. (1998). *Literature for All*. London, UK: David Fulton. **281**

Grove, N. and Dockrell, J. (2000). Multi-sign combinations by children with intellectual impairments: An analysis of language skills. *Journal of Language, Speech and Hearing Research, 43,* 309–23. **18, 147, 149, 233, 234, 249, 251, 302**

Grove, N., Dockrell, J. and Woll, B. (1996). The two-word stage in manual signs: Language development in signers with intellectual impairments. In S. von Tetzchner and M.H. Jensen (Eds), *Augmentative and Alternative Communication: European Perspectives* (pp. 101–18). London, UK: Whurr. **4, 10, 18, 19, 78, 86, 91, 120, 148, 149, 233, 249, 251**

Grove, N. and McDougall, S. (1989). *An exploration of the communication skills of Makaton students: Part II. Interviews with teachers and speech therapists. Report to Leverhulme Trust*. London, UK: Saint George's Hospital Medical School. **154**

Grove, N. and McDougall, S. (1991). Exploring sign use in two settings. *British Journal of Special Education, 18,* 149–56. **12, 13, 120, 147, 152, 233**

Grove, N. and Park, K. (1996). *Odyssey now*. London, UK: Jessica Kingsley. **281**

Grove, N. and Walker, M. (1990). The Makaton Vocabulary: Using manual signs and graphic symbols to develop interpersonal communication. *Augmentative and Alternative Communication, 6,* 15–28. **204, 234**

Grunwell, P. (Ed.) (1990). *Developmental Speech Disorders*. Edinburgh, UK: Churchill Livingstone. **3**

Guralnick, M.J. (Ed.) (2001). *Early Childhood Inclusion: Focus on Change*. Baltimore, Maryland: Paul H. Brookes. **293**

Guttentag, R.E. (1984). The mental effort requirement of cumulative rehearsal: a developmental study. *Journal of Experimental Child Psychology, 37,* 92–106. **44**

Guttentag, R.E. (1995). Mental effort and motivation: Influences on children's strategy use. In F.E. Weinert and W. Schneider (Eds), *Memory Performance and Competencies: Issues in Growth and Development* (pp. 283-300). Mahwah, New Jersey: Lawrence Erlbaum. **63**

Hammersley, M. (1974). The organisation of pupil participation. *Sociological Review, 22,* 355-68. **343, 347**

Hammersley, M. (1981). Putting competence into action: Some sociological notes on a model of classroom interaction. In P. French and M. Maclure (Eds), *Adult-child Conversation* (pp. 47-58). London, UK: Croom Helm. **338**

Harrington, K. (1984a). Lucky Me, Part 1. *Communicating Together, 2* (1), 9. **378**

Harrington, K. (1984b). Lucky Me, Part 2. *Communicating Together, 2* (2), 9. **378**

Harrington, K. and Harrington, R. (1988, October). Kari: Communicating, creating and learning. Presented at the Third Biennial Conference of the International Society for Augmentative and Alternative Communication, Anaheim, California, USA. **362, 364, 370, 378**

Harris, D. (1978). Descriptive analysis of communicative interaction processes involving nonvocal physically handicapped children. Unpublished PhD dissertation, University of Wisconsin, Madison, USA. **300**

Harris, D. (1982). Communicative interaction processes involving nonvocal physically handicapped children. *Topics in Language Disorders, 2,* 21-37. **9, 177, 204, 226**

Harris, M. (1992). *Language Experience and Early Language Development: From Input to Uptake.* Cambridge, Massachusetts: MIT Press. **79, 157**

Harris, M. and Beech, J. (1995). Reading development in pre-lingually deaf children. In K. Nelson and Z. Reger (Eds), *Children's Language, Volume 8* (pp. 181-202). Hillsdale, New Jersey: Lawrence Erlbaum. **233**

Harris, M., Clibbens, J., Chasin, J. and Tibbitts, R. (1989). The social context of early sign language development. *First Language, 9,* 81-97. **31–34**

Harris, M., Jones, D., Brookes, S. and Grant, J. (1986). Relations between the non-verbal context of maternal speech and rate of language development. *British Journal of Developmental Psychology, 4,* 261-8. **29, 31**

Harris, M., Jones, D. and Grant, J. (1983). The nonverbal context of mothers' speech to children. *First Language, 4,* 21-30. **29**

Harris, M., Jones, D. and Grant, J. (1984/85). The social-interactional context of maternal speech to children: An explanation for the event-bound nature of early word use? *First Language, 5,* 89-100. **29, 30**

Harris, S., Kasari, C. and Sigman, M.D. (1996). Joint attention and language gains in children with Down syndrome. *American Journal on Mental Retardation, 100,* 608-19. **33, 118**

Hasselhorn, M. (1995). Beyond production deficiency and utilization inefficiency: Mechanisms and emergence of strategic categorization in episodic memory tests. In F.E. Weinert and W. Schneider (Eds), *Memory Performance and Competencies: Issues in Growth and Development* (pp. 141-59). Mahwah, New Jersey: Lawrence Erlbaum. **46**

Hehner, B. (1980). *Blissymbols for Use.* Toronto, Canada: Blissymbolics Communication Institute. **370**

Heim, J.M. and Baker-Mills, A. (1996). Early development of symbolic communication and linguistic complexity through augmentative and alternative communication. In S. von

Tetzchner and M.H. Jensen (Eds), *Augmentative and Alternative Communication: European Perspectives* (pp. 232-48). London, UK: Whurr. **4**

Helfman, E.S. (1967). *Signs and Symbols around the World.* New York: Lothrop, Lee & Shepard. **365**

Hendrickson, J.M. and Frank, A.R. (1993). Engagement and performance feedback. In R.A. Gable and S.F. Warren (Eds), *Strategies for Teaching Students with Mild to Severe Mental Retardation* (pp. 11-48). Philadelphia, Pennsylvania: Jessica Kingsley. **347, 352**

Hesselberg, F. (Ed.) (1998). *Habiliteringsplaner: Et hjelpemiddel for å skape kontinuitet og stabilitet i tilbudet til mennesker med omfattende hjelpebehov: Noen artikler og eksempler (Habilitation Plans: An Aid to Create Continuity and Stability in the Services for People with a Large Need for Help: Some Articles and Examples).* Oslo, Norway: The Autism Centre, University of Oslo. **178**

Hildebrand-Nilshon, M. (1980). *Die Entwicklung der Sprache: Phylogenese und Onthogenese (The Development of Language: Phylogenesis and Ontogenesis).* Frankfurt am Main, Germany: Campus Verlag. **74**

Hirsh-Pasek, K., Treiman, R. and Schneiderman, M. (1984). Brown and Hanlon revisited: mothers' sensitivity to ungrammatical form. *Journal of Child Language, 11,* 81-8. **332**

Hitch, G.J. and Towse, J.N. (1995). Working memory: What develops? In F.E. Weinert and W. Schneider (Eds), *Memory Performance and Competencies: Issues in Growth and Development* (pp. 283-300). Mahwah, New Jersey: Lawrence Erlbaum. **43, 44**

Hjelmquist, E. (1999). Form and meaning in alternative language development. In F. Loncke, J. Clibbens, H. Arvidson and L. Lloyd (Eds), *Augmentative and Alternative Communication: New Directions in Research and Practice* (pp. 31-9). London, UK: Whurr. **172**

Hobson, P. (1993). Understanding persons: The role of affect. In S. Baron-Cohen, H. Tager-Flusberg and D. Cohen (Eds), *Understanding other Minds: Perspectives from Autism* (pp. 204-27). Oxford, UK: Oxford Medical Publications. **252**

Hoff-Ginsberg, E. (1990). Maternal speech and the child's development of syntax: A further look. *Journal of Child Language, 17,* 85-99. **24**

Hömberg, N., Burtscher, R. and Ginnold, A. (2001). Framing the future: Zukunftskonferenzen und Wege zur beruflichen Integration (Future conferences and way toward the occupational integration). In J. Boenisch and C. Bünk (Eds), *2001: Forschung und Praxis der Unterstützten Kommunikation* (pp. 170-82). Karlsruhe, Germany: von Loeper. **81**

Hooper, J., Connell, T.M. and Flett, P.J. (1987). Blissymbols and manual signs: A multimodal approach to intervention in a case of multiple disability. *Augmentative and Alternative Communication, 3,* 68-76. **177**

Horowitz, P.D. (1987). *Exploring Developmental Theories.* London, UK: Lawrence Erlbaum. **84**

Hudson, J.A. (1993). Understanding events: The development of script knowledge. In M. Bennett (Ed.), *The Child as Psychologist* (pp. 142-67). London, UK: Harvester Wheatsheaf. **208**

Hudson, J.A. and Nelson, K. (1986). Repeated encounters of a similar kind: Effects of familiarity on children's autobiographical memory. *Cognitive Development, 1,* 253-71. **230**

Hudson, J.A. and Shapiro, L.R. (1991). From knowing to telling: The development of children's scripts, stories and personal narratives. In A. McCabe and C. Peterson (Eds),

Developing Narrative Structure (pp. 89-136). Hillsdale, New Jersey: Lawrence Erlbaum. **230, 257**

Hunt, P., Alwell, M., Farron-Davis, F. and Goetz, L. (1996). Creating socially supportive environments for fully included students who experience multiple disabilities. *Journal of the Association for Persons with Severe Handicaps, 21,* 53-71. **297, 299**

Hunt, P., Alwell, M. and Goetz, L. (1991). Interacting with peers through conversation turntaking with a communication book adaptation. *Augmentative and Alternative Communication, 7,* 117-26. **297, 299**

Hunt, P., Soto, G., Maier, J. and Müller, E. (2002). Collaborative teaming to support students with augmentative and alternative needs in general education classrooms. *Augmentative and Alternative Communication, 18,* 20-35. **288, 292, 295-7, 299**

Hymes, D. (1971). Competence and performance in linguistic theory. In R. Huxley and E. Ingram (Eds), *Language Acquisition: Models and Methods* (pp. 3-28). New York: Academic Press. **300**

Iacono, T.A. (1994). Language development research: Theoretical concerns and future challenges. In J. Brodin and E. Björck-Åkesson (Eds), *Methodological Issues in Research in Augmentative and Alternative Communication* (pp. 11-17). Jönköping: Jönköping University Press. **302**

Iacono, T.A. and Parsons, C.L. (1986). A comparison of techniques for teaching signs to intellectually disabled individuals using an alternating treatment design. *Australian Journal of Human Communication Disorders, 14,* 23-34. **114**

Johnson, J.M. and Rash, S.J. (1990). A method for transcribing signed and spoken language. *American Annals of the Deaf, 135,* 343-51. **234**

Johnson, R. (1981). *The Picture Communication Symbols.* Solana Beach, California: Mayer-Johnson. **162, 176, 275**

Johnson, R. (1985). *The Picture Communication Symbols - Book II.* Solana Beach, California: Mayer-Johnson. **162, 176, 275**

Johnson, R. (1992). *The Picture Communication Symbols - Book III.* Solana Beach, California: Mayer-Johnson. **176, 275**

Jones, J. (2000) A total communication approach towards meeting the communication needs of people with learning disabilities. *Tizard Learning Disability Review, 5* (1), 20-26. **80**

Jones, O.H.M. (1980). Prelinguistic communication skills in Down's syndrome and normal infants. In T. Field, S. Goldberg, D. Stern and A. Sostek (Eds), *High-risk Infants and Children: Adult and peer interactions* (pp. 205-224). New York: Academic Press. **84-5**

Juvonen, J. (1997). Peer relations. In G.G. Bear, K.M. Minke and A. Thomas (Eds), *Children's Needs II: Development, Problems and Alternatives* (pp. 101-13). Bethesda, Maryland: National Association of School Psychologists. **274**

Kachru, Y. (1980). *Aspects of Hindi Grammar.* New Delhi, India: Manohar Publishers. **303**

Karlsson, F. (1987). *Finnish Grammar.* Second edition. Juva, Finland: WSOY. **140**

Kasari, C., Mundy, P., Yirmiya, N. and Sigman, M. (1990). Affect and attention in children with Down syndrome. *American Journal on Mental Retardation, 95,* 55-67. **84**

Kaul, S. (1993). An investigation into the emergence of patterns of syntax in the language of Hindi speaking children: A developmental study of children aged 18 months to 48 months. Unpublished Master's thesis, Department of Clinical Communication Studies, City University, London, UK. **303, 308, 324-5**

Kaul, S. (1999). *Picture Test of Receptive Language (Hindi)*. Calcutta, India: Indian Institute of Cerebral Palsy. **304**

Kauppinen, A. (1998). *Puhekuviot, tilanteen ja rakenteen liitto. Tutkimus kielen omaksumisesta ja suomen konditionaaleista (Speech Formulae, a Union of Context and Structure. A Study on Language Acquisition and Finnish Conditionals)*. Helsinki, Finland: Suomalaisen Kirjallisuuden Seura. **120**

Keating, D.P. (1990). Charting pathways to the development of expertise. *Educational Psychologist, 25*, 243-67. **360**

Kegan, R. (1980). Making meaning: The constructive developmental approach to persons and practice. *The Personal and Guidance Journal, 58*, 373-80. **194**

Kegan, R. (1982). *The Evolving Self: Problem and Process in Human Development*. Cambridge, Massachusetts: Harvard University Press. **194**

Keiler, P. (1997). *Feuerbach, Wygotski und Co. Studien zur Grundlegung einer Psychologie des gesellschaftlichen Menschen (Feuerbach, Vygotsky and Co. Studies for the Foundation of a Psychology of the Social Human Being)*. Berlin, Germany: Argument Verlag. **72**

Kelly, J.F. and Barnard, K.E. (2000). Assessment of parent-child interaction: Implications for early intervention. In J.P. Shonkoff and S.J. Meisels (Eds), *Handbook of Early Childhood Intervention* (pp. 258-89). Cambridge, UK: Cambridge University Press. **113**

Kernan, K.T. and Sabsay, S. (1996). Linguistic and cognitive ability of adults with Down syndrome and mental retardation of unknown etiology. *Journal of Communication Disorders, 29*, 401-22. **150**

Kile, J.E. (1996). Audiologic assessment of children with Down syndrome. *American Journal of Audiology, 5*, 44-52. **150**

Kimble, G.A. (1961). *Conditioning and Learning*. Second edition. New York: Appleton, Kimble & DuFort. **6**

Klima, E. and Bellugi, U. (1979). *The Signs of Language*. London, UK: Harvard University Press. **17**

Knowles, W. and Masidlover, M. (1982). *The Derbyshire Language Scheme*. Ripley, Derbyshire, UK: Education Office. **304**

Koppenhaver, D.A., Evans, D.A. and Yoder, D.E. (1991). Childhood reading and writing experiences of literate adults with severe speech and motor impairments. *Augmentative and Alternative Communication, 7*, 20-33. **362**

Koppenhaver, D.A. and Yoder, D.E. (1993). Classroom literacy instruction for children with severe speech and physical impairments (SSPI): What is and what might be. *Topics in Language Disorders, 13*, 1-15. **362**

Kouri, T. (1989). How manual sign acquisition relates to the development of spoken language: A case study. *Language, Speech, and Hearing Services in Schools, 20*, 50-62. **3, 4, 118, 119, 149**

Kraat, A.W. (1985). *Communication Interaction between Aided and Natural Speakers: A State of the Art Report*. Toronto, Canada: Canadian Rehabilitation Council for the Disabled. **42, 177, 204, 226, 386**

Krasnegor, N.A. Rumbaugh, D.M., Schiefelbusch, R.L. and Studdert-Kennedy, M. (Eds) (1991). *Biological and Behavioral Determinants of Language Development*. Hillsdale, New Jersey: Lawrence Erlbaum. **3**

Kuczaj, S. (Ed.) (1982). *Language Development, Volume 1: Syntax and demantics*. Hillsdale, New Jersey: Lawrence Erlbaum. **3**

Kuhn, D. (1999). Metacognitive development. In L. Balter and C.S. Tamis–LeMonda (Eds), *Child Psychology: A Handbook of Contemporary Issues* (pp. 259–86). Philadelphia, Pennsylvania: Psychology Press. **44, 48, 50**

Kunnari, S. (2000). *Characteristics of Early Lexical and Phonological Development in Children acquiring Finnish.* Oulu, Finland: Oulu University Press. **85**

Kyle, J. and Woll, B. (1985). *Sign Language: The Study of Deaf People and their Language.* Cambridge, UK: Cambridge University Press. **149**

Labov, W. (1972). *Language in the Inner City.* Philadelphia, Pennsylvania: University of Pennsylvania Press. **257**

Lage, D. and Antener, G. (2000, August). Knowledge management in AAC: Training AAC disseminators in social service systems. Presented at the 8th Biennial Conference of the International Society for Augmentative and Alternative Communication, Washington DC, USA. **80**

Lane, H. (1984). *When the Mind Hears.* Harmondsworth, UK: Penguin. **72, 101, 214**

Lange, S. and Larson, K. (1973). *Syntactical Development of a Swedish Girl, Embla, between 20 and 42 Months of Age.* Stockholm, Sweden: University of Stockholm. **3**

Launonen, K. (1996). Enhancing communication skills of children with Down syndrome: Early use of manual signs. In S. von Tetzchner and M.H. Jensen (Eds), *Augmentative and Alternative Communication: European perspectives* (pp. 213–32). London, UK: Whurr. **3, 34, 86, 87, 88, 109, 119, 146, 150**

Launonen, K. (1998). *Eleistä sanoihin, viittomista kieleen. Varhaisviittomisohjelman kehittäminen, kokeilu ja pitkäaikaisvaikutukset Downin syndrooma -lasten varhaiskuntoutuksessa (From Gestures to Words, from Signs to Language. Development, Application, and Long-term Effects of an Early Signing Programme in the Early Intervention of Children with Down Syndrome).* Helsinki, Finland: Kehitysvammaliittory. **3, 16, 146, 150**

Layton, T.L. (1988). Language training with autistic children using four different modes of presentation. *Journal of Communication Disorders, 21,* 333–50. **20**

Leekam, S.R., López, B. and Moore, C. Attention and joint attention in preschool children with autism. *Developmental Psychology, 36,* 261–73. **35**

Lenneberg, E.H. (1967). *Biological Foundations of Language.* New York: Wiley. **16, 18**

Leonard, L. (1992). The use of morphology by children with specific language impairment: Evidence from three different languages. In R.S. Chapman (Ed.), *Processes in Language Acquisition and Disorders* (pp. 186–201). Saint Louis, Missouri: Mosby Year Book. **300**

Leopold, W.F. (1939). *Speech Development of a Bilingual Child: A Linguist's Record, Volume 1.* Evanston, Illinois: Northwestern University Press. **3**

Leopold, W.F. (1947). *Speech Development of a Bilingual Child: A Linguist's Record. Volume 2. Sound-learning in the First Two Years.* Evanston, Illinois: Northwestern University Press. **3**

le Prevost, P. (1983). Using the Makaton vocabulary in early language learning with a Down's baby. *Mental Handicap, 11,* 28–9. **3, 16, 86**

Levy, E. and Nelson, K. (1994). Words in discourse: A dialectical approach to the acquisition of meaning and use. *Journal of Child Language, 21,* 367–89. **219**

Levy-Shiff, R. (1986). Mother-father-child interactions in families with a mentally retarded young child. *American Journal of Mental Deficiency, 91,* 141–9. **85**

Light, J. (1985). *The Communicative Interaction Patterns of Non-speaking Physically Disabled Children and their Primary Caregivers.* Toronto, Canada: Blissymbolics Communication Institute. **4, 19, 177**

Light, J. (1988). Interaction involving individuals using augmentative and alternative communication systems: State of the art and future directions. *Augmentative and Alternative Communication, 4,* 66–82. **207, 256, 300**

Light, J. (1989). Toward a definition of communication competence for individuals using augmentative and alternative communication. *Augmentative and Alternative Communication, 5,* 137–44. **24, 300, 330, 336, 341, 362**

Light, J. (1993). A three-tiered model of data analysis: Reconciling group results and individual performances. Unpublished manuscript, Pennsylvania State University, USA. **304**

Light, J. (1997). 'Let's go star fishing': Reflections on the contexts of language learning for children who use aided AAC. *Augmentative and Alternative Communication, 13,* 158–71. **9, 10, 16, 36, 201, 233**

Light, J., Binger, C. and Kelford-Smith, A. (1994). Story reading interactions between preschoolers who use AAC and their mothers. *Augmentative and Alternative Communication, 10,* 255–68. **51, 233**

Light, J. and Lindsay, P. (1991). Cognitive science and augmentative and alternative communication. *Augmentative and Alternative Communication, 7,* 186–203. **4, 61**

Light, J. and Lindsay, P. (1992). Message-encoding techniques for augmentative communication systems: The recall performances of adults with severe speech impairments. *Journal of Speech and Hearing Research, 35,* 853–64. **4, 62**

Light, J., Lindsay, P., Siegel, L. and Parnes, P. (1990). The effects of message and coding techniques on recall by literate adults using AAC systems. *Augmentative and Alternative Communication, 6,* 184–201. **62**

Light, J., McNaughton, D. and Parnes, P. (1994). *A protocol for the assessment of the communication interaction skills of nonspeaking severely handicapped adults and their facilitators.* Toronto, Canada: Sharing to Learn. **386**

Light, P., Watson, J. and Remington, B. (1990). Beyond the single sign: the significance of sign order in a matrix based approach to teaching productive sign combinations. *Mental Handicap Research, 3,* 161–78. **302**

Liles, B.Z. (1993). Narrative discourse in children with language disorders and children with normal language: A critical review of the literature. *Journal of Speech and Hearing Research, 36,* 868–82. **231**

Lincoln, A.J., Courchesne, E., Kilman, B.A. and Galambos, R. (1985). Neuropsychological correlates of information-processing by children with Down syndrome. *American Journal of Mental Deficiency, 89,* 403–14. **85, 150**

Lindblom, B. (1990). On the communication process: Speaker-listener interaction and the development of speech. *Augmentative and Alternative Communication, 6,* 220–30. **383, 384**

Lock, A. (Ed.) (1978). *Action, Gesture and Symbol: The Emergence of Language.* London, UK: Academic Press. **3**

Lock, A. (1980). *The Guided Reinvention of Language.* London, UK: Academic Press. **14, 176, 225**

Locke, J.L. (1994). Gradual emergence of developmental language disorders. *Journal of Speech and Hearing Research, 37,* 608–16. **18**

Locke, J.L. (1995). *The Child's Path to Spoken Language.* London, UK: Harvard University Press. **157**

Locke, J.L. (1997). A theory of neurolinguistic development. *Brain and Language, 58,* 265–326. **19**

Locke, P.A. and Mirenda, P. (1988). A computer-supported approach for a child with severe communication, visual and cognitive impairments: A case study. *Augmentative and Alternative Communication, 4*, 15–22. **177**

Locke, P.A. and Mirenda, P. (1992). Roles and responsibilities of special education teachers serving on teams delivering augmentative and alternative communication services. *Augmentative and Alternative Communication, 8*, 200–14. **339**

Loeding, B.L., Zangari, C. and Lloyd, L. (1990). A 'working party' approach to planning in-service training in manual signs for an entire public school staff. *Augmentative and Alternative Communication, 6*, 38–49. **336**

Loew, R. (1980). Learning American sign language as a first language: Roles and reference. Presented at Third International Symposium on Sign Language Research and Teaching, Boston, USA. **3**

Loncke, F. and Bos, H. (1997). Unaided AAC symbols. In L.L. Lloyd, D.R. Fuller and H.H. Arvidson (Eds), *Augmentative and Alternative Communication: A handbook of principles and practices* (pp. 80–106). London, UK: Allyn & Bacon. **22**

Lord, C. (1993). The complexity of social behaviour in autism. In S. Baron-Cohen, H. Tager-Flusberg and D. Cohen (Eds), *Understanding other Minds: Perspectives from Autism* (pp. 292–316). Oxford, UK: Oxford Medical Publications. **232**

Loveland, K.A., McEvoy, R.E., Tunali, B. and Kelley, M.L. (1990). Narrative story telling in autism and Down's syndrome. *British Journal of Developmental Psychology, 8*, 9–23. **232**

Loveland, K.A. and Tunali, B. (1993). Narrative language in autism and the theory of mind hypothesis: a wider perspective. In S. Baron-Cohen, H. Tager-Flusberg, and D. Cohen (Eds), *Understanding Other Minds: Perspectives from Autism* (pp. 247–66). Oxford, UK: Oxford Medical Publications. **232**

Luria, A.R. and Vygotsky, L.S. (1992). *Ape, Primitive Man and Child: Essays in the History of Behaviour.* New York: Harvester Wheatsheaf. **11**

Lyons, J. (1968). *Introduction to Theoretical Linguistics.* Cambridge, UK: Cambridge University Press. **18**

Lyons, J. (1977). *Semantics.* Cambridge, UK: Cambridge University Press. **205**

McCabe, A. and Peterson, C. (1991). Getting the story: A longitudinal study of parental styles in eliciting narratives and developing narrative skill. In A. McCabe and C. Peterson (Eds), *Developing Narrative Structure* (pp. 217–53). Hillsdale, New Jersey: Lawrence Erlbaum. **249**

McCabe, A. and Rollins, P.R. (1994). Assessment of preschool narrative skills. *American Journal of Speech and Language Pathology, 4*, 45–56. **229**

McCabe, P., Rosenthal, J.B. and McLeod, S. (1998). Features of developmental dyspraxia in the general speech-impaired population? *Clinical Linguistics and Phonetics, 12*, 105–26. **133**

McCathren, R., Yoder, P. and Warren, S. (1995). The role of directives in early language intervention. *Journal of Early Intervention, 19*, 99–101. **160**

McConachie, H. (1986). *Parents and Young Mentally Handicapped Children.* London, UK: Croom Helm. **116**

McDade, H.L. and Adler, S. (1980). Down syndrome and short-term memory impairment: A storage or retrieval deficit? *American Journal of Mental Deficiency, 84*, 561–7. **151**

McDonald, E.T. (1987). *Treating Cerebral Palsy: For Clinicians by Clinicians.* Austin, Texas: PRO-Ed. **312**

McDonald, E.T. and Schultz, A.R. (1973). Communication boards for cerebral-palsied children. *Journal of Speech and Hearing Disorders, 38*, 73–88. **359**

McGilly, K. and Siegler, R.S. (1989). How children choose among serial recall strategies. *Child Development, 60,* 172-82. **50**

McIntire, M. (1977). The acquisition of American sign language hand configuration. Sign Language Studies, 16, 247-66. **3**

McNaughton, S. (1973). *Report on Bliss Project Educational Programme. Symbol Communication Research Project, 1972-1973* (pp. 21-41). Toronto, Canada: Ontario Crippled Children's Centre. **366, 370, 373**

McNaughton, S. (1992a). Parents and symbols: Charting the language pathway together. *Communicating Together, 10* (2), 20-1. **362**

McNaughton, S. (1992b). Independence along the developmental pathway. *Communicating Together, 10* (3), 20-1. **362**

McNaughton, S. (1995). Responding to 'What is your latest thinking on Bliss?' *Communicating Together, 12* (4), 22-3. **387**

McNaughton, S. (1998). Reading acquisition of adults with severe congenital speech and physical impairments: Theoretical infrastructure, empirical investigation, educational application. Unpublished PhD thesis. University of Toronto, Canada. **202, 205, 209, 362, 379, 381-2**

McNaughton, S. (in press). The AAC literacy ramp. In L. L. Lloyd and H.H. Arvidson (Eds), *AAC from A to Z*. New York: Academic Press. **361**

McNaughton, S. and Lindsay, P.H. (1995). Approaching literacy with AAC graphics. *Augmentative and Alternative Communication, 11,* 212-28. **360, 362**

McNeill, D. (1992). *Hand and Mind.* Chicago: University of Chicago Press. **153**

Maharaj, S.C. (1980). *Pictogram Ideogram Communication.* Regina, Canada: The George Reed Foundation for the Handicapped. **110, 176**

Mannle, S. and Tomasello, M. (1987). Fathers, siblings and the bridge hypothesis. In K.E. Nelson and A. van Kleeck (Eds), *Children's Language.* Volume six. (pp. 23-42). Hillsdale, New Jersey: Lawrence Erlbaum. **159**

Marcell, M., Busby, E., Mansker, J. and Whelan, M. (1998). Confrontation naming of familiar sounds and pictures by individuals with Down Syndrome. *American Journal on Mental Retardation, 102,* 485-99. **151**

Markman, E. (1990). Constraints children place on word meanings. *Cognitive Science, 14,* 57-77. **155**

Martinsen, H. (1980). Biologiske forutsetninger for kulturalisering (Biological prerequisites for culturalization). *Tidsskrift for Norsk Psykologforening, Monografiserien, 6,* 122-9. **113**

Martinsen, H., Nordeng, H. and von Tetzchner, S. (1985). *Tegnspråk (Sign language).* Oslo, Norway: Universitetsforlaget. **22**

Martinsen, H. and von Tetzchner, S. (1989). Imitation at the onset of speech. In S. von Tetzchner, L.S. Siegel and L. Smith (Eds), *The Social and Cognitive Aspects of Normal and Atypical Language Development* (pp. 51-68). New York: Springer-Verlag. **249**

Martinsen, H. and von Tetzchner, S. (1996). Situating augmentative and alternative communication intervention. In S. von Tetzchner and M.H. Jensen (Eds), *Augmentative and Alternative Communication: European Perspectives* (pp. 37-48). London: Whurr. **10, 12, 20, 35, 80, 203, 273**

Masataka, N. (2000). The role of modality and input in the earliest stage of language acquisition: Studies of Japanese sign language. In C. Chamberlain and J. Morford (Eds), *Language Acquisition by Eye* (pp. 3-24). Mahwah, New Jersey: Lawrence Erlbaum. **157**

Masur, E. (1997). Maternal labelling of novel and familiar objects: Implications for children's development of lexical constraints. *Journal of Child Language, 24*, 427-39. **23, 79**

Mayer-Johnson, R. (1981). *The Picture Communication Symbols.* Solana Beach, California: Mayer-Johnson. **162**

Mayer-Johnson, R. (1985). *The Picture Communication Symbols: Volume II.* Solana Beach, California: Mayer-Johnson. **162**

Mead, G. H. (1955). *Mind, Self and Society.* Chicago, Illinois: University of Chicago Press. **337**

Meier, R. and Newport, E. (1990). Out of the mouths of babes: On a possible sign advantage in language acquisition. *Language, 66,* 1-23. **123**

Meisel, J. M. (1995). Parameters in acquisition. In P. Fletcher and B. MacWhinney (Eds), *The Handbook of Child Language* (pp. 10-35). Cambridge, Massachusetts: Basil Blackwell. **24**

Meng, K. (1992). Narrating and listening in kindergarten. *Journal of Narrative and Life History, 2,* 235-52. **257, 258**

Merritt, D.D. and Culatta, B. (1998). *Language Intervention in the Classroom.* San Diego, California: Singular. **295**

Miller, J.F. (1988). The developmental asynchrony of language development in children with Down syndrome. In L. Nadel (Ed.), *The Psychobiology of Down Syndrome* (pp. 167-98). Cambridge, Massachusetts: MIT Press. **85, 150**

Miller, J.F. (1992). Development of speech and language in children with Down syndrome. In I.T. Lott and E.E. McCoy (Eds), *Down Syndrome: Advances in medical care* (pp. 39-50). Chichester, UK: John Wiley. **34**

Miller, J.F., Leddy, M. and Leavitt, L.A. (1999). A view toward the future. Improving the communication of people with Down syndrome. In J.F. Miller, M. Leddy and L.A. Leavitt (Eds), *Improving the Communication of People with Down Syndrome* (pp. 241-260). Baltimore, Maryland: Paul H. Brookes. **119**

Miller, P. and Coyle, T.R. (1999). Developmental change: Lessons from microgenesis. In E.K. Scholnick, K. Nelson, S.A. Gelman and P. Miller (Eds), *Conceptual Development: Piaget's Legacy* (pp. 209-39). Mahwah, New Jersey: Lawrence Erlbaum. **49**

Miller, P.H. (1990). The development of strategies of selective attention. In D.F. Bjorklund (Ed.), *Children's Strategies. Contemporary Views of Cognitive Development* (pp. 157-84). Hillsdale, New Jersey: Lawrence Erlbaum. **48**

Miller, P.J. and Sperry, L.L. (1988). Early talk about the past: The origins of conversational stories of personal experience. *Journal of Child Language, 15,* 293-315. **230, 231, 234, 238, 239, 249, 257**

Mills, J. and Higgins, J. (1984). An environmental approach to delivery of microcomputer-based and other communication systems. *Seminars in Speech and Language, 5,* 35-45. **14**

Mirenda, P. and Datillo, J. (1987). Instructional techniques in alternative communication for students with severe intellectual handicap. *Augmentative and Alternative Communication, 3,* 143-52. **10**

Mirenda, P. and Locke, P. (1989). A comparison of symbol transparency in nonspeaking persons with intellectual disabilities. *Journal of Speech and Hearing Disorders, 54,* 131-40. **57**

Mirenda, P. and Mathy-Laikko, P. (1989). Augmentative and alternative communication applications for persons with severe congenital communication disorders: An introduction. *Augmentative and Alternative Communication, 5,* 3-13. **312**

Mogford, K., Gregory, S., Hartley, G. and Bishop, J. (1980). Deaf children of deaf parents and deaf children of hearing parents: a study of child-adult interaction. Presented at the International Congress of Psychology, Leipzig, Germany. **114**

Møller, S. and von Tetzchner, S. (1996). Allowing for developmental potential: A case study of intervention change. In S. von Tetzchner and M.H. Jensen (Eds), *Augmentative and Alternative Communication: European Perspectives* (pp. 249-69). London, UK: Whurr. **181**

Morehead, D.M. (Ed.) (1976). *Normal and Deficient Language*. Baltimore, Maryland: University Park Press. **3**

Morgan, G. and Woll, B. (Eds) (in press). *Directions in Sign Language Research*. Amsterdam, The Netherlands: John Benjamins. **3**

Morley, M.E. (1972). *The Development and Disorders of Speech in Childhood*. London, UK: Churchill Livingstone. **152**

Morris, S.E. (1981). Communication/interaction development at mealtimes for the multiple handicapped child: implications for the use of augmentative communication systems. *Language, Speech, and Hearing Services in Schools, 12*, 216-32. **14**

Morss, J.R. (1985). Early cognitive development: Difference or delay? In D. Lane and B. Stratford (Eds), *Current Approaches to Down's Syndrome* (pp. 242-59). London, UK: Holt, Rinehart & Winston. **85**

Morton, J. and Marshall, J.C. (Eds) (1977). *Psycholinguistic Series, Vol 1. Developmental and Pathological*. London, UK: Elek Science. **3**

Mundy, P., Kasari, C., Sigman, M. and Ruskin, E. (1995). Nonverbal communication and early language acquisition in children with Down syndrome and in normally developing children. *Journal of Speech and Hearing Research, 38*, 157-67. **84**

Murray, L. and Trevarthen, C. (1986). The infant's role in mother-infant communications. *Journal of Child Language, 13*, 15-29. **112**

Myklebust, H. (1967). *Development and Disorders of Written Language, Volume 1*. New York: Grune & Stratton. **359**

Nakamura, K., Newell, A. , Alm, N. and Waller, A. (1998). How do members of different language communities compose sentences with a picture-based communication system? A cross-cultural study of picture-based sentences constructed by English and Japanese speakers. *Augmentative and Alternative Communication, 14*, 71-80. **302**

Nakanishi, K. (1994). The influence of Japanese word order on Japanese Sign Language. In M. Brennan and G. Turner (Eds), *Word Order Issues in Sign Language:* Working papers presented at a workshop in Durham, 18-22 September 1991 (pp. 171-189). Durham, UK: International Sign Linguistics Association. **332**

Namir, L. and Schlesinger, I.M. (1978). The grammar of sign language. In I.M. Schlesinger and L. Namir (Eds), *Sign Language of the Deaf* (pp. 97-110). New York: Academic Press. **18, 25**

Nelson, K. (1985). *Making Sense: The Acquisition of Shared Meaning*. London, UK: Academic Press. **208, 289**

Nelson, K. (1994). Long-term retention of memory for preverbal experience: Evidence and implications. *Memory, 2*, 467-75. **248**

Nelson, K. (1996). *Language in Cognitive Development. The Emergence of the Mediated Mind*. New York: Cambridge University Press. **78, 84, 123, 192, 207, 208, 225, 226, 230**

Nelson, K. (1997). Cognitive change as collaborative construction. In E. Amsel and K.A. Renninger (Eds), *Change and Development: Issues of Theory, Method and Application* (pp. 99-115). London, UK: Lawrence Erlbaum. **155, 156, 157, 160**

Nelson, K. (1999). Levels and models of representation: Issues for the theory of conceptual change and development. In E.K. Scholnick, K. Nelson, S.A. Gelman and P. Miller

(Eds), *Conceptual Development: Piaget's Legacy* (pp. 269-91). Mahwah, New Jersey: Lawrence Erlbaum. **42, 46**

Nelson, K. and Gruendel, J.M. (1981). Generalized event representations: Basic building blocks of cognitive development. In M.E. Lamb and A.L. Brown (Eds), *Advances in Developmental Psychology, Volume 1* (pp. 131-58). Hillsdale, New Jersey: Lawrence Erlbaum. **230**

Nelson, K.E. (1991). On differentiated language-learning models and differentiated interventions. In N. Krasnegor, D. Rumbaugh and R. Schiefelbusch (Eds), *Biological and Behavioral Determinants of Language Development* (pp. 399-428). London, UK: Lawrence Erlbaum. **156, 160, 162**

Nelson, N.W. (1998). *Childhood Language Disorders in Context: Infancy through Adolescence.* Boston, Massachusetts: Allyn & Bacon. **229**

Newport, E.L. and Supalla, T. (1980). Clues from the acquisition of signed and spoken language. In U. Bellugi and M. Studdert-Kennedy (Eds), *Signed and Spoken Language: Biological Constraints on Linguistic Form* (pp. 187-211). Weinheim, Germany: Verlag Chemie. **17**

Ninio, A. (1992). The relation of children's single word utterances to single word utterances in the input. *Journal of Child Language, 19,* 87-110. **158**

Nunes, T., Schlieman, A.D. and Carraher, D.W. (1993). *Street Mathematics and School Mathematics.* Cambridge, UK: Cambridge University Press. **51**

Ochs, E. and Capps, L. (2001). *Living Narrative: Creating Lives in Everyday Storytelling.* Cambridge, Massachusetts, Harvard University Press. **226**

Odom, S. and Bailey, D.B. (2001). Inclusive preschool programs: Classroom ecology and child outcomes. In M. Guralnick (Ed.), *Early Childhood Inclusion: Focus on Change* (pp. 253-76). Baltimore, Maryland: Paul H. Brookes. **293**

Oliver, M. (1996). *Understanding Disability: From Theory to Practice.* Basingstoke, UK: Macmillan. **1**

Ornstein, P.A., Naus, M.J. and Liberty, C. (1975). Rehearsal and organizational processes in children's memory. *Child Development, 46,* 818-30. **41, 52, 54**

Owens, R. (1996). *Language Development: An Introduction.* Boston, Massachusetts: Allyn & Bacon. **229**

Oxley, J.D. (1995). The effect of developmental factors on the use of an electronic communication device. Doctoral dissertation, Louisiana State University. **59**

Oxley, J.D. and Norris, J.A. (2000). Children's use of memory strategies: Relevance to voice output communication aid. *Augmentative and Alternative Communication, 16,* 79-94. **53, 61**

Oxley, J.D. and von Tetzchner, S. (1999). Reflections on the development of alternative language forms. In F.T. Loncke, J. Clibbens, H.H. Arvidson and L.L. Lloyd (Eds), *Augmentative and Alternative Communication: New Directions in Research and Practice* (pp. 62-74). London, UK: Whurr. **86**

Pan, B.A. and Snow, C.E. (1999). The development of conversational and discourse skills. In M. Barrett (Ed.), *Development of Language* (pp. 229-49). Hove, UK: Psychology Press. **281, 298**

Papousek, H. (1969). Elaborations of conditioned head-turning. Paper presented at the symposium Learning of Human Infants, London, UK. **78**

Papousek, H. and Papousek, M. (1989). *Frühe Kommunikationsentwicklung und körperliche Beeinträchtigung (Early Communication Development and Body Impairment).* In A.A. Fröhlich (Ed.), *Kommunikation und Sprache körperbehin-*

derter Kinder (pp. 29-44). Düsseldorf, Germany: Verlag Modernes Lernen. **76**

Parker, J.G. and Asher, S.R. (1993). Friendship and friendship quality in middle childhood: links with peer group acceptance and feelings of loneliness and social dissatisfaction. *Developmental Psychology, 29,* 611-21. **293**

Paul, R. (2001). *Language Disorders from Infancy through Adolescence,* Second edition. Saint Louis, Missouri: Mosby. **40**

Pecyna, P.M. (1988). Rebus symbol communication training with a severely handicapped preschool child: a case study. *Language, Speech, and Hearing Services in Schools, 19,* 128-43. **177**

Peeters, T. (1997). *Autism: From Theoretical Understanding to Educational Intervention.* London, UK: Whurr. **26**

Peters, A. (1983). *The Units of Language Acquisition.* Cambridge, UK: Cambridge University Press. **120**

Peterson, C. and McCabe, A. (1983). *Developmental Psycholinguistics: Three Ways of Looking at a Child's Narrative.* New York: Plenum. **231, 258**

Peterson, C. and McCabe, A. (1991). Linking children's connective use and narrative microstructure. In A. McCabe and C. Peterson (Eds), *Developing Narrative Structure* (pp. 29-53). Hillsdale, New Jersey: Lawrence Erlbaum. **230**

Peterson, S.L., Bondy, A.S., Vincent, Y. and Finnegan, C.S. (1995). Effects of altering communicative input for students with autism and no speech: two case studies. *Augmentative and Alternative Communication, 11,* 93-100. **8**

Petitto, L.A. (1992). Modularity and constraints in early lexical acquisition: Evidence from children's early language and gesture. In M.R. Gunnar and M. Maratsos (Eds), *Minnesota Symposium on Child Psychology, Volume 25* (pp. 25-58). Hillsdale, New Jersey: Lawrence Erlbaum. **10**

Piaget, J. (1932). *The Moral Judgement of the Child.* London. UK: Kegan Paul. **274**

Piaget, J. (1950). *The Psychology of the Child.* London, UK: Routledge & Kegan Paul. **67**

Piaget, J. (1959). *The Language and Thought of the Child.* London, UK: Routledge & Kegan Paul. **67, 358**

Piaget, J. (1965). *Etudes sociologiques (Sociological Studies).* Geneva, Switzerland: Librairie Droz. **274**

Piaget, J. (1977). *The Origin of Intelligence in Children.* Harmondsworth, UK: Penguin. **155**

Pine, J. (1994). The language of primary caregivers. In C. Gallaway and B. Richards (Eds), *Input and Interaction in Language Acquisition* (pp. 15-37). London, UK: Cambridge University Press. **157, 173**

Pine, J. and Lieven, E. (1993). Reanalysing rote learned phrases: individual differences in the transition to multi-word speech. *Journal of Child Language, 20,* 551-74. **120**

Plunkett, K., Karmiloff-Smith, A., Bates, E., Elman, J.L. and Johnson, M.H. (1997). Connectionism and developmental psychology. *Journal of Child Psychology and Psychiatry, 38,* 53-80. **11**

Popich, E. and Alant, E. (1997). The frequency and quality of interaction between a teacher and the speaking and children with little or no speech in the class. *South African Journal of Disorders of Communication, 44,* 31-43. **341**

Popich, E. and Alant, E. (1999). The impact of a digital speaker on a teacher's interaction with a child with limited functional speech. *The South African Journal of Communication Disorders, 44,* 73-82. **341**

Powell, G. and Clibbens, J. (1994). Actions speak louder than words: signing and speech intelligibility in adults with Down's syndrome. *Down's Syndrome: Research and Practice, 2,* 127-9. **150**

Prechtl, H.F.R. (1993). Principles of early motor development in the human. In A.F. Kalverboer, B. Hopkins and R. Geuze (Eds), *Motor Development in Early and Later Childhood: Longitudinal Approaches* (pp. 35-50). Cambridge, UK: Cambridge University Press. **92**

Preece, A. (1987). The range of narrative forms conversationally produced by young children. *Journal of Child Language, 14,* 353-73. **240**

Pressley, M., Borkowski, J.G. and O'Sullivan, J. (1985). Children's metamemory and the teaching of memory strategies. In D.L. Forrest-Pressley, G.E. MacKinnon and T.G. Waller (Eds), *Metacognition, Cognition and Human Performance. Volume 1: Theoretical Perspectives* (pp. 111-53). Orlando, Florida: Academic Press. **50, 66**

Pressley, M., Forrest-Pressley, D.L., Elliott-Faust, D. and Miller, G. (1985). Children's use of cognitive strategies, how to teach strategies and what to do if they can't be taught. In M. Pressley and C.J. Brainerd (Eds), *Cognitive Learning and Memory in Children* (pp. 1-48). New York: Springer-Verlag. **47**

Pressman, L.J., Pipp-Siegel, S., Yoshinaga-Itano, C. and Deas, A. (1999). Maternal sensitivity predicts language gain in preschool children who are deaf and hard of hearing. *Journal of Deaf Studies and Deaf Education, 4,* 294-304. **30**

Pueschel, S.M., Gallagher, P.L., Zartler, A.S. and Pezzullo, J.C. (1987). Cognitive and learning processes in children with Down syndrome. *Research of Developmental Disabilities, 8,* 21-37. **85, 150**

Ratcliff, A. (1994). Comparison of relative demands implicated in direct selection and scanning: Considerations from normal children. *Augmentative and Alternative Communication, 10,* 67-74. **52**

Raven, J.C. (1956). *Coloured Progressive Matrices.* London, UK: H.K. Lewis. **304, 318**

Rayner, K. and Pollatsek, A. (1989). *The Psychology of Reading.* Englewood Cliffs, New Jersey: Prentice-Hall. **374**

Redmond, S. and Johnston, S. (2001). Evaluating the morphological competence of children with severe speech and physical impairments. *Journal of Speech, Hearing and Language Research, 44,* 1362-75. **302**

Reichle, J. (1991). Defining the decisions involved in designing and implementing augmentative and alternative communication systems. In J. Reichle, J. York and J. Sigafoos (Eds), *Implementing Augmentative and Alternative Communication: Strategies for Learners with Severe Disabilities* (pp. 39-60). Baltimore, Maryland: Paul H. Brookes. **57**

Reichle, J. and Ward, M. (1985). Teaching discriminative use of an encoding electronic communication device and Signing Exact English to a moderately handicapped child. *Language, Speech, and Hearing Services in Schools, 16,* 58-63. **10**

Reilly, J. (1992). How to tell a good story: the intersection of language and affect and in children's narratives. *Journal of Narrative and Life History, 2,* 355-77. **251, 258**

Reilly, J., Klima, E.S. and Bellugi, U. (1990). Once more with feeling: Affect and language in atypical populations. *Development and Psychopathology, 2,* 367-91. **231-2**

Remington, B. (1994). Augmentative and alternative communication and behavior analysis: A productive partnership. *Augmentative and Alternative Communication, 10,* 3-13. **10**

Remington, B. and Clarke, S. (1983). Acquisition of expressive signing by autistic children: An evaluation of the relative effects of simultaneous communication and sign-alone training. *Journal of Applied Behavior Analysis, 16,* 3154-328. **3, 10**

Remington, B. and Clarke, S. (1996). Alternative and augmentative systems of communication for children with Down's syndrome. In J.A. Rondal, J. Perera, L. Nadel and A. Comblain (Eds), *Down Syndrome: Psychological, Psychobiological and Socio-educational Perspectives* (pp. 129–43). London, UK: Whurr. **86**

Reynell, J. and Huntley, M. (1987). *Reynell Developmental Language Scales.* Revised edition. Windsor, UK: NFER-Nelson. **18, 89, 102, 106, 110–11**

Richardson, K. and Klecan-Aker, J.S (2000). Teaching pragmatics to language learning disabled children: a treatment outcome study. *Child Language Teaching and Therapy, 16,* 23-29. **332**

Ripich, D.N. and Griffith, P.L. (1988). Narrative abilities of children with learning disabilities and nondisabled children: Story structure, cohesion and propositions. *Journal of Learning Disabilities, 21,* 165-73. **231**

Rivarola, A., Schiaffino, A., Veruggio, G., Oldrini, S., Scarioni, M.G. and Chiari, A. (2000, August). CAA: Play activities and communication. Presented at the Ninth Biennial Conference of the International Society for Augmentative and Alternative Communication, Washington DC, USA. **335**

Rogoff, B. (1993). Guided participation in cultural activity by toddlers and caregivers. *Monographs of the Society for Research in Child Development, Volume 236.* **289–90, 294**

Rogoff, B., Goodman, C. and Bartlett, L. (2001). *Learning Together: Children and Adults in a School Community.* New York: Oxford University Press. **289, 290**

Romaine, S. (1999). Bilingual language development. In M. Barrett (Ed.), *Development of Language* (pp. 251-75). Hove, UK: Psychology Press. **20**

Romski, M.A. and Sevcik, R.A. (1996). *Breaking the Speech Barrier: Language Development through Augmented Means.* Baltimore, Maryland: Paul H. Brookes. **20–1, 36, 86, 298**

Romski, M.A., Sevcik, R.A. and Adamson, L.B. (1997). Framework for studying how children with developmental disabilities develop language through augmented means. *Augmentative and Alternative Communication, 13,* 172-8. **36**

Romski, M.A., Sevcik, R.A. and Pate, J.L. (1988). The establishment of symbolic communication in persons with severe retardation. *Journal of Speech and Hearing Disorders, 53,* 94-107. **118, 150**

Romski, M.A., Sevcik, R.A., Robinson, B.F., Mervis, C.B. and Bertrand, J. (1995). Mapping the meanings of novel visual symbols by youth with moderate or severe mental retardation. *American Journal on Mental Retardation, 100,* 391-402. **41**

Romski, M.A., White, R.A., Millen, C.E. and Rumbaugh, D.M. (1984). Effects of computer-keyboard teaching on the symbolic communication of severely retarded persons: five case studies. *The Psychological Record, 34,* 39-54. **177**

Rondal, J. (1980). Father's and mother's speech in early language development. *Journal of Child Language, 7,* 353-69. **158–9**

Rondal, J.A. and Edwards, S. (1997). *Language in Mental Retardation.* London, UK: Whurr. **19, 151, 232**

Rosenberg, S. and Abbeduto, L. (1993). *Language and Communication in Mental Retardation.* Hillsdale, New Jersey: Lawrence Erlbaum. **18–9**

Rostad, A.M. (1989). Erfaringer med tegnopplæring av psykisk utviklingshemmede småbarn (Experiences with sign teaching in intellectually disabled todlers). Levanger, Norway: Unpublished manuscript. **118–9**

Rotenberg, K.J. (1995). Moral development and children's differential disclosure to adults versus peers. In K.J. Rotenberg (Ed.), *Disclosure Processes in Children and Adolescents* (pp. 135–47). Cambridge, UK: Cambridge University Press. **273, 296**

Roth, F.P. and Spekman, N. (1986). Narrative discourse: spontaneously generated stories of learning-disabled and normally achieving students. *Journal of Speech and Hearing Disorders, 51,* 8–23. **231**

Rowland, C. and Schweigert, P. (1993). Analyzing the communication environment to increase functional communication. *Journal for the Association for Persons with Severe Handicaps,* 18, 161–76. **339**

Ruder, K.F. and Smith, M.D. (Eds) (1984). *Developmental Language Intervention.* Baltimore, Maryland: University Park Press. **3**

Ryan, J. (1974). Early language development: Towards a communication analysis. In M.P.M. Richards (Ed.), *The Integration of a Child into a Social World* (pp. 185–213). London, UK: Cambridge University Press. **14**

Ryan, J. (1977). The silence of stupidity. In J. Morton and J.C. Marshall (Eds), *Psycholinguistic Series, Vol 1. Developmental and Pathological* (pp. 99–124). London, UK: Elek Science. **84, 113**

Sachs, J. (1983). Talking about the there and then: The emergence of displaced reference in parent-child discourse. In K.E. Nelson (Ed.), *Children's language, Volume 4* (pp. 1–28). New York: Gardner Press. **257**

Sackett, G.P. (1978). *Observing Behaviour, Volume 2: Data Collection and Analysis Methods.* Baltimore, Maryland: University Park Press. **308**

Salvia, J. and Hughes, C. (1990). Curriculum-based Assessment: Testing What is Taught. New York: Macmillan. **362, 383**

Sameroff, A.J. (1987). The social context of development. In N. Eisenberg (Ed.), *Contemporary Topics in Developmental Psychology* (pp. 273–91). New York: John Wiley. **69, 286**

Sameroff, A.J. and Chandler, M.J. (1975). Reproductive risk and the continuum of caretaking causality. In P.D. Horowitz (Ed.), *Review of Child Development Research.* Volume 4 (pp. 187–244). Chicago, Illinois: Chicago University Press. **8, 358, 382**

Sameroff, A.J. and Fiese, B.H. (2000). Models of development and developmental risk. In C.H. Zeanah (Ed.), *Handbook of Infant Mental Health.* Second edition (pp. 3–19). London, UK: Guildford Press. **112**

Sampaio, D. (2000). *Ninguém morre sozinho: O adolescente e o suicídio.* Lisbon, Portugal: Caminho. **273**

Sampaio, D. (2001). *Vozes e ruídos: Diálogos com adolescentes.* Lisbon, Portugal: Caminho. **274**

Sandberg, A.D. and Hjelmquist, E. (1996). Phonological awareness and literacy abilities in nonspeaking preschool children with cerebral palsy. *Augmentative and Alternative Communication, 12,* 138–54. **56**

Sandberg, A.D. and Hjelmquist, E. (1997). Language and literacy in nonvocal children with cerebral palsy. *Reading and Writing: An Interdisciplinary Journal, 9,* 107–33. **202**

Saville-Troike, M. (1982). *The Ethnography of Communication.* Baltimore, Maryland: University Park Press. **347**

Schaeffer, B., Kollinzas, G., Musil, A. and McDowell, P. (1977). Spontaneous verbal language for autistic children through signed speech. *Sign Language Studies, 17,* 287–328. **8**

Schaffer, H.R. (1989). Language development in context. In S. von Tetzchner, L.S. Siegel and L. Smith (Eds), *The Social and Cognitive Aspects of Normal and Atypical Language Development* (pp. 1-22). New York: Springer-Verlag. **23, 79, 211, 225, 226**

Schank, R.C. and Abelson, R.P. (1977). *Script, Plans, Goals and Understanding*. Hillsdale, New Jersey: Lawrence Erlbaum. **208**

Scherer, N. and Olswang, L. (1984). The role of mothers' expansions in stimulating children's language production. *Journal of Speech and Hearing Research, 27*, 387-96. **332**

Schieffelin, B.B. (1979). Getting it together: An ethnographic approach to the study of the development of communicative competence. In E. Ochs and B.B. Schieffelin (Eds), *Developmental Pragmatics* (pp. 73-108). New York: Academic Press. **24**

Schlinger, H.D. (1995). *A Behavior Analytic View of Child Development*. New York: Plenum Press. **7, 10**

Schmidt, C.R., Ollendick, T.H. and Stancowicz, L.B. (1988). Developmental changes in the influence of assigned goals on cooperation and competition. *Developmental Psychology, 24*, 574-9. **51**

Schneider, W. (1985). Developmental trends in the metamemory-memory behavior relationship: An integrative review. In D.L. Forrest-Pressley, G.E. MacKinnon and T.G. Waller (Eds), *Metacognition, Cognition and Human Performance. Volume 1: Theoretical Perspectives* (pp. 57-109). Orlando, Florida: Academic Press. **63**

Schneider, W. and Pressley, M. (1989). *Memory Development between 2 and 20*. New York: Springer-Verlag. **59, 61**

Schober-Peterson, D. and Johnson, C.J. (1991). Non-dialogue speech during preschool interactions. *Journal of Child Language, 18*, 153-70. **258**

Schuler, A.L. and Wolfberg, P.J. (2000). Promoting peer play and socialization: The art of scaffolding. In A.M. Wetherby and B. Prizant (Eds), *Autism Spectrum Disorders: A Transactional Developmental Perspective* (pp. 251-77). Baltimore, Maryland: Paul Brookes. **292, 294**

Scollon, R. (1976). *Conversations with a One Year Old*. Honolulu, Hawaii: University Press of Hawaii. **169, 185**

Scollon, R. (1979). A real early stage: an unzippered condensation of a dissertation on child language. In E. Ochs and. B. Schieffelin (Eds), *Developmental Pragmatics* (pp. 215-27). New York, UK: Academic Press. **231**

Scribner, S. (1997). Three developmental paradigms. In E. Tobach, L.M.W. Martin, R. Falmagne, A.S. Scribner and M.B. Parlee (Eds), *Mind and Social Practice: Selected Writings of Sylvia Scribner* (pp. 281-8). Cambridge, UK: Cambridge University Press. **172**

Service, V., Lock, A. and Chandler, P. (1989). Individual differences in early communicative development: A social constructivist perspective. In S.v. Tetzchner, L.S. Siegel and L. Smith (Eds), *The Social and Cognitive Aspects of Normal and Atypical Language Development* (pp. 23-49). New York: Springer-Verlag. **11**

Sevcik, R. A. and Romski, M. A. (1997). Comprehension and language acquisition: Evidence from youth with severe disabilities. In L.B. Adamson and M.A. Romski (Eds), *Communication and Language Acquisition: Discoveries from Atypical Development* (pp. 187-202). Baltimore, Maryland: Paul H. Brookes. **41**

Sevcik, R.A., Romski, M.A. and Wilkinson, K. (1991). Roles of graphic symbols in the language acquisition process for persons with severe cognitive disabilities. *Augmentative and Alternative Communication, 7*, 161-70. **300**

Siegler, R.S. (1996). *Emerging Minds: The Process of Change in Children's Thinking.* New York: Oxford University Press. **48**

Siegler, R.S. (2000). The rebirth of children's learning. *Child Development, 71,* 26–35. **66**

Siewierska, A. (1988). *Word Order Rules.* London, UK: Croom Helm. **301, 302**

Silverman, H., McNaughton, S. and Kates, B. (1978). *Handbook of Blissymbolics.* Toronto, Canada: Blissymbolics Communication Institute. **362, 371, 372, 381**

Singleton, J., Goldin-Meadow, S. and McNeill, D. (1995). The cataclysmic break between gesticulation and sign: Evidence against a unified continuum of gestural communication. In K. Emmory and J. Reilly (Eds), *Language, Gesture and Space* (pp. 287–312). Hove, UK: Lawrence Erlbaum. **81, 153**

Singleton, J., Morford, J. and Goldin-Meadow, S. (1993). Once is not enough: Standards of well-formedness in manual communication created over three timespans. *Language, 69,* 683–715. **149**

Skinner, B.F. (1957). *Verbal Behavior.* New York: Appleton-Century-Crofts. **10**

Slobin, D.I. (1967). Imitation and grammatical development in children. In N.S. Endler, L.R. Boulter and H. Osser (Eds), *Contemporary Issues in Developmental Psychology* (pp. 437–43). New York: Holt, Rinehart & Winston. **300**

Slobin, D.I. (Ed.) (1985a). *The Crosslinguistic Study of Language Acquisition.* Hillsdale, New Jersey: Lawrence Erlbaum. **3**

Slobin, D.I. (1985b). Crosslinguistic evidence for the language-making capacity. In D.I. Slobin (Ed.), *The Crosslinguistic Study of Language Acquisition* (pp. 1157–256). Hillsdale, New Jersey: Lawrence Erlbaum. **300**

Smith, B.L. and Stoel-Gammon, C. (1983). A longitudinal study of the development of stop consonant production in normal and Down's syndrome children. *Journal of Speech and Hearing Disorders 48,* 114–18. **85**

Smith, F. (1971). *Understanding Reading.* New York: Holt, Rinehart & Winston. **360, 374**

Smith, F. (1973). *Psycholinguistics and Reading.* New York: Holt, Rinehart & Winston. **360**

Smith, F. (1979). *Reading without Nonsense.* New York: Teachers College Press. **360**

Smith, L. and von Tetzchner, S. (1986). Communicative, sensorimotor, and language skills of young children with Down syndrome. *American Journal of Mental Deficiency, 91,* 57–66. **84**

Smith, M.M. (1991). Assessment of interaction patterns and AAC use – A case study. *Journal of Clinical Speech and Language Studies, 1,* 76–102. **171**

Smith, M.M. (1994). Speech by any other name: the role of communication aids in interaction. *European Journal of Communication, 29,* 225–40. **312**

Smith, M.M. (1996). The medium or the message: a study of speaking children using communication boards. In S. von Tetzchner and M.H. Jensen (Eds), *Augmentative and Alternative Communication: European Perspectives* (pp. 119–36). London, UK: Whurr. **24, 74, 177, 225, 301, 385**

Smith, M.M. (1997). The bimodal situation of children developing alternative modes of language. In E. Björck-Åkesson and P. Lindsay (Eds), *Communication Naturally. Theoretical and Methodological Issues in Augmentative and Alternative Communication* (pp. 12–18). Västerås, Sweden: Mälardalen University Press. **78**

Smith, M.M. and Blischak, D.M. (1997). Literacy. In L.L. Lloyd, D.R. Fuller and H.H. Arvidsson (red), *Augmentative and Alternative Communication: A handbook of principles and practices* (pp. 414–44). Boston, Massachusetts: Allyn & Bacon. **205, 209**

Smith, M.M. and Grove, N. (1996, July). Input/output asymmetry: Language development in AAC. Presented at the Biennial Conference of the International Society for Augmentative and Alternative Communication, Vancouver, Canada. **301**

Smith, M.M. and Grove, N. (1999). The bimodal situation of children learning language using manual and graphic signs. In F.T. Loncke, J. Clibbens, H.H. Arvidson and L.L. Lloyd (Eds), *Augmentative and Alternative Communication: New Directions in Research and Practice* (pp. 8-30). London, UK: Whurr. **2, 24, 39, 78, 86, 171, 203, 205, 249**

Smith, M.M. and Grove, N. (2001). Determining utterance boundaries: Problems and strategies. In S. von Tetzchner and J. Clibbens (Eds), *Understanding the Theoretical and Methodological Bases of Augmentative and Alternative Communication* (pp. 15-41). Toronto, Canada: International Society for Augmentative and Alternative Communication. **74, 169, 301, 302**

Snow, C.E. (1991). Diverse conversational contexts for the acquisition of various language skills. In J. Miller (Ed.), *Research on Child Language Disorders: A Decade of Progress* (pp. 105-24). Austin, Texas: Pro-ed. **360**

Snow, C.E. (1995). Issues in the study of input: Finetuning, universality, individual and developmental differences, and necessary causes. In P. Fletcher and B. MacWhinney (Eds), *The Handbook of Child Language* (pp. 180-193). Oxford, UK: Blackwell Press. **24, 157, 158, 159, 160, 203, 298, 332**

Snow, C.E. and Ferguson, C.A. (Ed.) (1977), *Talking to Children*. Cambridge, UK: Cambridge University Press. **3**

Snow, C.E. and Goldfield, B.A. (1983). Turn the page, please: Situation-specific language acquisition. *Journal of Child Language, 10,* 551-70. **114**

Sodian, B. and Schneider, W. (1999). Memory strategy development – gradual increase, sudden insight or roller coaster? In F.E. Weinert and W. Schneider (Eds), *Individual Development from 3-12: Findings from the Munich Longitudinal Study* (pp. 61-77). Cambridge, Massachusetts: Cambridge University Press. **48**

Soto, G. (1997a). Multi-unit utterances and syntax in graphic communication. In E. Björck-Åkesson and P. Lindsay (Eds), *Communicating Naturally* (pp. 26-32). Västerås, Sweden: Mälardalen University Press. **301**

Soto, G. (1997b). Special education teacher attitudes toward AAC: Preliminary survey. *Augmentative and Alternative Communication, 13,* 186-97. **339**

Soto, G. (1999). Understanding the impact of graphic sign use on the message formulation structure. In F. Loncke, J. Clibbens, H. Arvidson and L. Lloyd (Eds), *Augmentative and Alternative Communication: New directions in research and practice* (pp. 40-8). London, UK: Whurr. **171, 275, 287, 300, 301, 312, 385**

Soto, G., Müller, E., Hunt, P. and Maier, J. (2001). Critical issues in the inclusion of students who use AAC: An educational team perspective. *Augmentative and Alternative Communication, 17,* 62-72. **288**

Soto, G., and Toro-Zambara, W. (1995). Investigation of Blissymbol use from a language research paradigm. *Augmentative and Alternative Communication, 11,* 118-30. **301**

Sperber, D. and Wilson, D. (1986). *Relevance: Communication and Cognition.* Cambridge, Massachusetts: MIT Press. **28, 332**

Sperber, D. and Wilson, D. (1995). *Relevance, Communication and Cognition.* Second edition. Oxford, UK: Blackwell. **58**

Spiegel, B.B., Benjamin, B.J. and Spiegel, S.A. (1993). One method to increase spontaneous use of assistive communication: A case study. *Augmentative and Alternative Communication, 9,* 111-18. **177**

Spiker, D. and Hopmann, M.R. (1997). The effectiveness of early intervention for children with Down syndrome. In M.J. Guralnick (Ed.), *The Effectiveness of Early Intervention* (pp. 271-305). Baltimore, Maryland: Paul H. Brookes. **86, 119**

Stanovich, K.E. (1984). The interactive-compensatory model of reading: A confluence of developmental, experimental, and educational psychology. *Remedial and Special Education,* 5, 11-19. **374**

Stanovich, K.E. (1986). Matthew effects in reading: Some consequences of individual differences in the acquisition of literacy. *Reading Research Quarterly,* 21, 360-407. **374**

Stein, N. and Albro, E. (1997). Building complexity and coherence: children's use of goal-structured knowledge in telling stories. In M. Bamberg (Ed.), *Narrative Development* (pp. 5-44). London, UK: Lawrence Erlbaum. **251**

Stein, N. and Glenn, C. (1982). Children's concept of time: The development of a story schema. In W.J. Friedman (Ed.), *The Developmental Psychology of Time* (pp. 255-82). New York: Academic Press. **230**

Stokes, T. and Baer, D. (1977). An implicit technology of generalisation. *Journal of Applied Behavior Analysis,* 10, 349-67. **356**

Stokoe, W., Casterline, D. and Cronenburg, C. (1965). *A Dictionary of American Sign Language on Linguistic Principles.* Washington DC: University of Gallaudet Press. **125, 234**

Stoloff, L. and Dennis, Z. (1978). Matthew. *American Annals of the Deaf, 123,* 442-51. **3**

Sutton, A. (1997). Language theory and intervention practice. In E. Björck-Åkesson and P. Lindsay (Eds), *Communication Naturally: Theoretical and Methodological Issues in Augmentative and Alternative Communication* (pp. 33-47). Västerås, Sweden: Mälardalen University Press. **74, 301, 314**

Sutton, A. (1999). Linking language learning experiences and grammatical acquisition. In F. Loncke, J. Clibbens, H. Arvidson and L. Lloyd (Eds). *Augmentative and Alternative Communication: New Directions in Research and Practice* (pp. 49-61). London, UK: Whurr. **171, 205, 385**

Sutton, A.E. and Gallagher, T.M. (1993). Verb class distinctions and AAC language-encoding limitations. *Journal of Speech and Hearing Research, 36,* 1216-26. **302**

Sutton, A., Gallagher, T., Morford, J. and Shahnaz, N. (2000). Relative clause production using augmentative and alternative communication systems. *Applied Psycholinguistics, 21,* 473-8. **20, 25, 305**

Sutton, A. and Morford, J. (1998). Constituent order in picture pointing sequences produced by speaking children using augmentative and alternative comm systems. *Applied Psycholinguistics, 19,* 525-36. **301, 332**

Sutton-Spence, R. and Woll, B. (1999). *The Linguistics of British Sign Language: An Introduction.* Cambridge, UK: Cambridge University Press. **230**

Sweeney, L.A. (1999). Moving forward with families: Perspectives on augmentative and alternative communication research and practice. In F.T. Loncke, J. Clibbens, H.H. Arvidson and L.L. Lloyd (Eds), *Augmentative and Alternative Communication: New Directions in Research and Practice* (pp. 231-54). London, UK: Whurr. **273**

Tager-Flusberg, H. (Ed.) (1994). *Constraints on Language Acquisition: Studies of Atypical Children.* Hillsdale, New Jersey: Lawrence Erlbaum. **300**

Thelen, E. and Smith, L.B. (1994). *A Dynamic Systems Approach to the Development of Cognition and Action.* London, UK: MIT Press. **6, 152**

Thomas, R.M. (1996). *Comparing Theories of Child Development.* Fourth edition. London, UK: Brooks/Cole. **291**

Thoonen, G., Maassen, B., Gabreels, F. and Schreuder, R. (1994). Feature analysis of singleton consonant errors in developmental verbal dyspraxia. *Journal of Speech and Hearing Research, 37,* 1424-40. **133**

Thousand, J.S. and Villa, R.A. (1992). Collaborative teams: A powerful tool in school restructuring. In R.A. Villa, J.S. Thousand, W.C. Stainback and S.B. Stainback (Eds), *Restructuring for Caring and Effective Education: An Administrative Guide to Creating Heterogeneous Schools* (pp. 73-108). Baltimore, Maryland: Paul H. Brookes. **288**

Tiedemann, T. (1787). Beobachtungen über die Entwicklung der Seelesfähigkeiten bei Kindern (Observations on the mental development in children). *Hessische Beiträge zur Gelehrsamkeit und Kunst, 2* (6-7). **3**

Tiilikka, P. and Hautamäki, J. (1986). *Portaat - varhaiskasvatusohjelma (Portage Guide to Early Education)*. Helsinki, Finland: Kehitysvammaliitto. **89**

Todman, J., Alm, N. and File, P. (1999). Modelling pragmatics in AAC. In F.T. Loncke, J. Clibbens, H.H. Arvidson and L.L. Lloyd (Eds), *Augmentative and Alternative Communication: New Directions in Research and Practice* (pp. 84-91). London, UK: Whurr. **74**

Tomasello, M. (1992). The social bases of language acquisition. *Social Development, 1,* 67-87. **42**

Tomasello, M. (1996). Piagetian and Vygotskian approaches to language acquisition. *Human Development, 39,* 269-76. **42**

Tomasello, M. (1999). *The Cultural Origins of Human Cognition*. London, UK: Harvard University Press. **23, 79, 84, 123, 176, 225, 289**

Tomasello, M. and Akhtar, N. (1995). Two-year-olds use pragmatic cues to differentiate reference to objects and actions. *Cognitive Development, 10,* 201-24. **289**

Tomasello, M. and Barton, M. (1994). Learning words in nonostensive contexts. *Developmental Psychology, 30,* 639-50. **289**

Tomasello, M., Conti-Ramsden and Ewert, B. (1990) Young children's conversations with their mothers and fathers - differences in breakdown and repair. *Journals of Child Language, 17,* 115-130 **158, 159**

Tomasello, M. and Farrar, M.J. (1986). Joint attention and early language. *Child Development, 57,* 1454-63. **29, 33**

Tomasello, M., Kruger, A.C. and Ratner, H.H. (1993). Cultural learning. *Behavioral and Brain Sciences, 16,* 540-52. **42**

Tomasello, M. and Merriman, W.E. (Eds) (1995). *Beyond Names for Things: Young Children's Acquisition of Verbs*. Hillsdale, New Jersey: Lawrence Erlbaum. **3**

Tomasello, M., Striano, T. and Rochat, P. (1999). Do children use objects as symbols? *British Journal of Developmental Psychology, 17,* 563-84. **57**

Tomlin, R.S. (1986). *Basic Word Order: Functional Principles*. London, UK: Croom Helm. **301**

Turnbull, A.P., Turbiville, V. and Turnbull, H.R. (2000). Evolution of family-professional relationship: Collective empowerment as the model for the early twenty-first century. In J.P. Shonkoff and S.J. Meisels (Eds), *Handbook of Early Childhood Intervention* (pp. 630-50). Cambridge, UK: Cambridge University Press. **113**

Udwin, O. and Yule, W. (1990). Augmentative communication systems taught to cerebral palsy children – A longitudinal study. 1: The acquisition of signs and symbols and syntactic aspects of their use over time. *British Journal of Disorders of Communication, 25,* 295-309. **4, 19, 120, 312**

Valsiner, J. (1987). *Culture and the Development of Children's Action*. New York: John Wiley. **295**

van Balkom, H. and Donker-Gimbrère, M.W. (1996). A psycholinguistic approach to graphic language use. In S. von Tetzchner and M. H. Jensen (Eds), *Augmentative and Alternative Communication: European Perspectives* (pp. 153-70). London, UK: Whurr. **4, 301**

Vanderheiden, G.G. and Grilley, K. (1976). *Non-verbal Communication Techniques and Aids for the Severely Physically Handicapped.* Baltimore: University Park Press. **359**

van Oosterom, J. and Devereux, K. (1985). *Learning with Rebus Glossary. Back Hill, UK: Earo, The Resource Centre.* **206**

Varnhagen, C.K., Das, J.P. and Varnhagen, S. (1987). Auditory and visual memory span: cognitive processing by TMR individuals with Down syndrome and other etiologies. *American Journal of Mental Deficiency, 91*, 398-405. **85, 151**

Vaughn, B. and Horner, R.H. (1995). Effects of concrete versus verbal choice systems on problem behavior. *Augmentative and Alternative Communication, 11*, 89-92. **8**

Veneziano, E., Sinclair, H. and Berthoud, I. (1990). From one word to two words: repetition patterns on the way to structured speech. *Journal of Child Language, 17*, 633-50. **130**

Vickers, B. (1974). *Non-oral Communication System Project, 1964-73, Iowa University Hospital School.* Iowa: University of Iowa. **359**

Villa, R.A. and Thousand, J.S. (1996). Student collaboration: An essential for curriculum delivery in the 21st century. In S. Stainback and W. Stainback (Eds), *Inclusion: A guide for Educators* (pp. 171-92). Baltimore, Maryland: Paul H. Brookes. **297**

Volterra, V. and Erting, C.J. (1990). *From Gesture to Language in Deaf Children.* Berlib, Germany: Springer-Verlag. **3**

von Tetzchner, S. (1984a). First signs acquired by a Norwegian deaf child of hearing parents. *Sign Language Studies, 44*, 225-57. **3**

von Tetzchner, S. (1984b). Tegnspråksopplæring med psykotiske/autistiske barn: Teori, metode og en kasusbeskrivelse (Sign language intervention for psychotic/autistic children: Theory, methodology and a case story). *Tidsskrift for Norsk Psykologforening, 21*, 3-15. **8, 118, 207**

von Tetzchner, S. (1984c). Facilitation of early speech development in a dysphatic child by use of signed Norwegian. *Scandinavian Journal of Psychology, 25*, 265-75. **118, 150**

von Tetzchner, S. (1985). Words and chips - pragmatics and pidginization of computer-aided communication. *Child Language Teaching and Therapy, 1*, 295-305. **2, 22, 24, 25, 225, 301**

von Tetzchner, S. (1988, October). Becoming an aided speaker. Presented at the Third Biennial Meeting of the International Society for *Augmentative and Alternative Communication,* Anaheim, California, USA. **171, 213, 358**

von Tetzchner, S. (1996, August). The contexts of early aided language acquisition. Presented at the 7th Biennial Conference of the International Society for Augmentative and Alternative Communication, Vancouver, Canada. **79, 123**

von Tetzchner, S. (1997). The use of graphic language intervention among young children in Norway. *European Journal of Disorders of Communication, 18*, 217-34. **16, 73, 201, 380**

von Tetzchner, S. (1999, April). The acquisition of atypical language forms. Invited keynote at The 1999 Annual Conference of the British Psychological Society, Belfast, UK. **13**

von Tetzchner, S. (2001a). *Utviklingspsykologi:* Barne- og ungdomsalderen (Developmental Psychology: Childhood and Adolescence). Oslo, Norway: Gyldendal Akademisk. **70, 84, 114, 296** von Tetzchner, S. (2001b). Aspectos evolutivos de la intervención an comunicación aumentiva y alternative (Developmental perspectives on augmentative and alternative communication). In F. Alcantud Marín and M. Lobato Galindo (Eds), *2001: Odisea de la Comunicación* (pp. 13-27). Valencia, Spain: Sociedad Española de Comunicación Aumentiva y Alternativa. **78**

von Tetzchner, S. (2001c, March). Theoretical perspectives on alternative communication. Intervention with severely disabled children: Implications for assessment and intervention. Workshop of the German-speaking section of the International Society of Augmentative and Alternative Communication, 8-9 March, 2001, Bielefeld, Germany. **81**

von Tetzchner, S. (2001d, June). Inclusion in normal school: Experiences from Norway, particularly related to children without speech. Lecture at the Technical University of Berlin, 6 June, 2001, Berlin, Germany. **81**

von Tetzchner, S. (2001e, February). Issues in the development of alternative modes of communication. Instructional course, Centre for Cerebral Palsy, Porto, Portugal. **274**

von Tetzchner, S., Dille, K., Jørgensen, K.K., Ormhaug, B.M., Oxholm, B. and Warme, R. (1998). From single signs to relational meanings. *Proceedings of the 8th Biennial Conference of the International Society of Augmentative and Alternative Communication* (p. 204). Dublin, Ireland: International Society for Augmentative and Alternative Communication. **4, 18, 21, 74**

von Tetzchner, S., Grove, N., Loncke, F., Barnett, S., Woll, B. and Clibbens, J. (1996). Preliminaries to a comprehensive model of augmentative and alternative communication. In S. von Tetzchner and M.H. Jensen (Eds), *Augmentative and Alternative Communication: European perspectives* (pp. 19-36). London, UK: Whurr. **20, 80, 86, 385**

von Tetzchner, S. and Jensen, M.H. (1996). Introduction. In S. von Tetzchner and M.H. Jensen (Eds), *Augmentative and Alternative Communication: European Perspectives* (pp. 1-18). London, UK: Whurr. **2, 201, 383**

von Tetzchner, S. and Martinsen, H. (1996). Words and strategies: Conversations with young children who use aided language. In S. von Tetzchner and M.H. Jensen (Eds), *Augmentative and Alternative Communication: European Perspectives* (pp. 65-88). London, UK: Whurr. **4, 9, 18, 19, 35, 58, 166, 169, 171, 177, 185, 204, 205, 221, 226, 233, 249, 256, 259, 261, 273**

von Tetzchner, S. and Martinsen, H. (2000). *Augmentative and Alternative Communication*. Second edition. London, UK: Whurr. **2, 18, 34, 38, 39, 76, 77, 80, 124, 140, 146, 171, 180, 203, 213, 275, 283**

von Tetzchner, S., Martinsen, H. and Ottem, E. (1983, June). Asymmetries in letter confusions among dyslectic, deaf, and normally reading and hearing children. Presented at the Second World Congress on Dyslexia, Halkidiki, Greece. **209**

von Tetzchner, S., Rogne, S.O. and Lilleeng, M.K. (1997). Literacy intervention for a deaf child with severe reading disorder. *Journal of Literacy Research, 29,* 25-46. **124, 209**

von Tetzchner, S. and Smith, L. (1986). Mødres tale til tre år gamle barn med Down syndrom (Mothers' speech to three-year-old children with Down syndrome). In P.E. Mjaavatn and L. Smith (Eds), *Barnespråk* (pp. 43-58). Trondheim, Norway: NAVF's Senter for Barneforskning. **112**

Vygotsky, L.S. (1962). *Thought and Language.* Cambridge, Massachusetts: MIT Press. **11, 67, 84, 289, 359**

Vygotsky, L.S. (1978). *Mind in Society: The Development of Higher Psychological Processes.* Cambridge, Massachusetts: Harvard University Press. **11, 38, 67, 84, 289, 294**

Vygotsky, L.S. (1987). Das Problem der Altersstufen (The problem of the steps of age).

Ausgewählte Schriften, Volume 2: Arbeiten zur Psychischen Entwicklung der Persönlichkeit (pp. 53-90). Berlin, Germany: Verlag Volk und Wissen. **70, 71, 72**

Vygotsky, L.S. (1993). *Collected Works, Volume. 2: The fundamentals of defectology.* New York: Plenum Press. **71, 156**

Waller, A. (1992). Providing narratives in an augmentative communication system. Unpublished PhD Thesis, University of Dundee, UK. **257**

Waller, A., O'Mara, D., Tait, L., Booth, L. and Hood, H. (2001). Conversational narrative and AAC: A case study. *Augmentative and Alternative Communication, 17,* 221-32. **256, 262, 270**

Wanner, E. and Gleitman, L.R. (Eds) (1982). *Language Acquisition: The State of the Art.* Cambridge, UK: Cambridge University Press. **3**

Warren, S. and Rogers-Warren, A. (1985). *Teaching Functional Language.* Austin, Texas: Pro-ed. **356**

Warrick, A. (1989). Sociocommunicative considerations with augmentative and alternative communication. *Augmentative and Alternative Communication, 4,* 45-51. **330**

Watkins, R.V. and Rice, M.L. (Eds) (1994). *Specific Language Impairments in Children.* Baltimore, Maryland: Paul H. Brookes. **3**

Watson, J.B. (1928). *Psychological Care of Infant and Child.* London, UK: Allen & Unwin. **7**

Wechsler, D. (1949). *Wechsler Intelligence Test for Children.* New York: The Psychological Corporation. **371**

Wells, G. (1987). *The Meaning Makers: Children Learning Language and Using Language to Learn.* London, UK: Hodder & Stoughton. **13**

Werker, J.F. and Tees, R.C. (1984). Cross-language speech perception: Evidence for the perceptual reorganization during the first year of life. *Infant Behavior and Development, 7,* 49-63. **17**

Werner, H. (1948). *Comparative Psychology of Mental Development, Revised edition.* New York: International Universities Press. **6**

Westby, C. (1998). Communicative refinement in school age and adolescence. In W.O. Haynes, B.B. Shulman (Eds), *Communication Development: Foundations, Processes and Clinical Applications* (pp. 311-60). Baltimore, Maryland: Williams & Wilkins. **63**

Westby, C., Dongen, R. and Maggart, Z. (1989). Assessing narrative competence. *Seminars in Speech and Language, 10,* 63-75. **231**

Wetherby, A.M., Reichle, J. and Pierce, P.L. (1998). The transition to symbolic communication. In A.M. Wetherby, S.F. Warren and J. Reichle (Eds), *Transitions in Prelinguistic Communication* (pp. 197-230). Baltimore, Maryland: Paul H. Brookes. **227**

Wetherby, A.M., Yonclas, D.G. and Bryan, A.A. (1989). Communicative profiles of preschool children with handicaps: Implications for early identification. *Journal of Speech and Hearing Disorders, 54,* 148-58. **84**

Whitehead, R.L., Schiavetti, N., Whitehead, B.H. and Metz, D.E. (1997). Effect of sign task on speech timing in simultaneous communication. *Journal of Communication Disorders, 30,* 439-55. **113, 118**

Wilbur, R.B. (1979). *American Sign Language and Sign Systems.* Baltimore, Maryland: University Park Press. **22**

Wilkinson, K.M. and Albert, A.G. (2001). Adaptations of fast mapping for vocabulary intervention with augmented language users. *Augmentative and Alternative Communication, 17,* 120-32. **41**

Wilkinson, K.M. and Green, G. (1998). Implications of fast mapping for vocabulary expansion in individuals with mental retardation. *Augmentative and Alternative Communication, 14,* 162-70. **41**

Wilkinson, K.M., Romski, M.A. and Sevcik, R.A. (1994). Emergence of visual-graphic symbol combinations by youth with moderate or severe mental retardation. *Journal of Speech and Hearing Research, 37*, 883-95. **4**

Williams, M.B. (1991). A comment on Light et al. *Augmentative and Alternative Communication, 7*, 133-4. **65**

Windsor, J. and Fristoe, M. (1989). Key word signing: listeners' classifications of signed and spoken narratives. *Journal of Speech and Hearing Disorders, 54*, 374-82. **113, 118**

Wishart, J.G. (1987). Performance of young nonretarded children and children with Down syndrome on Piagetian infant search tasks. *American Journal of Mental Deficiency, 92*, 169-77. **85**

Wittgenstein, L. (1953). *Philosophical Investigations*. New York: Macmillan. **176**

Woll, B. and Barnett, S. (1998). Toward a sociolinguistic perspective on augmentative and alternative communication. *Augmentative and Alternative Communication, 14*, 200-11. **15, 78, 80, 172**

Woll, B. and Kyle, J.G. (1989). Communication and language development in children of deaf parents. In S. von Tetzchner, L.S. Siegel and L. Smith (Eds), *The Social and Cognitive Aspects of Normal and Atypical Language Development* (pp. 129-44). New York: Springer-Verlag. **3**

Wood, D. (1998). *How Children Learn and Think,* Second edition. Oxford, UK: Basil Blackwell. **24**

Wood, D., Bruner, J. and Ross, G. (1976). The role of tutoring in problem solving. *Journal of Child Psychology and Psychiatry, 17*, 89-100. **5, 23, 78**

Woodcock, R.W., Clark, C.R. and Davies, C.O. (1969). *Peabody Rebus Reading Program.* Circle Pines, MN: American Guidance Service. **206, 227**

World Health Organisation (1980). *International Classification of Impairments, Disabilities and Handicaps.* Geneva, Switzerland. **81**

World Health Organisation (2001). *International Classification of Functioning, Disability and Health.* Geneva, Switzerland. **81**

Wragg, E. and Brown, G. (1993). *Explaining*. London, UK: Routledge. **24**

Wygotski, L.S. [Vygotsky, L.S.] (1975). Zur Psychologie und Pädagogik der kindlichen Defektivität (On the psychology and pedagogy of childhood defectivity). *Die Sonderschule, 20*, 65-72. **71**

Wyke, M.A. (1978). *Developmental Dysphasia*. London, UK: Academic Press.

Yoder, D.E. and Kraat, A. (1983). Intervention issues in nonspeech communication. In J. Miller, D.E. Yoder and R.L. Schiefelbusch (Eds), *Contemporary Issues in Language Intervention* (pp. 27-51). Rockville, Maryland: American Speech and Hearing Association. **2, 24**

Yorkston, K.M., Honsinger, M.J., Dowden, P.A. and Marriner, N. (1989). Vocabulary selection: A case report. *Augmentative and Alternative Communication, 5*, 101-9. **74, 204**

Zangari, C., Lloyd, L. and Vicker, B. (1994). Augmentative and Alternative Communication: An historic perspective. *Augmentative and Alternative Communication, 10*, 27-59. **2**

Index

Printed in the United Kingdom
by Lightning Source UK Ltd.
117218UKS00001B/60

9 781861 563316